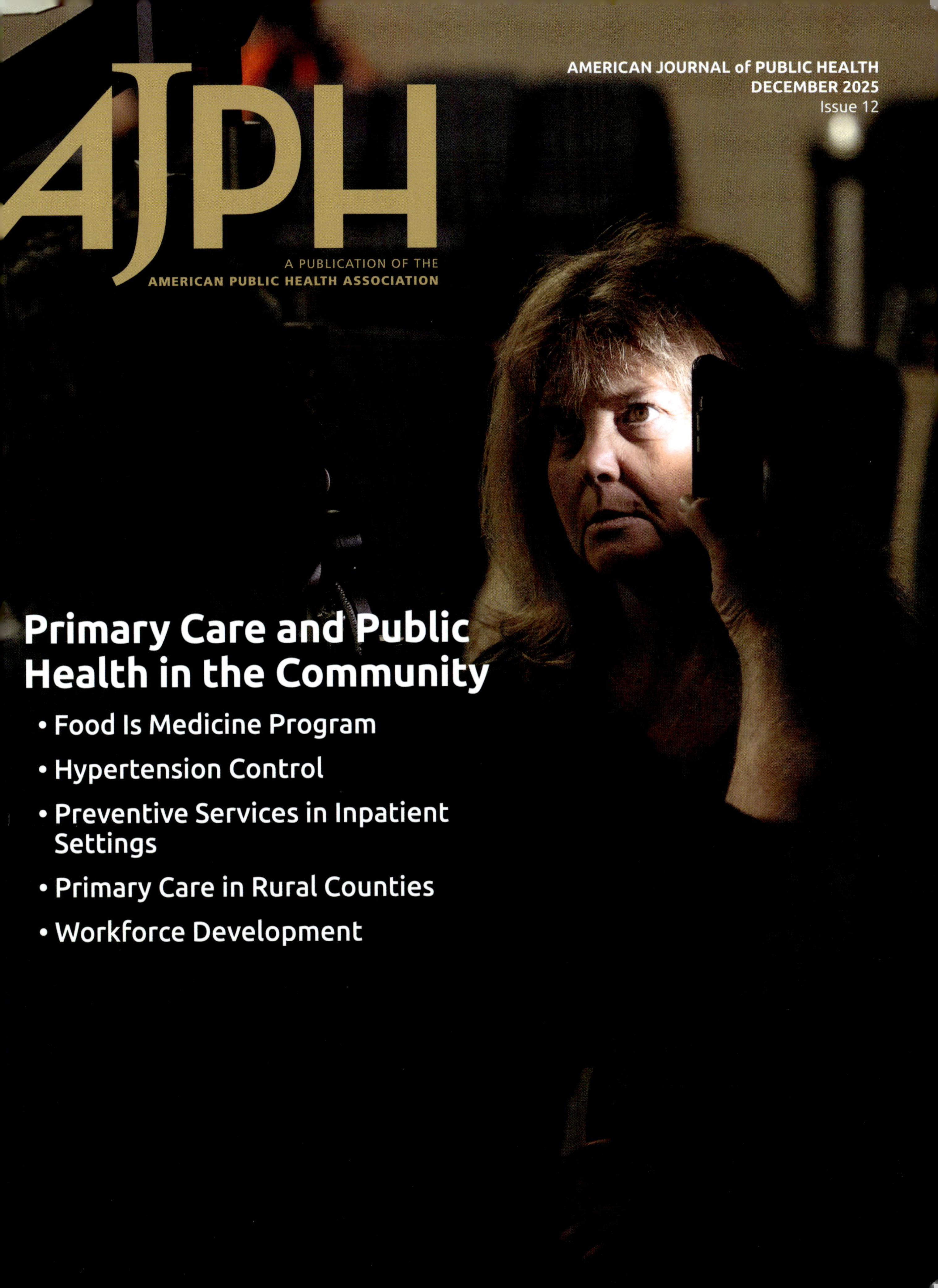

AMERICAN JOURNAL of PUBLIC HEALTH
DECEMBER 2025
Issue 12

AJPH

A PUBLICATION OF THE
AMERICAN PUBLIC HEALTH ASSOCIATION

Primary Care and Public Health in the Community

- Food Is Medicine Program
- Hypertension Control
- Preventive Services in Inpatient Settings
- Primary Care in Rural Counties
- Workforce Development

APHA
AMERICAN PUBLIC HEALTH ASSOCIATION
For science. For action. For health.

AJPH®, published monthly, is the official Journal of the American Public Health Association®, 800 I St NW, Washington, DC 20001-3710; (202) 777- APHA; TDD (202) 777-2500. APHA is a nongovernmental professional society founded in 1872, representing all disciplines and specialties in public health.

The *American Journal of Public Health*® (*AJPH*) (print ISSN: 0090-0036; electronic ISSN: 1541- 0048), first published in 1911, is the official journal of the American Public Health Association® (APHA). The oldest and largest organization of public health professionals in the world, APHA represents approximately 30 000 members from more than 50 occupations of public health.

Submissions: Visit www.editorialmanager.com/ajph or ajph.edmgr.com for online manuscript preparation and submission guidelines. Contributions of original unpublished research, social science analyses, scholarly essays, critical commentaries, departments, and letters to the editor are welcome. Questions? Write ajph.submissions@apha.org or call APHA at (202) 777-2469.

Print plus online subscriptions: Institutional price (print copy with online access for a single institution and all authorized users, regardless of geographic location) varies by size of organization and ranges from $993–$1445 for US organizations, and $1073–$1526 for international organizations (air delivery); multiple campuses not permitted without special arrangement. Details of the tiered pricing system at https://subscriptionoffice.com/pages/apha-landing-page. To order, write apha.subscriptions@apha.org.

Online-only subscriptions: Institutional price for one institution and its authorized users (regardless of geographic location) is $878–$1307. To order, write apha.subscriptions@apha.org. For academic consortia or multisite corporate subscriptions, contact apha.subscriptions@apha.org.

Print-only subscriptions: Institutional price is US $701, $782 international.

Back print issues: A limited number of print issues are for sale. Single copies are US $65, $75 international (air delivery). Shipping included; prepay only. To order, write apha.subscriptions@apha.org.

Reprints: For prices and ordering information on 50 or more reprints, check the Reprints section at www.ajph.org. To order smaller quantities of reprints (rush delivery), use the "Purchase Article" link on the article site itself.

Electronic access: Online articles more than 10 years old are available free for personal use at www.ajph.org. Recent articles are available through pay-per-view: single PDF article for $24, single issue access for 24 hours for $33, or entire site access for 24 hours for $38.

Postal information: Periodicals postage paid at Washington, DC, and additional mailing offices. Postmaster: Send address changes to American Journal of Public Health, 800 I St NW, Washington, DC 20001-3710.

Address changes: Send to AJPH, Membership Department (members) or AJPH Subscriptions (subscribers), APHA, 800 I St NW, Washington, DC 20001-3710. Or write to membership.mail@apha.org (members) or apha.subscriptions@apha.org (subscribers).

Advertising: For pricing and other information, see www.ajph.org. Please write to brian.selzer@apha.org or call (202) 777-2470 for other advertising opportunities. Ask about special exhibit packages and sponsorships. Acceptance of advertising by the *Journal* does not imply endorsement of products.

Indexes: Publications that index or abstract articles from *AJPH* include the following: Ageline, Assia (Applied Social Science Index and Abstracts), Biological Abstracts, Chemical Abstracts, CINAHL, Criminal Justice Abstracts, EMBASE, EMCare, Environmental Abstracts, e-psyche, ERIC, ETOH (Alcohol and Alcohol Problems Science Database), Excerpta Medica, Food Science and Technology, General Science Index, Grateful Med, Hospital Literature Index, Human Resources Abstracts, International Pharmaceutical Abstracts (IPA), Medline, Physical Education Index, Pollution Abstracts, Psychological Abstracts, PsychINFO, Safety Science Abstracts, Sage Family Studies Abstracts, Sage Human Resources Abstracts, Science Citation Index, SCOPUS, SIIC Data Bases, Social Work Research and Abstracts, and Statistical Reference Index (SRI)/LexisNexis.

AJPH

A PUBLICATION OF THE
AMERICAN PUBLIC HEALTH ASSOCIATION

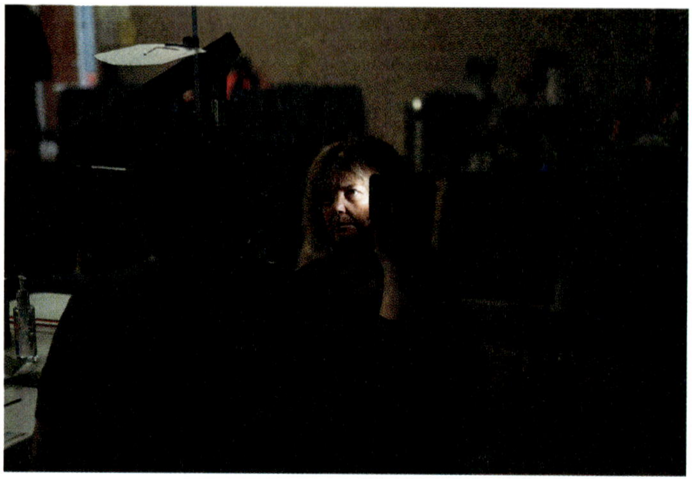

COVER: A doctor looks at a patient's eye using an iPhone flashlight at a free AMEN (Adventist Medical Evangelism Network) health clinic at the Asheville Foster Seventh-day Adventist Church on June 27, 2025, in Asheville, NC. The health clinic, which includes vision, dental, and other medical services at no cost in various parts of the United States on select dates, is available to everybody regardless of health insurance, employment, income, ID, or immigration status. Services are on a first-come, first-served basis, and appointments cannot be made in advance.

Cover concept and selection by Aleisha Kropf. Photo by Allison Joyce/AFP via Getty Images. Printed with permission.

APHA
AMERICAN PUBLIC HEALTH ASSOCIATION
For science. For action. For health.

Promoting public health research, policy, practice, and education is the *AJPH* mission. As we widen our scope to embrace global issues, we also sharpen our focus to support the needs of public health practitioners. We invite contributions of original unpublished research, opinion and commentary, and letters to the editor.

The *Journal* is printed on acid-free recycled paper.

AJPH December 2025, Vol. 115, No. 12

OPEN ACCESS ONLINE ONLY PODCAST DATA SUPPLEMENT AVAILABLE

EDITOR'S CHOICE

1949 Shooting at the CDC: Tragedy, Turmoil, and Resilience
D. T. Lau

BOOKS & MEDIA

1951 The Saga of Particulate Matter Air Pollution: Review of *Particles of Truth: A Story of Discovery, Controversy, and the Fight for Healthy Air*
J. M. Samet

OPINIONS, IDEAS, & PRACTICE

EDITORIALS

1954 Universal Unconditional Cash Transfers for Pregnant and Postpartum Women: Necessary but Insufficient
B. D. Kerker

1957 Air Pollution and Breast Cancer Risk: More Than Just Hot Air
M. B. Terry

1960 Traditional Risk Factors Plus Prevalence-Based Screening for Syphilis: Time for a Dual Approach
S. E. Rowan, M. Wallace, and K. Wendel

NOTES FROM THE FIELD

1963 An Individualized TTM-Based Intervention Promotes Child Safety Seat Purchase Among Pregnant Women: A Randomized Controlled Trial in Shantou, China
W. Yao, F. Wu, J. Yang, Y. Chen, Z. Tan, and L. Li

1967 Disarming Intimate Partner Violence Perpetrators: Stakeholder Perspectives on Enforcement Gaps and the Consequences of Federal Funding Cuts
J. A. Wagman and W. H. Hammett

1971 Evaluation of ShootSafe, an Interactive, Sequential Website to Teach Youths Firearms Safety: A Randomized Clinical Trial
D. C. Schwebel, D. L. Long, A. Johnston, Y. He, C. H. Morgan, J. Severson, G. Taylor, and K. Trullinger

1978 Building EXCITEment for Vaccines in Rural Communities
M. S. Rodgers, L. H. Downey, T. M. Gregory, E. W. Austin, D. E. Burton, L. Clark, R. Hursman, P. Peters, K. A. Stofer, J. Wilkins, and E. L. DeWald

1982 "I Didn't Have to Struggle": Caregivers' Perspectives on the Synergistic Interplay of WIC and SNAP on Family Health
C. M. Gago, M. M. Lee, N. M. Hammad, J. O. Wynne, M. K. Poole, M. Zimmer, R. S. Mozaffarian, R. Colchamiro, K. May, E. B. Rimm, and E. L. Kenney

PRIMARY CARE AND PUBLIC HEALTH IN THE COMMUNITY

1988 Integrating Primary Care and Public Health: Promising Pathways to Building Infrastructure and Delivering Services
K. M. Anderson, L. N. Borrell, and L. Thorpe

1992 Improving Hypertension Control in Southern Arizona: A Collaboration Between Community Health Centers and Local Health Departments
L. Soltani, A. Saal, and T. Cullen

1997 Advancing Equity in Preventive Care: Leveraging Hospital Admissions for Vulnerable Populations
N. Allaudeen, D. B. Huberman, and E. Le

2002 Integration of Health Care, Public Health, and Communities: A New Model for Rural Public Health
D. A. Mills

RESEARCH & ANALYSIS

PRIMARY CARE AND PUBLIC HEALTH IN THE COMMUNITY

2006 Retooling the Workforce for Collaboration: Centering Collective Efficacy in Public Health and Primary Care Leadership Development
J. Z. Martelino and B. Bekemeier

2015 Characteristics of the People and Communities Served by GusNIP Produce Prescriptions: United States, 2020–2024
C. Byker Shanks, V. A. Zigmont, R. Quattro, C. R. Long, C. A. Parks, H. Fricke, E. Mitchell, B. Houghtaling, H. Seligman, S. Stotz, and A. L. Yaroch

OPEN-THEMED RESEARCH

2020 Hardship and Hope: The Relationship Between Unconditional Prenatal and Infant Cash Transfers, Economic Stability, and Maternal Mental Health and Well-Being
M. Hanna, H. L. Shaefer, E. Finegood, S. Agarwal, Y. Zamani-Hank, and J. LaChance

2030 Air Pollutants and Breast Cancer Risk: A Parallel Analysis of Five Large US Prospective Cohorts
A. J. White, J. E. Hart, S. M. Quraishi, D. B. Bookwalter, M. R. Sweeney, E. W. Spalt, M. S. Hendryx, V. L. Irvin, D. S. Lane, A. H. Shadyab, S. Sealy-Jefferson, M. L. Neuhouser, E. A. Whitsel, J. D. Kaufman, F. Laden, and D. P. Sandler

2044 Examining Trends in Substance Use Behaviors Among Women With Primary and Secondary Syphilis: United States, 2018–2023
J. Rushmore, D. A. Jackson, J. A. Grey, E. A. Torrone, and E. R. Learner

2053 The Prevalence of Chronic Diseases Among Older Chinese Adults in the Past 2 Decades: A Study Based on the Chinese Longitudinal Healthy Longevity Survey, 2002–2022
K. Cao, Q. Feng, W. Tian, M. Liu, D. Tang, T. Feng, X. Sun, Y. Zeng, and Z. Wang

2062 Temporal Trends in Sexual Identity and Sociodemographic Disparities in Stockholm, Sweden, 2010–2021
W. Zhang, P. Tynelius, M. B. Mathur, M. Quartagno, G. Brandén, F. Liljeros, and K. Kosidou

2072 Crash-Related Protective and Risky Behaviors Among Micromobility Riders: A Nationally Representative Survey
N. Ni, M. Duren, and J. P. Ehsani

BACKMATTER

ERRATA

2077 Erratum In: "Emergency Food Support Preference and Usage During COVID-19: A Neighborhood Study of Low-Income Black Mothers' Use of School-Based Food Distribution and P-EBT"

2078 Erratum In: "Navigating Dual-Harm: Integrating Self- and Other-Harm Into Public Health Inquiry"

OTHER DEPARTMENTS

2080 Subscription Form

PEER REVIEWERS

e1 *AJPH* Peer Reviewers 2024–2025: Thank You for Your Services
M. Henry, B. Selzer, A. Ferguson, and K. Crocker

Shooting at the CDC: Tragedy, Turmoil, and Resilience

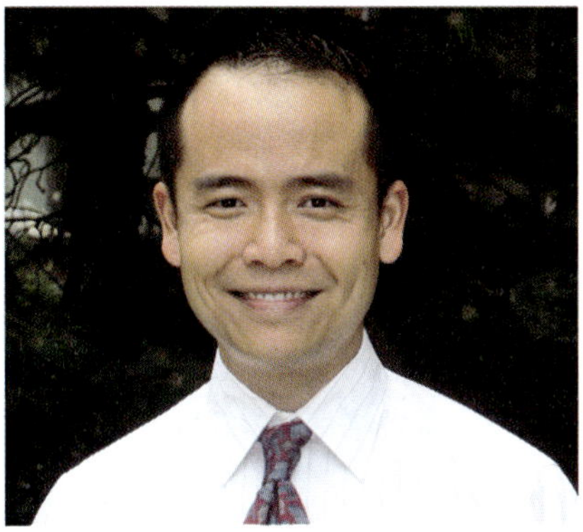

Denys T. Lau, PhD
Editor-in-Chief, *AJPH*

In early August 2025, a gunman fired about 500 rounds at the Centers for Disease Control and Prevention (CDC) headquarters, striking six buildings on campus with 200 rounds and tragically killing the responding local police officer. This act of violence was no ordinary one. The attack occurred at the very agency that is charged with protecting Americans from health threats. Moreover, four months earlier, the Trump administration's extensive layoffs significantly reduced CDC divisions responsible for gun violence research and prevention.

The shooter reportedly acted out of discontent with the COVID-19 vaccine, believing the vaccine had caused his mental health struggles. Law enforcement found that his grievance was based on misinformation on vaccines (https://nyti.ms/420sBuX). Scientific research does not support the idea that the COVID-19 vaccine causes depression or other mental health disorders. A vast body of evidence, including systematic reviews, meta-analyses, and population-level observation studies, has found no such link. More than 13 billion doses have been administered globally, and a recent systematic review found that, in very rare cases, temporary psychiatric symptoms have been reported following COVID-19 vaccination (https://bit.ly/4pufqMX). Even so, a causal relationship between COVID-19 vaccination and mental health cannot be inferred because case reports do not adequately account for preexisting history of mental health conditions or stress related to the pandemic or the vaccination process.

The crisis of public distrust in our nation's public health institutions, unfortunately, is growing, fueled by years of antiscience rhetoric and conspiracy theories. Vaccines are particularly susceptible to politicization because they involve public health measures that affect entire communities and, for many vaccines, children. Distrust in public health reached new heights during the COVID-19 pandemic when immediate guidance was in demand but research-informed public health recommendations were slow in coming and conflicted early in the pandemic on issues such as mask wearing and social distancing. Critics raised safety concerns about the unprecedented rapid development of new vaccines, and government-mandated lockdowns, for which many opponents blamed public health officials, contributed to economic and social hardship.

Social media also played a critical role in spreading false information about vaccines globally and almost instantly. Despite initial shortcomings, the CDC established extensive monitoring systems to track the spread and evolution of SARS-CoV-2 (severe acute respiratory syndrome coronavirus 2) across the nation and played a key role in widely distributing and administering COVID-19 vaccines and treatments, significantly decreasing the risk of death among those infected with SARS-CoV-2.

Does the shooting incident at the CDC mark a pivotal moment for meaningful change, or is it a warning of worse things to come if inaction continues? Condemning violence and addressing antivaccine and anti-CDC sentiments, especially among policymakers, are crucial to combating misinformation, rebuilding trust in public health institutions, and discrediting the use of violence for political or ideological purposes. Staying silent and not denouncing the attacker's vaccine-related motive imply complicity and allow vaccine misinformation to continue spreading, potentially inspiring more acts of violence.

Protecting the health of the people in the United States should never come with violence as an occupational hazard. Public health leaders and workers should not receive death threats or require security protection (https://bit.ly/4gsoYnr). Ironically, around the time of the shooting, major budget cuts and staffing reductions had led to the elimination of entire CDC divisions that were responsible for preventing workplace injuries, illnesses, and fatalities.

In a climate of turmoil and despondency, many CDC employees returned to their offices, showing remarkable

AJPH December 2025, Vol. 115, No. 12

resilience and an unwavering commitment to the public's health. In a rare move, more than 750 current and former Department of Health and Human Services (HHS) employees sent a signed letter to the HHS Secretary, asking him to stop spreading inaccurate health information, stand up for the CDC's scientific integrity, and ensure the HHS workforce's safety (http://bit.ly/4nduahl).

Less than three weeks after the letter was sent, another poignant example of dedication to public health occurred. While the buildings' facade still bore the marks of hundreds of bullets, the CDC director, Susan Monarez, was fired after less than one month on the job. She testified in a Senate Committee on Health, Education, Labor, and Pensions hearing that she had refused to comply with a request from the HHS Secretary to preapprove vaccine policy changes that contradicted scientific evidence (http://bit.ly/3VZnmrS). Weeks earlier, the HHS Secretary had denied these claims in a Senate Finance Committee hearing.

Although the CDC needs to operate in line with the policy priorities of the presidential administration, the lead US public health agency also must use the best scientific evidence as the basis for its recommendations and actions. Monarez's refusal to preapprove vaccine policy changes that went against scientific evidence and the protest resignations of several senior CDC officials reflected their conviction that science and integrity must guide public health decisions. As the political and social landscape shifts, the resolution of public health leaders and workers to uphold rigorous science remains even more essential—especially in times when these leaders and workers are facing ideologies that do not align with the principles of public health. AJPH

DOI: https://doi.org/10.2105/AJPH.2025.308294

The Saga of Particulate Matter Air Pollution: Review of *Particles of Truth: A Story of Discovery, Controversy, and the Fight for Healthy Air*

Jonathan M. Samet, MD, MS

ABOUT THE AUTHOR

Jonathan M. Samet is with the Colorado School of Public Health, Aurora.

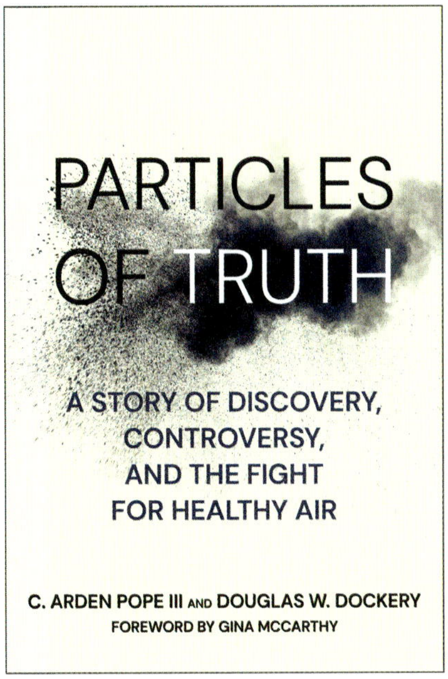

Particles of Truth: A Story of Discovery, Controversy, and the Fight for Healthy Air
By C. Arden Pope III and Douglas W. Dockery
Cambridge, MA: MIT Press; 2025
264 pp; $29.95
ISBN: 9780262551670

In 1997, Environmental Protection Agency (EPA) Administrator Carol M. Browner promulgated a National Ambient Air Quality Standard (NAAQS) for small airborne particles, $PM_{2.5}$ (particles less than 2.5 microns in aerodynamic diameter).[1] The new NAAQS included 24-hour and annual standards, reflecting epidemiological evidence of increased risk from time-series studies of daily mortality and particulate matter (PM) concentrations and from longer-term cohort studies of mortality and time-averaged PM concentrations, respectively. Previously, the NAAQS for PM used only PM_{10} as the index, which includes particles extending up to 10 microns in aerodynamic diameter, encompassing both $PM_{2.5}$ and particles ranging from 2.5 to 10 microns. The new $PM_{2.5}$ NAAQS was motivated by emerging epidemiological evidence on health risks of particles in this smaller size range and understanding that these small particles penetrated deeply into the lung. Some industries, particularly the fossil fuel sector, opposed a NAAQS for $PM_{2.5}$, concerned by cost and other implications. One strategy for derailing the $PM_{2.5}$ NAAQS was questioning the credibility of the underlying scientific evidence, an approach long followed by the tobacco industry.[2]

CONTROVERSIES AROUND THE AIR QUALITY STANDARD

In *Particles of Truth*, C. Arden Pope III and Douglas W. Dockery, two of the principals in developing the epidemiological evidence supporting the $PM_{2.5}$ NAAQS, chronicle their work and that of others interlaced with the efforts to create doubt about the epidemiological findings and steps taken to counter the attacks.[3] They tell the story in 12 chapters, each titled with a question, spanning from the Industrial Revolution and its introduction of profligate burning of fossil fuels to persisting concerns about airborne particles and health and rising concern about climate change. Much of the story is personalized as their research figured centrally in the evidence base supporting the $PM_{2.5}$ NAAQS, and they were caught up in responding to abundant unfriendly critiques of their work. Two of their studies were pivotal in motivating the $PM_{2.5}$ NAAQS: the Harvard Six Cities Study and the American Cancer Society Cancer Prevention Study II, both addressing longer-term exposure to PM and increased risk of dying.[4,5]

Per Pope and Dockery, the book has three objectives: (1) to present the scientific evidence on air pollution and health, (2) to address the controversies spawned by the $PM_{2.5}$ research, and (3) to tell this science history. They note the futility of the first objective, given the scope of the scientific evidence on air pollution and health. In a recent general PubMed search on

AJPH December 2025, Vol. 115, No. 12

"air pollution and health," I identified a cumulative total of around 70 000 articles. However, for the 1997 promulgation of the $PM_{2.5}$ NAAQS, a few studies were key and are described by Pope and Dockery.

The first wave of these studies were time-series analyses of daily mortality and 24-hour average PM levels in various cities.[6] These analyses from the 1980s showed positive associations (i.e., mortality was greater on days with higher PM levels). In interpreting the findings of these studies, one proposed explanation was that the timing of death had been advanced by a brief interval; in other words, susceptible people died some days earlier than they might have, absent exposure to PM air pollution, a phenomenon initially and inappropriately labeled "harvesting" (later referred to more neutrally as "mortality displacement"). This interpretation was dismissive of significant public health implications of the time-series studies. The findings of the Harvard and the American Cancer Society's studies countered the mortality displacement argument by showing that mortality was increased by fine particle pollution over the longer term. Pope's study of health in the Utah Valley, heavily polluted by a steel mill, further indicted PM air pollution.[7] He used a quasi-experimental design that took advantage of the research opportunity posed by a strike-related closure of the steel mill to show the effect of air pollution on child respiratory health.

THE HEALTH EFFECTS INSTITUTE AND STUDY REANALYSIS

In developing the new NAAQS, the EPA used a relatively transparent approach for moving from evidence gathering, synthesis, and integration to policy formulation that highlighted the reliance on the findings of these and some other studies. Because the studies' importance could be pinpointed, targeted criticisms were launched and controversy resulted. The findings of the time-series studies were the first target; the critiques centered on the analytical methods and the validity of the data. A response to these critiques came with a 1994 funding call from the Health Effects Institute, a foundation supported by the EPA and the vehicle manufacturers, to validate the time-series data and replicate the analyses. My Johns Hopkins colleague Scott Zeger and I took on the task, independently recreating the data sets and finding the same results with new analytical methods applied transparently. The model of independent replication of key research supporting regulation was launched.[6]

It was soon applied to the Six Cities and American Cancer Society studies as well, again with the Health Effects Institute funding and overseeing the work. As described in *Particles of Truth*, a mechanism was worked out for providing the data from the two studies to the selected reanalysis team, led by Daniel Krewski at the University of Ottawa. For these studies, the data validation and analytical replication tasks were more complex, but the reanalysis report in 2000 confirmed original findings.[8] More than a decade later, the two studies were labeled as "secret science" and efforts were made by several senators to block the EPA from relying on findings of studies with data not publicly available. Beyond the successful reanalysis project, *Particles of Truth* compiles the findings of the many cohort studies since the initial publications that have been confirmatory.

The spillover from the $PM_{2.5}$ story, well described by Pope and Dockery, has had broad implications for formulating evidence-based regulations. Consistent with the general strategy of doubt creation, the $PM_{2.5}$ example includes targeted attacks on methods of epidemiology (i.e., the time-series studies) and on specific studies (e.g., the Harvard Six Cities Study). Legislation was launched (e.g., the HONEST [Honest and Open New EPA Science Treatment] Act). In 1999, the data access controversy also sparked the so-called Shelby Amendment to Office of Management and Budget Circular A-110 (concerned with federally funded research). Circular A-110 was amended to require agencies to ensure that "all data produced under a [federally funded] award will be made available to the public through the procedures established under the Freedom of Information Act."[9(p54926)] In the ensuing decades, the movement toward open data access and adherence to the FAIR principles (guidelines aimed at improving the findability, accessibility, interoperability, and reusability of data) makes these earlier discussions seem anachronistic.

WHO SHOULD READ *PARTICLES OF TRUTH*?

As a participant in the story, I read the book as an insider, and memories were triggered of research and controversy, contentious meetings of the EPA review panel, and the complexities of offering guidance in the face of uncertainty on a national regulatory standard. In fact, the opinions of the panel members for the EPA Clean Air Scientific Advisory Committee on the $PM_{2.5}$ NAAAQS were quite varied.[10] For the noninsiders, the book offers a comprehensive accounting of an important step toward improving air quality and an in-depth look at how scientific evidence supports regulation. For insiders and noninsiders, the book captures the principled positions taken by Pope, Dockery, and others in contending with the diverse actions taken to obstruct the $PM_{2.5}$ NAAQS by undermining its scientific foundation. Particulate matter air pollution has declined progressively as the process of evidence-based standard-setting has supported ever-tighter standards. AJPH

CORRESPONDENCE

Correspondence should be sent to Jonathan M. Samet, 13001 E 17th Place, Aurora, CO 80045 (e-mail: jon.samet@cuanschutz.edu). Reprints can be ordered at https://www.ajph.org by clicking the "Reprints" link.

PUBLICATION INFORMATION

Full Citation: Samet JM. The saga of particulate matter air pollution: review of *Particles of Truth: A Story of Discovery, Controversy, and the Fight for Healthy Air*. *Am J Public Health*. 2025;115(12): 1951–1953.

Acceptance Date: July 30, 2025.

DOI: https://doi.org/10.2105/AJPH.2025.308260

ORCID iD:

Jonathan M. Samet https://orcid.org/0000-0001-5676-9175

CONFLICTS OF INTEREST

The author has no conflicts of interest to disclose.

REFERENCES

1. *Revised Ozone and Particulate Matter (PM) National Ambient Air Quality Standards*. Washington, DC: Environmental Protection Agency; 1998.
2. Michaels D. *Doubt Is Their Product: How Industry's Assault on Science Threatens Your Health*. New York, NY: Oxford University Press; 2008.
3. Pope CA III, Dockery DW. *Particles of Truth: A Story of Discovery, Controversy, and the Fight for Healthy Air*. Cambridge, MA: The MIT Press; 2025.
4. Dockery DW, Pope CA III, Xu X, et al. An association between air pollution and mortality in six US cities. *N Engl J Med*. 1993;329(24):1753–1759. https://doi.org/10.1056/NEJM199312093292401
5. Pope CA III, Thun MJ, Namboodiri MM, et al. Particulate air pollution as a predictor of mortality in a prospective study of US adults. *Am J Respir Crit Care Med*. 1995;151(3_pt_1):669–674. https://doi.org/10.1164/ajrccm.151.3.7881654
6. *Particulate Air Pollution and Daily Mortality: Replication and Validation of Selected Studies (The Phase IA Report of the Particle Epidemiology Evaluation Project). Special Report*. Boston, MA: Health Effects Institute; 1995.
7. Pope CA III. Respiratory disease associated with community air pollution and a steel mill, Utah Valley. *Am J Public Health*. 1989;79(5):623–628. https://doi.org/10.2105/ajph.79.5.623
8. Krewski D, Burnett RT, Goldberg MS, et al. *Reanalysis of the Harvard Six Cities Study and the American Cancer Society Study of Particulate Air Pollution and Mortality. Investigators' Reports Parts I and II*. Health Effects Institute. 2000. Available at: https://www.healtheffects.org/publication/reanalysis-harvard-six-cities-study-and-american-cancer-society-study-particulate-air. Accessed July 7, 2025.
9. Congressional Research Service. Public access to data from federally funded research: provisions in OMB Circular A-110. 2013. R42983. March 1, 2013. Available at: https://www.congress.gov/crs_external_products/R/PDF/R42983/R42983.3.pdf. Accessed July 7, 2025.
10. Wolff GT. Closure letter on draft OAQPS staff paper on particulate matter from chairman of Clean Air Scientific Advisory Committee to EPA administrator. EPA-SAB-CASAC-LTR-96-008. Washington, DC: Environmental Protection Agency; June 13, 1996.

Universal Unconditional Cash Transfers for Pregnant and Postpartum Women: Necessary but Insufficient

Bonnie D. Kerker, PhD

ABOUT THE AUTHOR

Bonnie D. Kerker is with the Departments of Population Health and Child and Adolescent Psychiatry, NYU Grossman School of Medicine, New York, NY.

See also Hanna et al., p. 2020.

Economic hardship is often exacerbated during pregnancy, childbirth, and infancy. This period is laden with additional expenses at a time when women might be reducing work hours. Purchasing and eating healthy food is particularly important during pregnancy but can be costly. Once the baby is born, increased expenses include health care and childcare, as well as material goods such as diapers. As a result, pregnancy can both lead to and worsen financial burden among expectant and new parents.[1]

DISPARITIES IN PERINATAL HEALTH

Poverty is highly correlated with multiple conditions that can harm pregnant and postpartum women and their children. Low income is associated with food insecurity, unstable housing, and unhealthy neighborhood conditions, all of which can be detrimental to maternal and infant health. Moreover, poverty, particularly during the perinatal period, can increase maternal stress, which can lead to mental health disorders and physical chronic disease, thus increasing the risk of maternal morbidity and mortality.[2] This is of great concern given that in recent years maternal deaths because of cardiovascular disease and other medical conditions have increased in the United States. Overall, women giving birth in the United States suffer from higher rates of morbidity and mortality than those in similarly large and developed countries, and large racial/ethnic disparities exist.[3]

The pregnancy-related death rate among Black women is almost three times higher than among White women, and more than three times higher than among Hispanic women.[3] Disparities are evident even after controlling for social and economic factors, highlighting the role that racism and discrimination likely play in these differences.[3] In this issue of *AJPH*, Hanna et al. (p. 2020) describe how Rx Kids, a community-wide, universal, and unconditional prenatal and infant cash transfer program, addresses these disparities by investing in families in Flint, Michigan, a community consisting mostly of Black residents with high rates of poverty.

WHAT WE LEARNED FROM RX KIDS

Women enrolled in Rx Kids receive a one-time sum of $1500 during pregnancy and $500 per month postnatally for 12 months. The authors present evidence of the effectiveness of the Rx Kids program in alleviating economic hardship and improving maternal health and well-being. Specifically, participation in Rx Kids was associated with decreases in not having enough food, owing past due rent or mortgage, and eviction after childbirth. Furthermore, the program was linked to decreases in postpartum depression and increases in mothers' feelings of being valued, respected, and hopeful, as well as trust in health care and government.

The findings of Hanna et al. suggest that in addition to increasing income and reducing hardship, unconditional cash programs during pregnancy and postpartum may be effective at improving maternal health and well-being, which can have an impact on child outcomes in the long term. This is notable, given that a recent large study on an unconditional cash transfer program during the first four years of the baby's life, Baby's First Years (BFY), did not find significant associations with maternal health outcomes.[4] There are several important differences between BFY and Rx Kids. BFY distributed a lower amount, $333 per month, but for a longer duration than the Rx Kids program. In addition, BFY was implemented during the height of the COVID-19 pandemic, and it is possible that economic and health hardships outweighed the impact of the program or that other government programs during the pandemic washed out meaningful effects.[5] Rx Kids was launched in 2024, after the height of the pandemic, and—unlike BFY—begins cash distribution prenatally, which is when the stress of motherhood starts for many women.

Moreover, while BFY was a means-tested program, Rx Kids is universal within a low-income community, where 59% of children live in poverty and 57% of the community identify as Black or African American. Black women, in particular, experience great economic and health inequalities in the United States; universal programs may be more effective at addressing racial and income inequalities because they are associated with less stigma than means-tested programs.[6] Inequalities are believed to erode trust,[7] so the universal nature of Rx Kids could have led to increases in trust, which may have contributed to enhanced civic and social engagement,[7] increased social connectedness, and, ultimately, improved maternal mental health outcomes. Furthermore, means-tested benefits can lead to feelings of disempowerment and a lack of autonomy. In contrast, the universal nature of Rx Kids may have been responsible for participants' enhanced feelings of value and respect. As Hanna et al. point out, feelings of love, respect, hope, and trust "capture the underpinning of a reimagined social contract—what it means to be part of a society and community that cares and provides for each other" (p. 2026). The full benefits of such a "reimagined society" may extend beyond the outcomes reported in this article.

INCREASING THE SAFETY NET

Importantly, many other countries have long histories supporting universal programs that guarantee living wages; in fact, the United States is the only developed country that does not guarantee a period of paid and job-protected leave for new mothers.[8] In 2021, the United States expanded the Child Tax Credit in what was tantamount to a near-universal, unconditional child cash benefit. The US Census Bureau recorded large drops in poverty, which rose when the tax credit was rescinded at the end of that year.[9]

In lieu of a national policy, the Rx Kids program is funded through a public–private partnership, leveraging the Temporary Assistance for Needy Families (TANF) block grant dollars to states via a mechanism that does not trigger time limits or work requirements.[6] This is a creative use of federal funds, and other states might consider following suit. Unfortunately, the current federal administration is on track to reduce the US safety net. Accordingly, states will likely soon receive fewer dollars to spend on benefits, including Medicaid, Supplemental Nutrition Assistance Program, and TANF.[10] Given the medical importance of addressing poverty in the perinatal period and the potential effectiveness of cash-benefit programs in improving maternal health, this is the exact opposite of what should be done. We should identify ways to use universal or near-universal programs to increase the safety net and ensure living wages to entire communities.

NECESSARY BUT NOT SUFFICIENT

Programs like Rx Kids are an important start, but even universal programs are not enough. Cash is necessary but not sufficient to support families in ways that enable them to thrive. Cash does not instantly provide social support, which is critical to mental health and the ability to care for a newborn, or actionable strategies for integrating play, storytelling, and reading into daily routines. Reduced poverty may help women initiate mental health care, but those services need to be available, part of comprehensive primary care, and aligned with language and culture.[11] Increased income can give women flexibility and time to attend medical appointments, but mothers need to have insurance to obtain quality care. Universal health insurance that includes mental and physical health care would enable all women to receive necessary medical care and use their income to support their families in other ways. Systems reform must be a part of any comprehensive approach to address perinatal and infant health.

A supportive US system would incorporate all of this—unconditional cash benefits during the perinatal period; effective programming to support pregnancy, postpartum, and early childhood development; and equitable systems able to address the real needs of families. As advocates Aisha Nyandoro and Kathy Spillar write, "By addressing the improvements necessary to our broader economic systems, we can create a society where all women, particularly Black women, have the opportunity to thrive."[12] AJPH

CORRESPONDENCE

Correspondence should be sent to Bonnie D. Kerker, NYU Grossman School of Medicine, 180 Madison Ave, 6th Floor, New York, NY 10016 (e-mail: bonnie.kerker@nyulangone.org). Reprints can be ordered at https://www.ajph.org by clicking the "Reprints" link.

PUBLICATION INFORMATION

Full Citation: Kerker BD. Universal unconditional cash transfers for pregnant and postpartum women: necessary but insufficient. *Am J Public Health*. 2025;115(12):1954–1956.

Acceptance Date: September 7, 2005.
DOI: https://doi.org/10.2105/AJPH.2025.308292
ORCID iD:
Bonnie D. Kerker https://orcid.org/0000-0002-2962-1666

ACKNOWLEDGMENTS

The author is grateful to Laurie Brotman and Peter Ephross for their thoughtful review of this article.

CONFLICTS OF INTEREST

The author has no conflicts of interest to disclose.

REFERENCES

1. Doser M. Pregnancy and poverty: forging a path forward for families. American Public Human Services Administration. September 26, 2022. Available at: https://aphsa.org/resources/pregnancy-and-poverty-forging-a-path-forward-for-families. Accessed July 15, 2025.
2. Agorastos A, Chrousos GP. The neuroendocrinology of stress: the stress-related continuum of chronic disease development. *Mol Psychiatry.* 2022;27(1):502–513. https://doi.org/10.1038/s41380-021-01224-9
3. Ranji U, Diep K, Gomez I, Sobel L, Salganicoff A. Health policy issues in women's health. In: Altman D, ed. *Health Policy 101.* KFF. July 2024 Available at: https://www.kff.org/health-policy-101-health-policy-issues-in-womens-health. Accessed July 15, 2025.
4. Duncan GJ, Magnuson K, Kunin-Batson AS, et al. Cash transfers and their effect on maternal and young children's health: a randomized clinical trial. *JAMA Pediatr.* 2025;179(8):867–875. https://doi.org/10.1001/jamapediatrics.2025.1612
5. DeParle J. 2025, July 30. Study may undercut idea that cash payments to poor families help child development. *New York Times.* July 28, 2025. Available at: https://www.nytimes.com/2025/07/28/us/politics/cash-payments-poor-families-child-development.html. Accessed August 6, 2025.
6. Hanna M, Shaefer HL, Fogle H, et al. 2024, December. Scaling up prenatal and infant cash prescriptions to eradicate deep infant poverty in the United States. Brookings. December 20, 2024. Available at: https://www.brookings.edu/articles/prenatal-and-infant-cash-prescriptions-to-eradicate-deep-infant-poverty-united-states. Accessed July 15, 2025.
7. Onifade E, Shishane K, Elonge F, Glover L. Guaranteed income: experiences of African American mothers in the Magnolia Mother's Trust Project. *J Community Pract.* 2023;31(1):105–120. https://doi.org/10.1080/10705422.2023.2190327
8. Doran EL, Bartel AP, Ruhm CJ, Waldfogel J. California's paid family leave law improves maternal psychological health. *Soc Sci Med.* 2020;256:113003. https://doi.org/10.1016/j.socscimed.2020.113003
9. Sy S, Cuevas K. 2023, September 12. Child poverty increases sharply following expiration of expanded tax credit. *PBS News Hour.* Available at: https://www.pbs.org/newshour/show/child-poverty-increases-sharply-following-expiration-of-expanded-tax-credit. Accessed August 7, 2025.
10. Kallins L, Katz E. How proposed changes to federal safety net programs could affect the states. National Conference of State Legislatures. Available at: https://www.ncsl.org/events/details/how-proposed-changes-to-federal-safety-net-programs-could-affect-the-states. Accessed August 7, 2025.
11. Kerker BD, Barajas-Gonzalez RG, Rojas NM, Norton JM, Brotman LM. Enhancing immigrant families' mental health through the promotion of structural and community-based support. *Front Public Health.* 2024;12:1382600. https://doi.org/10.3389/fpubh.2024.1382600
12. Nyandoro A, Spiller K. 2024 Front & Center's next phase: how we fix systems designed to fail Black women. *Ms.* August 13, 2024. Available at: https://msmagazine.com/2024/08/13/front-center-magnolia-mothers-trust-jackson-mississippi-black-women-poverty-childcare. Accessed July 30, 2025.

Air Pollution and Breast Cancer Risk: More Than Just Hot Air

Mary Beth Terry, PhD

ABOUT THE AUTHOR

Mary Beth Terry is with the Herbert Irving Comprehensive Cancer Center and the Department of Epidemiology, Columbia University Mailman School of Public Health, New York, NY; she is executive director of Silent Spring Institute, Newton, MA.

See also White et al., p. 2030.

For more than three decades, epidemiological studies have investigated environmental exposures and breast cancer risk. The bulk of these studies, however, has been conducted in postmenopausal women, and when premenopausal women are included, the subgroup is usually too small to analyze separately. From a public health perspective, this focus seems reasonable, as most cases occur later in life. However, over the past two decades we have learned that exposures affect breast cancer risk most during windows of susceptibility (e.g., when the breast tissue is changing). Evidence generated during these windows of susceptibility shows stronger and more consistent associations with exposures such as endocrine-disrupting chemicals and metals.[1] We also have found that evidence is stronger and more consistent in susceptible populations, including younger women with a family history of cancer and women with alterations in cancer genes.[2] As with genetic research, studying more susceptible populations can help identify environmental exposures that are also relevant to individuals at average risk.

Studies limited to postmenopausal women at average risk, without considering susceptibility, have produced inconsistent results, especially for exposures that are difficult to measure. Unlike risk factors (e.g., alcohol) that can be measured by questionnaires, environmental chemical exposures have been difficult to measure because of both the ubiquity of exposures and the resources needed to measure them through biospecimens and monitoring devices. This has made it easy for skeptics to dismiss associations by focusing on the data from postmenopausal women and overlooking how study biases in measurement and selection underestimate effects.

The pooled analysis by White et al., in this issue of *AJPH* (p. 2030), reflects these same challenges: data from these cohorts lacked information on windows of susceptibility, and only one of the five cohorts was enriched for susceptibility. Using data from more than 28 000 breast cancer cases and approximately 400 000 individuals, they observed a 3% linear increase per 10–parts-per-billion (ppb) increase in nitrogen dioxide (NO_2) and a 14% and 10% increase in estrogen receptor– and progesterone receptor–negative breast cancer per 5–micrograms per cubic meter ($\mu g/m^3$) increase in fine particulate matter ($PM_{2.5}$) and 10–ppb increase in ozone, respectively.

The pooled study was rigorous, with a mean follow-up of 17.5 years, and it adjusted for multiple confounders. Adjusted and unadjusted results were similar, suggesting little confounding bias, at least in the covariates as measured. The large sample size also enabled subgroup analyses by menopausal status, race/ethnicity, census region, body mass index, and neighborhood socioeconomic status.

White et al. did not test for interactions with smoking, but previous work found that polycyclic aromatic hydrocarbon exposure, a constituent of air pollution, during two windows of susceptibility (prenatal and pregnancy) may interact with cigarette smoke exposure to increase adolescent and adult breast density, respectively.[3] Assessing synergistic effects among multiple constituents of air pollution will be important both to quantify total exposure and to improve individual risk assessment. Furthermore, the authors did not measure indoor air pollution, and as most people spend the majority of time indoors, failure to capture indoor air exposures and exposures during windows of susceptibility means that their estimates are conservative. This is what makes their results so striking.

Two of the studies excluded premenopausal women, and only two enrolled participants younger than 40 years. This is notable because we would hypothesize that individuals with more exposures to environmental chemicals may have other cancers or comorbidities and may not be included in studies that skew toward older ages. Such an approach may produce the "deleting the susceptible" phenomenon,[4] whereby vulnerable individuals develop diseases or die before enrollment. We hypothesized and observed

AJPH December 2025, Vol. 115, No. 12

this with polycyclic aromatic hydrocarbon,[5] and our findings were later supported by a systematic review of environmental chemicals and breast cancer.[2] This phenomenon has broader implications; individuals who are more biologically sensitive to pollutants may develop chronic diseases, including aggressive cancers, and are excluded from eligibility or die before study screening. This highlights why the literature may appear inconsistent when most studies focus on postmenopausal women: the problem is not that environmental exposures are unimportant but that the populations in which effects are strongest are often missing from the data.

The pooled analysis also underscores the need to examine molecular subtypes. Their novel findings of 14% and 10% linear increases in progesterone receptor–negative breast cancer with $PM_{2.5}$ and ozone exposure suggest that breast cancer studies require enough power to detect subtype effects. Laboratory studies show that endocrine-disrupting chemicals may increase transformation of estrogen-sensitive cells into basal cells.[6] If confirmed, this mechanism could explain higher rates of triple-negative breast cancer in subgroups with elevated $PM_{2.5}$, ozone, or other endocrine-disrupting chemical exposures.

White et al. found stronger associations between NO_2 and $PM_{2.5}$ and breast cancer in the lowest quartile of neighborhood socioeconomic status. Although the cohorts had geographic diversity, they lacked sufficient racial/ethnic and socioeconomic status diversity. Findings may be stronger in a more representative US sample, particularly because Hispanic women—who made up only 0.9% to 4.5% of participants although Hispanic men and women are 19.6% of the US population—showed stronger associations with $PM_{2.5}$ and ozone (Table B, available as a supplement to the online version of this article at http://www.ajph.org), although the associations were not statistically significant because of power issues. It would be important to know whether these associations were even stronger when restricted by progesterone receptor–negative tumors or by younger age.

The lack of representation also obscures critical issues of environmental justice. Communities of color and low-income neighborhoods are disproportionately exposed to traffic-related air pollution, industrial emissions, and poor-quality housing conditions. Without adequate enrollment of these groups, pooled analyses will miss precisely the cancers that are most aggressive and clinically challenging. Recently, the multiethnic cohort study, 70% of whose cohort was Black or Hispanic individuals, reported associations with $PM_{2.5}$; the associations were stronger for women with a family history and for younger women.[7]

Two thirds of cancers diagnosed for those younger than 50 years occur in women.[8] To address early onset cancers, we must consider case-control studies and enriched cohorts.[4] More than 900 chemicals relevant to breast cancer have been identified in common products.[9] Case-control studies using exposomics and linking to chemical lists with known breast cancer mechanisms are urgently needed. Ecological and time-trend analyses can also complement cohort work and have the advantage of including all cancer cases for a geographic area. For example, using data from all cancers in New York State, we found positive associations between $PM_{2.5}$ and early onset breast cancer, as well as other cancers.[10]

For public health, the implications are significant. As White et al. note, their effect sizes are likely underestimates. Thus, their estimate of 9500 US breast cancer cases avoided is almost certainly conservative. Extrapolation globally is challenging, given higher pollution levels in other countries, but breast cancer remains the most common cancer in women and the leading cancer in those younger than 50 years. Early onset cancers disproportionately contribute to disability-adjusted life years and years of life lost.[11] For early onset breast cancer alone, the global burden is an estimated 5.34 million disability-adjusted life years annually. Air pollution levels in many low- and middle-income countries are severalfold higher than in the United States, meaning potential attributable risks could be far greater—although extrapolations from areas with lower levels may not be straightforward. Interventions to reduce emissions would provide wide-ranging cobenefits, lowering not only breast cancer risk but also risks of other cancers, cardiovascular disease, asthma, and other pollution-related conditions. Framing breast cancer prevention as part of broader clean air initiatives underscores its dual relevance to women's health and environmental justice worldwide. AJPH

CORRESPONDENCE

Correspondence should be sent to Mary Beth Terry, 320 Nevada St, Suite 302, Newton, MA 02460 (e-mail: terry@silentspring.org). Reprints can be ordered at https://www.ajph.org by clicking the "Reprints" link.

PUBLICATION INFORMATION

Full Citation: Terry MB. Air pollution and breast cancer risk: more than just hot air. *Am J Public Health*. 2025;115(12):1957–1959.

Acceptance Date: September 23, 2025.

DOI: https://doi.org/10.2105/AJPH.2025.308300

ORCID iD:
Mary Beth Terry https://orcid.org/0000-0002-4106-5033

ACKNOWLEDGMENTS

I wish to acknowledge the Breast Cancer Research Foundation.

CONFLICTS OF INTEREST

The author has no conflicts of interest to disclose.

REFERENCES

1. Terry MB, Michels KB, Brody JG; Breast Cancer and the Environment Research Program, et al. Environmental exposures during windows of susceptibility for breast cancer: a framework for prevention research. *Breast Cancer Res.* 2019;21(1):96. https://doi.org/10.1186/s13058-019-1168-2
2. Zeinomar N, Oskar S, Kehm RD, Sahebzeda S, Terry MB. Environmental exposures and breast cancer risk in the context of underlying susceptibility: a systematic review of the epidemiological literature. *Environ Res.* 2020;187:109346. https://doi.org/10.1016/j.envres.2020.109346
3. Kehm RD, Walter EJ, Oskar S, et al. Exposure to polycyclic aromatic hydrocarbons during pregnancy and breast tissue composition in adolescent daughters and their mothers: a prospective cohort study. *Breast Cancer Res.* 2022;24(1):47. https://doi.org/10.1186/s13058-022-01546-8
4. Kehm RD, Lloyd SE, Burke KR, Terry MB. Advancing environmental epidemiologic methods to confront the cancer burden. *Am J Epidemiol.* 2025;194(1):195–207. https://doi.org/10.1093/aje/kwae175
5. Shen J, Liao Y, Hopper JL, Goldberg M, Santella RM, Terry MB. Dependence of cancer risk from environmental exposures on underlying genetic susceptibility: an illustration with polycyclic aromatic hydrocarbons and breast cancer. *Br J Cancer.* 2017;116(9):1229–1233. https://doi.org/10.1038/bjc.2017.81
6. Schroeder J, Polemi KM, Tapaswi A, Svoboda LK, Sexton JZ, Colacino JA. Investigating phenotypic plasticity due to toxicants with exposure disparities in primary human breast cells in vitro. *Front Oncol.* 2024;14:1411295. https://doi.org/10.3389/fonc.2024.1411295
7. Wu AH, Wu J, Tseng C, et al. Air pollution and breast cancer incidence in the multiethnic cohort study. *J Clin Oncol.* 2025;43(3):273–284. https://doi.org/10.1200/JCO.24.00418
8. Kehm RD, Terry MB. Early onset cancer trends and the persistently higher burden of cancer in young women. *Oncologist.* 2025;30(5):oyaf084. https://doi.org/10.1093/oncolo/oyaf084
9. Kay JE, Brody JG, Schwarzman M, Rudel RA. Application of the key characteristics framework to identify potential breast carcinogens using publicly available in vivo, in vitro, and in silico data. *Environ Health Perspect.* 2024;132(1):17002. https://doi.org/10.1289/EHP13233
10. Yuan H, Kehm RD, Daaboul JM, et al. Cancer incidence trends in New York State and associations with common population-level exposures 2010–2018: an ecological study. *Sci Rep.* 2024;14(1):7141. https://doi.org/10.1038/s41598-024-56634-w
11. Yan W, Liu M, Jing W, et al. Disparities in the incidence, mortality, and disability-adjusted life years of 33 early-onset cancer groups globally, 2012–2021: a systematic analysis. *Exp Hematol Oncol.* 2025;14(1):38. https://doi.org/10.1186/s40164-025-00634-7

Traditional Risk Factors Plus Prevalence-Based Screening for Syphilis: Time for a Dual Approach

Sarah E. Rowan, MD, Meghan Wallace, DO, and Karen Wendel, MD

ABOUT THE AUTHORS

All authors are with the Public Health Institute at Denver Health, Denver Health Medical Center, Denver, CO. Sarah E. Rowan and Karen Wendel are also with the Division of Infectious Diseases, University of Colorado School of Medicine, Aurora. Meghan Wallace is with the Department of Family Medicine, University of Colorado School of Medicine.

See also Rushmore et al., p. 2044.

When the Centers for Disease Control and Prevention released *The National Plan to Eliminate Syphilis From the United States* in 1999, case counts were at historic lows.[1,2] The plan, which aimed to increase services in "high morbidity areas" and "potentially reemergent areas," was initially successful at reducing disparities and preventing congenital syphilis (CS). However, rather than decreasing, syphilis rates overall began a steady rise. The rates of primary and secondary syphilis are now the highest since 1990, with women constituting an increasing proportion of the epidemic and CS increasing from 304 cases in 2012 to 3882 cases in 2023.[2]

National strategies to combat syphilis focus on understanding epidemiologic and behavioral risk factors. The article by Rushmore et al. (p. 2044) in this issue of *AJPH* offers new data to inform tactical approaches. Using the Centers for Disease Control and Prevention's surveillance data for primary and secondary syphilis cases among Hispanic, non-Hispanic Black, and non-Hispanic White women from 2018 through 2023, the authors investigated whether substance use has contributed to an increase in syphilis cases among women. The authors tracked temporal trends in methamphetamine use, having sex while intoxicated or high, and having sex with individuals who inject drugs and assessed associations with syphilis, geography, race, and ethnicity.

Of 51 209 cases among the included groups, the prevalence of the specified substance use behaviors remained largely unchanged over six years. The data indicate that substance use has not been the overwhelming driver of increased primary and secondary syphilis among women, although it remains important for identifying key populations who may benefit from focused interventions. Notably, 36% of respondents reported having sex while intoxicated, 12% reported having sex with someone who injects drugs, and 18% reported having used methamphetamines in the previous year.

Recognizing that substance use is common among women with incident syphilis, but likely not the main reason for increasing cases, prompts a broader consideration of risk factors. Unlike HIV and hepatitis C for which injection drug use is a direct transmission pathway, the association between substance use and syphilis is indirect and occurs through behaviors that heighten transmission risk. These include having multiple or new sexual partners, concurrent sexual partnerships, anonymous or transactional sex, anal intercourse, and inconsistent condom use—activities that may be increasing regardless of substance use.[3] Additional challenges, such as lack of health care access, stigma, and medical mistrust, may limit health care utilization, contributing to worsening rates. Factors such as unstable housing, poverty, and incarceration disrupt access to testing and treatment, and changing sexual networks and increased use of dating apps may also drive transmission.[4]

As our understanding of syphilis risk factors evolves, screening guidelines must also adapt. An analysis of syphilis cases in Colorado revealed that the proportion of women with syphilis who had guideline-recommended indications for screening dropped from 88% in 2011 to 2012 to 59% from 2019 through 2020, suggesting that broader screening criteria are needed.[5] The current Centers for Disease Control and Prevention Sexually Transmitted Infections (STI) Treatment Guidelines and the US Preventive Services Task Force recommend screening based on a broad set of risk factors, including diagnosis of other STIs or HIV, transactional sex work, multiple or new sexual partners, incarceration history, military service, pregnancy, substance use, sexual partner exposure to an STI, and living in communities with high syphilis rates.[6,7] Recently, McDonald et al. suggested that community prevalence may be the most significant risk factor for many individuals and proposed a prevalence threshold aligning with Healthy People 2030 goals (4.6 cases per

AJPH December 2025, Vol. 115, No. 12

100 000 population) for the implementation of universal syphilis screening in sexually active women and girls aged 15 to 44 years and their partners.[8] Using this threshold, by 2023 data, 45% of US counties would meet the criteria for prevalence-based syphilis screening.[9]

Several US states and counties—including Colorado, California, New Mexico, Massachusetts, and others—began recommending universal or expanded screening in 2024 based on local prevalence data. Although it is too soon to assess the full impact of universal and expanded screening, early national data suggest that primary and secondary syphilis rates may finally be decreasing.[9]

Although Rushmore et al. appropriately suggest consideration of universal screening, it does not come without a price. The US Preventive Services Task Force cautions that "potential harms of screening include false-positive results that require clinical evaluation and unnecessary anxiety to the patient." They also note that screening in nonpregnant persons without risk factors is likely to be low yield and, given the imperfect nature of syphilis testing, may result in "high false-positive rates and overtreatment."[6(p1245)] Furthermore, equivocal results may generate stress in relationships or feelings of stigmatization. Lessons from HIV and hepatitis C initiatives show that uptake of nontargeted screening may be limited, and the cost-effectiveness of universal screening has not been evaluated in this context.[10–11] Moreover, as incidence decreases, clinicians may lack guidance on when to return to risk-based screening. A systematic analysis of both the benefits and harms of universal syphilis screening is needed.

Beyond screening, traditional public health approaches remain essential; surveillance, contact tracing, outbreak response, and STI clinical services must be sustained and strengthened. Additionally, universal one-time syphilis screening should not replace risk-based ongoing screening. Detailed sexual histories obtained by trained health care providers remain vital for proper testing and follow-up, and asking about alcohol and drug use during clinical encounters creates opportunities for discussions of STI prevention and substance use risks.

As some individuals access health care only through sexual health or substance treatment clinics, using these encounters to offer STI screening, substance use referrals, or harm reduction services at either venue should be evaluated. Similarly, embedding syphilis screening in community health centers, emergency departments, and correctional facilities could increase identification and treatment, as has been the case for HIV and hepatitis C.[10–12]

Major knowledge gaps remain. The Rushmore et al. study included only Black, White, and Hispanic/Latino individuals, limiting the generalizability of their findings. In particular, understanding the impact of substance use on syphilis rates among American Indian and Alaska Native individuals is crucial, as these populations had the highest CS rates in 2023.[9] Also, the study lacked data on other substances, such as alcohol, fentanyl, and cocaine, that may be relevant to syphilis transmission. Additionally, data about women of transgender experience, who face disproportionately high rates of substance use disorders and STIs, are not routinely collected and were not included, as only 26 states were reporting gender identity in syphilis surveillance by 2023, although this has increased annually since 2018.[9] It is unclear whether gains in the collection of gender identity data will continue to increase and support improved syphilis public health initiatives or whether changes in federal language mandates and gender definitions will hinder progress in understanding populations at risk.

Although total syphilis elimination is presently out of reach, we do have the tools to end the public health emergency of CS. Screening and treatment during pregnancy are imperative but must be accompanied by comprehensive, data-driven efforts to expand appropriate screening, guide outreach, ensure timely treatment and partner services, improve education, and strengthen access to both medical and social support to prevent reinfection and ongoing transmission. Going forward, expanded uptake of prevalence-based screening for sexually active individuals in high morbidity age groups should be prioritized, with clear public health guidance from experts at the national, state, and local levels. Success in syphilis control will depend on the rigorous evaluation of screening approaches and sustained efforts to provide holistic sexual health care to diverse patient populations. AJPH

CORRESPONDENCE

Correspondence should be sent to Sarah E. Rowan, MD, 601 Broadway, Denver, CO 80203 (e-mail: Sarah.rowan@dhha.org). Reprints can be ordered at https://www.ajph.org by clicking the "Reprints" link.

PUBLICATION INFORMATION

Full Citation: Rowan SE, Wallace M, Wendel K. Traditional risk factors plus prevalence-based screening for syphilis: time for a dual approach. *Am J Public Health*. 2025;115(12):1960–1962.

Acceptance Date: September 18, 2025.

DOI: https://doi.org/10.2105/AJPH.2025.308296

ORCID iDs:

Sarah E. Rowan https://orcid.org/0000-0003-2144-7410

Meghan Wallace https://orcid.org/0009-0008-6478-8323

CONTRIBUTORS

S. E. Rowan wrote the first draft of the editorial. M. Wallace and K. Wendel critically reviewed the editorial and added key intellectual content. All authors have approved the final version of the editorial and agree to be accountable for all aspects of the work.

CONFLICTS OF INTEREST

The authors have no conflicts of interest to disclose.

REFERENCES

1. Centers for Disease Control and Prevention. The national plan to eliminate syphilis from the United States. Available at: https://stacks.cdc.gov/view/cdc/149963. Accessed September 4, 2025.
2. Centers for Disease Control and Prevention. Table 1. Sexually transmitted infections—reported cases and rates of reported cases, United States. *STI Statistics*. November 4, 2024. Available at: https://www.cdc.gov/sti-statistics/data-vis/table-sticasesrates.html. Accessed September 4, 2025.
3. Strathdee SA, Bristow CC, Gaines T, Shoptaw S. Collateral damage: a narrative review on epidemics of substance use disorders and their relationships to sexually transmitted infections in the United States. *Sex Transm Dis*. 2021;48(7):466–473. https://doi.org/10.1097/OLQ.0000000000001341
4. Allen JE, Mansergh G, Mimiaga MJ, Holman J, Herbst JH. Mobile phone and internet use mostly for sex-seeking and associations with sexually transmitted infections and sample characteristics among Black/African American and Hispanic/Latino men who have sex with men in 3 US cities. *Sex Transm Dis*. 2017;44(5):284–289. https://doi.org/10.1097/OLQ.0000000000000590
5. Bianchini ML, Rowan SE, Frost HM, Valuck R, McQueen RB, Anderson HD. Trends in demographic characteristics and risk factors among individuals with syphilis in Colorado from 2011 to 2020. *Sex Transm Dis*. 2025;52(6):345–351. https://doi.org/10.1097/OLQ.0000000000002130
6. Mangione CM, Barry MJ, Nicholson WK; US Preventive Services Task Force, et al. Screening for syphilis infection in nonpregnant adolescents and adults: US Preventive Services Task Force reaffirmation recommendation statement. *JAMA*. 2022;328(12):1243–1249. https://doi.org/10.1001/jama.2022.15322
7. Centers for Disease Control and Prevention. STI screening recommendations. March 13, 2025. Available at: https://www.cdc.gov/std/treatment-guidelines/screening-recommendations.htm. Accessed September 4, 2025.
8. Centers for Disease Control and Prevention. Vital signs: missed opportunities for preventing congenital syphilis—United States, 2022. *MMWR Morb Mortal Wkly Rep*. 2023;72(46):1269–1274. https://doi.org/10.15585/mmwr.mm7246e1
9. Centers for Disease Control and Prevention. National overview of STIs in 2023. *STI Statistics*. November 7, 2024. Available at: https://www.cdc.gov/sti-statistics/annual/summary.html. Accessed September 4, 2025.
10. Haukoos JS, Lyons MS, Rothman RE; HIV TESTED Trial Investigators, et al. Comparison of HIV screening strategies in the emergency department: a randomized clinical trial. *JAMA Netw Open*. 2021;4(7):e2117763. https://doi.org/10.1001/jamanetworkopen.2021.17763
11. Haukoos J, Rothman RE, Galbraith JW; DETECT Hep C Screening Trial Investigators, et al. Hepatitis C screening in emergency departments: the DETECT Hep C randomized clinical trial. *JAMA*. 2025;334(6):497–507. https://doi.org/10.1001/jama.2025.10563
12. Stanford KA, Mason J, Friedman E, Hazra A, Augustine E, Schneider J. An opt-out emergency department screening intervention leads to major increases in diagnosis of syphilis. *Open Forum Infect Dis*. 2024;11(9):ofae490. https://doi.org/10.1093/ofid/ofae490

An Individualized TTM-Based Intervention Promotes Child Safety Seat Purchase Among Pregnant Women: A Randomized Controlled Trial in Shantou, China

Weichen Yao, MD, Feng Wu, MD, Jingzhen Yang, PhD, Yueliang Chen, MD, Ziyue Tan, and Liping Li, PhD

This study evaluated a transtheoretical model (TTM)-based intervention's effectiveness in improving child safety seat (CSS) purchasing behaviors. A randomized controlled trial assigned 414 pregnant women to TTM, child passenger safety education, and control groups. At three, six, and 12 months after the intervention, the intervention groups showed significant improvements in CSS purchase rates and behavioral stage progression from baseline compared with the control group, with the TTM group showing the greatest effect. These findings may inform future efforts to promote CSS use and behavioral change. (*Am J Public Health*. 2025;115(12):1963–1966. https://doi.org/10.2105/AJPH.2025.308248)

AJPH December 2025, Vol. 115, No. 12

Road traffic injuries are the second leading cause of death among children aged one to 14 years in China. The absence of child safety seats (CSS) significantly contributes to road traffic injuries and fatalities among children.[1,2] In 2021, China enacted national regulations requiring CSS use for children younger than six years, yet usage rates remain below 15%.[3] A key factor is the lack of effective education programs, highlighting the urgent need for interventions to boost CSS usage.[4] The transtheoretical model (TTM) outlines the process of behavioral change in five stages: precontemplation, contemplation, preparation, action, and maintenance. By tailoring interventions to an individual's specific behavioral stage and associated characteristics, TTM provides a more responsive approach to measuring progress than traditional methods, improving the adoption of healthy behaviors.[5] Motivational interviewing complements TTM by using stage-specific techniques to strengthen motivation and commitment, guiding individuals toward lasting behavior change.[6] Research shows that combining the TTM model with motivational interviewing effectively promotes healthy behavior change.[7,8] Tailoring CSS interventions for pregnant women using this framework may yield better results than traditional strategies.

INTERVENTION AND IMPLEMENTATION

We designed a three-arm, parallel-group randomized controlled trial. Participants were randomly assigned to one of three study groups at a ratio of 1:1:1 (Figure A in Appendix, available as a supplement to the online version of this article at http://www.ajph.org):

1. TTM-based intervention group: participants received customized interventions aligned with the five stages of change within the TTM. This included motivational interviewing–style messages, delivered either in person or remotely via WeChat or telephone, tailored to each participant's stage of behavioral change (see online Table A);
2. Child passenger safety education (CPSE) intervention group: participants received educational materials and videos on CSS usage, delivered digitally once every two

months for a total of six sessions during the 12-month study period;
3. Control group: participants received educational materials and videos on pregnancy health and care, unrelated to child car safety, with the same format and duration as the CPSE intervention group.

Data collection was conducted at three, six, and 12 months after the intervention via online electronic questionnaires (consistent with baseline surveys). We used the CSS Behavioral Stage Scale to assess the stage of change for pregnant women, and the effectiveness of the intervention was evaluated by assessing changes in behavioral stages before and after the intervention across three groups. We performed data analysis using SPSS 26.0 (SPSS, Inc, Chicago, IL). We used repeated-measures two-way analysis of variance and post hoc least significant difference tests to analyze differences in CSS purchasing behavior changes.

PLACE, TIME, AND PERSONS

The study was conducted between November 2022 and January 2024, recruiting pregnant women from three hospitals in Shantou City, China. Eligible participants were in good health throughout their pregnancy, owned a private car, and signed a written informed consent form. Women with a history of severe pregnancy-related illnesses or miscarriages or requiring prolonged bed rest were excluded from the study.

PURPOSE

We aimed to evaluate the effectiveness of the TTM-based intervention and standardized CPSE compared with the controls in improving CSS purchase behaviors among pregnant women and compare behavioral stage progression across three groups.

EVALUATION AND ADVERSE EFFECTS

A total of 414 pregnant women were included in the study. Baseline survey data showed that participants averaged 30.2 ±0.8 years old, with 59.2% having bachelor's degrees, 57.0% being first-time mothers, and 94.7% having heard of CSS (online Table B). There were no differences in demographics among the three groups. During the 12-month intervention period, 79 participants were lost to follow-up. Ultimately, we obtained outcome data from 335 participants, including 116 in the TTM intervention group, 111 in the CPSE intervention group, and 108 in the control group.

Changes in CSS Purchase Behaviors

Changes within the group postintervention over time. The CSS purchase rate in the TTM-based intervention group increased significantly, from 15.52% at baseline to 23.28% at three months (an increase of 7.76 percentage points), 31.03% at six months (an increase of 15.51 percentage points), and 51.72% at 12 months (an increase of 36.20 percentage points; $P < .001$ for all). In the CPSE intervention group, the CSS purchase rate increased, but not as significantly as in the TTM-based intervention group. The control group showed no significant change (online Table C).

Intergroup comparisons. Compared with the control group, the probability of purchasing CSS increased in both intervention groups as the intervention progressed. The TTM-based intervention group showed the best effect, with an odds ratio (OR) of 3.96 (95% confidence interval [CI] = 2.20, 7.12) at 12 months after the intervention, whereas the CPSE intervention group had an OR of 2.08 (95% CI = 1.14–3.80; see online Table D).

Behavioral Stage Changes

Changes within groups over time. In the TTM-based intervention group, the proportion of participants remaining in their original stage decreased significantly, from 72.41% at baseline to 26.72% at the 12-month follow-up. Meanwhile, participant stage progression was as follows: 27.59% of participants advanced one stage, 26.72% advanced two stages, 15.52% advanced three stages, and 3.45% advanced four stages ($\chi^2 = 63.14$; $P < .001$). The proportion of participants in each stage of the CPSE intervention group decreased to 47.75%, 27.03%, 18.02%, 5.40%, and 1.80%, respectively ($\chi^2 = 33.20$; $P < .001$; Table 1).

Between-group comparisons. Participants in both the TTM-based intervention group and the CPSE intervention group exhibited significant changes in behavioral stages after the intervention ($\chi^2 = 55.457$; $P < .001$), with the TTM-based intervention group showing the most optimal effects (online Table E).

SUSTAINABILITY

To ensure sustainability, future interventions should account for parity, as multiparous women may have greater child safety knowledge. A one-size-fits-all approach for primiparous and multiparous women may not yield

TABLE 1— Changes in Child Safety Seat Purchasing Behavior Among Pregnant Women Before and After Intervention: Shantou, China, 2023

Stages	TTM-Based Interventions, No. (%)	CPSE Intervention, No. (%)	Control Group, No. (%)	Total, No. (%)
Precontemplation	31 (26.7)	53 (47.8)	73 (67.6)	157 (46.9)
Contemplation	32 (27.6)	33 (27.0)	28 (25.9)	90 (26.9)
Preparation	31 (26.7)	20 (18.0)	6 (5.6)	57 (17.0)
Action	18 (15.5)	6 (5.4)	1 (0.9)	25 (7.5)
Maintenance	4 (3.5)	2 (1.8)	0 (0.0)	6 (1.8)

Note. CPSE = child passenger safety education; TTM = transtheoretical model. $\chi^2 = 55.457$; $P < .001$.

optimal results. Additionally, TTM-based interventions for pregnant women should ensure both evidence-based content and highly trained, empathetic staff, given the heightened physical and emotional vulnerability during pregnancy. Finally, future research should create stage-specific implementation guidelines to ensure consistent delivery of core components while addressing individual needs.

PUBLIC HEALTH SIGNIFICANCE

TTM-based interventions can activate self-reinforcing maintenance mechanisms, unlike purely educational approaches, significantly increasing pregnant women's CSS purchasing behavior. These interventions are simple, effective, and easy to implement. In China, the "Guidelines for Preconception and Prenatal Care (2018)" recommend seven to 11 prenatal checkups over an approximately 280-day pregnancy period, creating a consistent and ideal opportunity for TTM-based interventions. This study found that integrating TTM strategies into prenatal education programs not only increased CSS purchase rates but also drove meaningful progress in CSS-related behavioral stages, with the potential to further improve CSS usage. Given their operational feasibility, scalability, and socioeconomic benefits, such interventions align well with existing maternal and child health systems in China. *AJPH*

ABOUT THE AUTHORS

Weichen Yao is with the School of Public Health, Shantou University, Shantou, China. Feng Wu, Yueliang Chen, Ziyue Tan, and Liping Li are with the Injury Prevention Research Center, Shantou University Medical College, Shantou, China. Jingzhen Yang is with the Center for Injury Research and Policy, The Research Institute at Nationwide Children's Hospital, Columbus, OH.

CORRESPONDENCE

Correspondence should be sent to Liping Li, 243 University Road, Shantou, Guangdong, China (e-mail: lpli@stu.edu.cn). Reprints can be ordered at https://www.ajph.org by clicking the "Reprints" link.

PUBLICATION INFORMATION

Full Citation: Yao W, Wu F, Yang J, Chen Y, Tan Z, Li L. An individualized TTM-based intervention promotes child safety seat purchase among pregnant women: a randomized controlled trial in Shantou, China. *Am J Public Health*. 2025;115(12):1963–1966.

Acceptance Date: July 8, 2025.

DOI: https://doi.org/10.2105/AJPH.2025.308248

ORCID iDs:

Weichen Yao https://orcid.org/0009-0003-9294-856X

Ziyue Tan https://orcid.org/0009-0002-0195-9355

Liping Li https://orcid.org/0000-0003-3306-779X

CONTRIBUTORS

W. Yao designed the methodology, completed the data collection and processing, analyzed and graphed the data, wrote the original manuscript, and was responsible for subsequent revisions. F. Wu and J. Yang reviewed and revised the original manuscript. Y. Chen performed validation, review, and editing. Z. Tan supervised, reviewed, and edited. L. Li conceptualized and directed the design of the study framework.

ACKNOWLEDGMENTS

Funding for this work has been provided by the Reproductive Preservation and Fertility Protection Research Project of the Chinese Preventive Medicine Association (grant no. 836), and the Science and Technology Project of Shantou Medical and Health Care Category (STYL2022015).

All authors acknowledge the selected participants and all survey staff for their support. Thanks to the editors and reviewers for their precious time and constructive comments.

Note. The funders had no role in the design of the study; the collection, analysis, and interpretation of data; or the writing of the manuscript.

CONFLICTS OF INTEREST

The authors have no conflicts of interest to declare.

HUMAN PARTICIPANT PROTECTION

The authors declare that all methods were carried out in accordance with relevant guidelines and regulations, and all experimental protocols were approved by the Medical Ethics Committee, Shantou University Medical College (SUMC-2022-037).

REFERENCES

1. Lee G, Pope CN, Nwosu A, et al. Child passenger fatality: child restraint system usage and contributing factors among the youngest passengers from 2011 to 2015. *J Safety Res.* 2019;70:33–38. https://doi.org/10.1016/j.jsr.2019.04.001
2. Degeorge KC, Neltner CE, Neltner BT. Prevention of unintentional childhood injury. *Am Fam Physician.* 2020;102(7):411–417.
3. Zheng X, Li R, Yang H, et al. The rate of child restraint system use among children aged under six years in China. *Scand J Public Health.* 2022;50(8):1192–1198. https://doi.org/10.1177/14034948211036621

4. Sun YR, Liu T, Ran N, et al. Assessment of the effectiveness of parent-targeted interventions for the use of child restraint systems: a systematic review and meta-analysis. *Transl Pediatr.* 2022;11(12):1939–1948. https://doi.org/10.21037/tp-22-560
5. Prochaska JO, Velicer WF. The transtheoretical model of health behavior change. *Am J Health Promot.* 1997;12(1):38–48. https://doi.org/10.4278/0890-1171-12.1.38
6. Hoy J, Natarajan A, Petra MM. Motivational interviewing and the transtheoretical model of change: under-explored resources for suicide intervention. *Community Ment Health J.* 2016;52(5):559–567. https://doi.org/10.1007/s10597-016-9997-2
7. Magill M, Apodaca TR, Borsari B, et al. A meta-analysis of motivational interviewing process: technical, relational, and conditional process models of change. *J Consult Clin Psychol.* 2018;86(2):140–157. https://doi.org/10.1037/ccp0000250
8. Bischof G, Bischof A, Rumpf HJ. Motivational interviewing: an evidence-based approach for use in medical practice. *Dtsch Arztebl Int.* 2021;118(7):109–115. https://doi.org/10.3238/arztebl.m2021.0014

Disarming Intimate Partner Violence Perpetrators: Stakeholder Perspectives on Enforcement Gaps and the Consequences of Federal Funding Cuts

Jennifer A. Wagman, PhD, MHS, and Wilson H. Hammett, PhD, MPH

Firearm relinquishment laws aim to prevent intimate partner homicide, yet enforcement remains fragmented and underresourced. Drawing on 25 stakeholder interviews conducted in California in 2021 and 2024 to 2025, we examined implementation challenges related to domestic violence restraining orders and gun violence restraining orders and explored how recent federal funding cuts have impacted survivor access to legal protection. Findings reveal structural enforcement gaps, design misalignments, and the compounding effects of disinvestment, highlighting urgent needs for policy realignment, sustained investment, and survivor-centered systems. (*Am J Public Health*. 2025;115(12):1967–1970. https://doi.org/10.2105/AJPH.2025.308287)

AJPH December 2025, Vol. 115, No. 12

As firearm-related intimate partner violence (IPV) continues to threaten public health and safety, understanding the effectiveness of protective laws remains critical.

STUDY OBJECTIVE

We sought to examine how IPV and firearm policy stakeholders in California perceive the enforcement of firearm relinquishment laws—specifically domestic violence restraining orders (DVROs) and gun violence restraining orders (GVROs)[1,2]—and explore the impact of recent federal funding cuts—particularly from the Victims of Crime Act (VOCA) and Office on Violence Against Women (OVW)—on survivors' access to legal protections.[3–5] We highlight intersections between legal infrastructure, public health, and gender-based violence prevention.[6,7]

RESEARCH OR ASSESSMENT QUESTIONS

What are the primary barriers to enforcing firearm surrender in IPV cases in California? How do federal funding constraints affect the implementation of firearm relinquishment laws and survivor safety in California?

PARTICIPANTS, SAMPLE, GEOGRAPHIC LOCATION, SETTING, AND YEARS OF STUDY

We conducted 25 qualitative interviews with professionals across California. Fifteen were conducted in 2021 in Los Angeles County with law enforcement officers, legal advocates, and service providers, originally as part of a study assessing the feasibility of integrating the Lethality Assessment Program into a domestic violence response initiative.[8] Ten additional interviews, completed between December 2024 and March 2025, included legal aid attorneys, gun policy experts, city or county officials, and advocates for IPV survivors (i.e., professionals who support and represent the rights of IPV survivors). This dual-phase design allowed us to examine persistent enforcement barriers alongside emerging threats tied to federal disinvestment.

Participants were purposively selected on the basis of their involvement in IPV prevention, firearm policy, restraining order enforcement, or survivor services. The sample included stakeholders from urban and semirural areas working in law enforcement, advocacy, government, and legal services. Interviews were conducted via Zoom.

METHODS

We used semistructured interview guides tailored to each data collection phase. Topics included DVRO and GVRO enforcement, interagency coordination, survivor access to legal protections, and the consequences of federal funding reductions.

All interviews were transcribed verbatim and analyzed using inductive thematic analysis.[9] Coding matrices enabled comparisons across time, roles, and regions to distinguish persistent challenges from emergent concerns related to recent disinvestment.

KEY FINDINGS

Our analysis identified several key themes reflecting persistent and emerging barriers to the enforcement of firearm relinquishment laws in IPV contexts.

Gaps in Firearm Surrender Enforcement

Participants across roles described persistent limitations in enforcing firearm surrender following DVROs and GVROs. In most jurisdictions, enforcement is functionally dependent on the honor system: agencies often rely on self-reporting, asking the restrained person whether they still possess a firearm and accepting that response without verification. Stakeholders emphasized that many restrained individuals are deemed at risk for harming themselves or others and may intentionally conceal gun access:

> Judges may order the surrender of firearms, but without proper verification, it's essentially an honor system. If an abuser claims they don't have a gun, there's rarely an effort to prove otherwise.
>
> –Prosecutor (2024)

Even in jurisdictions where surrender orders are issued, enforcement rarely extends beyond the paperwork. Without clear follow-up mechanisms—such as home visits or centralized tracking—implementation depends on officer discretion and time:

> Unless the firearm is used in an actual crime, there's often no mechanism to ensure it was surrendered after a restraining order is issued. We just don't have the resources to follow up on every single case.
>
> –Law enforcement officer (2021)

Most jurisdictions lack personnel designated for firearm surrender. Officers unfamiliar with enforcement procedures may serve orders, and follow-up is inconsistent or absent.

Breakdowns in coordination between courts, law enforcement, and advocacy organizations further weaken implementation. Participants described delays, siloed systems, and confusion over agency roles—often when system readiness is most critical:

> We've had people located and ready to be served, but the person with authority wasn't available. Then the moment is lost.
>
> –Legal advocate (2021)

This moment, they explained, often represents the culmination of survivor courage, legal action, and multiagency effort. When it slips away because of scheduling gaps or lack of follow-through, opportunities for disarmament can be lost—and survivor trust severely damaged.

Limited Use of Gun Violence Restraining Orders

Participants reported that GVROs are rarely used in IPV cases. Survivors and advocates for survivors described the process as ill-suited to IPV dynamics, citing procedural delays, limited legal support, and safety risks:

> Even when survivors know about GVROs, they're afraid that filing one will escalate the violence before the gun can be removed. There's a huge safety gap in the process.
>
> –Advocate for IPV survivors (2024)

Stakeholders emphasized GVROs were originally created to prevent suicide or mass shootings—not to address domestic violence—and lack the trauma-informed design of DVROs. GVROs do not include confidentiality protections, safety planning, or linkage to services:

> The GVRO process wasn't built with domestic violence survivors in mind. It's missing the wraparound protections that survivors need to stay safe.
>
> –Legal aid attorney (2025)

We found no support for the idea that survivors should routinely pursue both GVROs and DVROs. California DVROs already include firearm surrender, and most participants viewed underenforcement—not legal gaps—as the core issue. Some, however, saw GVROs as a complementary option when survivors cannot safely pursue DVROs. Unlike DVROs, GVROs can be petitioned by family or law enforcement, offering a potential route in urgent cases.

Still, participants cautioned that without survivor-centered safeguards, promoting GVROs in IPV cases can be harmful. Survivors may be left to navigate a process without legal advocacy, trauma-informed procedures, or confidentiality. As one advocate warned, in 2024, "We can't just push GVROs in IPV cases without survivor protections in place. That's how you end up escalating violence or retraumatizing someone who's already at risk."

Others stressed the importance of judicial education and legal infrastructure reform to ensure GVROs, when used in IPV cases, do not replicate or reinforce systemic failures that already place survivors at risk. Most agreed that, as currently constructed, GVROs cannot substitute for the survivor-centered protections provided by DVROs in IPV contexts.

Funding Cuts and Legal Aid Shortages

Participants described how chronic underinvestment, intensified by recent cuts to federal programs such as VOCA and OVW, has weakened the infrastructure needed to enforce firearm relinquishment in IPV cases. One law enforcement officer explained, in 2021, "We used to have more dedicated resources for this, but those funds dried up. Now, it's really only happening if an officer has extra time, which isn't often." The absence of dedicated personnel was said to reduce follow-up on firearm surrender orders and limit cross-agency coordination.

Participants felt legal aid attorneys—who play a critical role in helping survivors navigate the complex restraining order system—were similarly impacted, particularly in cases involving firearm removal. Many legal aid organizations were said to be operating with reduced staff because of federal disinvestment. VOCA-related reductions were reported to have led to attorney layoffs, unstaffed legal clinics, and the cancellation of survivor-centered services such as court accompaniment and firearm-related advocacy. One legal aid attorney shared, in 2024, "When survivors call, we sometimes have to tell them no attorneys are available." These conditions were said to contribute to severe attorney burnout, reduced case preparation capacity, and delayed legal processing. In several jurisdictions, survivors were said to face long wait times or be turned away entirely—barriers that increase legal attrition and limit the likelihood of enforcement follow-through.

These disruptions burden survivors and compromise the public health intent of firearm relinquishment laws. Participants stressed that while additional funding is necessary, it is not sufficient on its own. Rather, disinvestment compounds entrenched structural failures—such as siloed communication systems, inconsistent judicial decision-making, and the absence of enforcement infrastructure. Even well-crafted firearm laws cannot function effectively in a system where the mechanisms for legal access and follow-through are eroded.

Participants also called for the development of scalable training programs for law enforcement, legal aid staff, and judges to support consistent implementation. These were viewed as essential for reducing jurisdictional variability and ensuring that both DVROs and GVROs are applied and enforced in ways that reflect survivor risk and legal intent.

EVALUATION, TRANSFERABILITY, AND ADVERSE EFFECTS

California is viewed as a leader in firearm regulation,[10] yet the challenges identified here—legal aid shortages, poor coordination, and inconsistent enforcement—are not unique to the state. Several stakeholders with experience in other jurisdictions affirmed the national relevance of these findings, including in other states with DVRO and GVRO laws. No adverse effects were reported.

SCALABILITY

Future research should evaluate enforcement practices across jurisdictions, examine court outcomes, and explore survivor experiences. Participants advocated scalable, role-specific training—particularly for judges—to clarify GVRO applicability in IPV contexts. Several emphasized that legislative refinement is needed so that survivors are not forced to navigate multiple legal systems to secure firearm relinquishment.

PUBLIC HEALTH SIGNIFICANCE

Firearms remain a leading method of intimate partner homicide.[6] This study shows that structural gaps, design mismatches, and institutional disinvestment undermine the protective intent of California's laws even though the laws offer strong statutory tools.[10] Without adequate investment in legal infrastructure, the system cannot enforce firearm laws effectively—and faces downstream consequences such as attorney burnout, case delays, and survivor attrition. Effective IPV firearm policy requires not only statutory authority but also investment in enforcement, legal services, and survivor access to justice. AJPH

ABOUT THE AUTHORS

Jennifer A. Wagman and Wilson H. Hammett are with the Department of Community Health

Sciences, Jonathan and Karin Fielding School of Public Health, University of California, Los Angeles.

CORRESPONDENCE

Correspondence should be sent to Jennifer A. Wagman, Jonathan and Karin Fielding School of Public Health, University of California, Los Angeles, 650 Charles E Young S, Los Angeles, CA 90095 (e-mail: jennwagman@ucla.edu). Reprints can be ordered at https://www.ajph.org by clicking the "Reprints" link.

PUBLICATION INFORMATION

Full Citation: Wagman JA, Hammett WH. Disarming intimate partner violence perpetrators: stakeholder perspectives on enforcement gaps and the consequences of federal funding cuts. *Am J Public Health*. 2025;115(12):1967–1970.

Acceptance Date: August 27, 2025.

DOI: https://doi.org/10.2105/AJPH.2025.308287

ORCID iDs:

Jennifer A. Wagman https://orcid.org/0000-0002-9957-1932

Wilson H. Hammett https://orcid.org/0000-0002-3904-8269

CONTRIBUTORS

J. A. Wagman conceptualized and designed the study and led the writing of the article. W. H. Hammett contributed to data collection, analysis, and interpretation. Both authors participated in drafting and revising the article for important intellectual content and approved the final version to be published.

ACKNOWLEDGMENTS

This work was supported by grants from the California Firearm Violence Research Center at the University of California, Davis, and from the National Collaborative on Gun Violence Research.

We thank Daphne Marvel for her assistance with the interviews, and we are especially grateful to all study participants for generously sharing their time and perspectives.

CONFLICTS OF INTEREST

The authors declare no conflicts of interest.

HUMAN PARTICIPANT PROTECTION

This study was approved by the University of California, Los Angeles, Office of the Human Research Protection Program (institutional review board protocols 20-001548 and 24-0654).

REFERENCES

1. Seave PL. Disarming batterers through restraining orders: the promise and the reality in California. *Eval Rev.* 2006;30(3):245–265. https://doi.org/10.1177/0193841X06287675
2. Oliphant SN, Zeoli AM. State efforts to enforce firearm dispossession through relinquishment laws. *Criminol Public Policy.* 2024;23(4):893–918. https://doi.org/10.1111/1745-9133.12677
3. Dodda TP. Funding cuts leave domestic violence survivors trapped with their abusers. *Ms. Magazine.* February 11, 2025. Available at: https://msmagazine.com/2025/02/11/trump-domestic-violence-funding-cuts-shelter-survivors. Accessed March 10, 2025.
4. Newmark LC. *Crime Victims' Needs and VOCA-Funded Services: Findings and Recommendations from Two National Studies.* Final Report to the National Institute of Justice. Alexandria, VA: Institute for Law and Justice; 2006. Report No. 214263. Available at: https://www.ojp.gov/pdffiles1/nij/grants/214263.pdf. Accessed October 16, 2025.
5. Wright E, Ponder Selib C. Cutting federal funding for victim service providers jeopardizes Americans' safety. Urban Institute. March 31, 2025. Available at: https://www.urban.org/urban-wire/cutting-federal-funding-victim-service-providers-jeopardizes-americans-safety. Accessed October 6, 2025.
6. Campbell JC, Webster D, Koziol-McLain J, et al. Risk factors for femicide in abusive relationships: results from a multisite case control study. *Am J Public Health.* 2003;93(7):1089–1097. https://doi.org/10.2105/ajph.93.7.1089
7. Goodyear A, Rodriguez M, Glik D. The role of firearms in intimate partner violence: policy and research considerations. *J Public Health Policy.* 2020;41(2):185–195. https://doi.org/10.1057/s41271-019-00198-x
8. Wagman JA, Nguyen G, Marvel D. Assessing the feasibility of integrating the lethality assessment program into the Los Angeles Domestic Abuse Response Team. *J Fam Viol.* 2024 https://doi.org/10.1007/s10896-024-00742-8
9. Braun V, Clarke V. Using thematic analysis in psychology. *Qual Res Psychol.* 2006;3(2):77–101. https://doi.org/10.1191/1478088706qp063oa
10. Zeoli AM, McCourt A, Buggs S, Frattaroli S, Lilley D, Webster DW. Analysis of the strength of legal firearms restrictions for perpetrators of domestic violence and their associations with intimate partner homicide. *Am J Epidemiol.* 2018;187(11):2365–2371. https://doi.org/10.1093/aje/kwy174

Evaluation of ShootSafe, an Interactive, Sequential Website to Teach Youths Firearms Safety: A Randomized Clinical Trial

David C. Schwebel, PhD, D. Leann Long, PhD, Anna Johnston, MA, Yefei He, PhD, Casie H. Morgan, PhD, Joan Severson, MS, Gregory Taylor, BA, and Katelyn Trullinger, MA, CMI

This randomized trial evaluated ShootSafe, a theory-based website using a graphic novel storyline, educational and testimonial videos, and games, to teach firearms safety to children aged 10 to 12 years. A total of 163 youths participated. Linear mixed models found that youths randomized to ShootSafe demonstrated greater knowledge, safer behavioral intentions, and safer simulated hunting behaviors following training and at four-month follow-up compared with the control condition. Broad dissemination could reduce risk of unintentional pediatric firearms injury and death.

Trial Registration. ClinicalTrials.gov identifier: NCT4622943. (*Am J Public Health*. 2025;115(12): 1971–1977. https://doi.org/10.2105/AJPH.2025.308267)

In this study, we implemented and evaluated ShootSafe, a theory-based, firearms safety Internet program to teach youths safe firearms storage, transport, and handling. The target age group was 10 to 12 years, an age when typically developing youths have cognitive capacity to learn requisite skills to make safe decisions[1,2] and may begin using firearms independently for recreational purposes.[3]

INTERVENTION AND IMPLEMENTATION

ShootSafe offers lessons through interactive and experiential learning,[4] delivering information via a sequential website design.[5] It is grounded in health behavior theory and designed to increase youths' self-efficacy to behave safely and alter perceptions about vulnerability to firearm injury, potential severity of firearms-related injury, and normative peer behavior to engage safely with firearms.[5]

The website offers games, instructional videos, and testimonial videos amid a graphic novel storyline.[5] Youths accompany animal characters through chapters to learn safe firearms storage, transport, and use (Appendix Figure A, available as a supplement to the online version of this article at https://ajph.org). Expert-narrated videos provide short lessons on topics like cleaning firearms and climbing tree stands. Testimonials present emotional and moving stories about serious firearms injuries and fatalities using real-world visuals and child actors (Appendix Figure B). Games reinforce knowledge and provide practice of relevant cognitive skills like impulse control and hypothetical thinking (Appendix Figure C).

We evaluated ShootSafe via a repeated-measures randomized parallel group, two-arm superiority trial with three assessment time points (baseline, postintervention, and four-month follow-up) and considered three primary outcomes: firearms safety knowledge, behavioral intention, and simulated behaviors. We compared ShootSafe with vHappy, an unpublished child nutrition and well-being website of similar size and scope.

PLACE, TIME, AND PERSONS

We recruited 163 youths and their parents from community sources in and around Birmingham, Alabama (mean age = 11.4 years; SD = 0.8). Appendix Table A presents demographic information. Inclusion criteria included English fluency and some exposure to firearms, defined as youths having firearms present in their primary residence and knowing where they were stored, engaging in hunting or shooting activities at least once in the past two years, or both.

Parents provided informed consent and youths provided informed assent. We collected baseline data from February 2022 through October 2023, until the desired sample size was reached; follow-up data collection continued through March 2024. Appendix Figure D presents the CONSORT diagram. We conducted analyses with intention-to-treat principles, assuming outcomes were missing at random. Sensitivity analyses used multiple imputation.

PURPOSE

Firearms kill more American youths than any other cause of death,[6] with approximately 17% of fatalities among children younger than 13 years being unintentional, the result of risky and preventable decisions while storing, transporting, and handling firearms.[7] Most prevention efforts target adults, urging safe firearms storage.[8–10] This strategy can be effective but fails when youths use firearms recreationally, a frequent occurrence.[3,11] ShootSafe takes a different approach, recognizing that youths use firearms recreationally and sometimes independently and, thus, teaching them to do so safely once they have requisite cognitive development capacity.

EVALUATION AND ADVERSE EFFECTS

Following recruitment and consenting but before randomization, parents completed baseline surveys and youths engaged in a structured battery. Random assignment, driven by computer-generated lists in a one-to-one allocation model, occurred at the end of that visit.

At separate appointments one and two weeks later, youths engaged in their randomly assigned website for 45-minute sessions. A week after training ended and again four months later, youths completed postintervention and follow-up assessments, respectively, each largely replicating baseline assessments.[5]

Training

Children were provided a tablet (ShootSafe) or desktop computer (vHappy) to engage in the assigned website. Researchers monitored youths through one-way mirrors and redirected if needed (e.g., wandering off assigned website; considerable inattention). Redirection was required on six occasions (< 2% training visits), all for youths randomized to vHappy. Following engagement, ShootSafe children provided opinions about the website.

Measures

We assessed demographics via parent report. We considered three primary outcomes, each assessed at all three time points: (1) firearms safety knowledge, (2) behavioral intention surrounding firearm use, and (3) firearm safety behaviors in simulated tasks.

We assessed knowledge through two strategies: (1) a self-administered 12-item firearm knowledge and safety questionnaire and (2) responses concerning safety of 13 photographs depicting unknown peers conducting either safe or dangerous behaviors with firearms (Appendix Figure E).

We assessed behavioral intention through two strategies: (1) the same set of photographs, with oral responses concerning whether youths would engage in that behavior themselves, and (2) response to intended action in 11 short storyboard-accompanied vignettes presented orally by researchers (Appendix Figure F).

We assessed behavior through laboratory simulations. The first simulated a hunting outing, including a fence-climbing obstacle. Youths selected deer-hunting attire and eye and ear protection from many choices, then removed a realistic-looking and -feeling toy rifle from a storage locker. They were instructed to traverse a wooden fence placed in a laboratory doorway while carrying their rifle and ammunition. Following negotiation of the fence, youths entered a large room decorated like a forest. On one wall, animated images of moving prey were projected. Youths could shoot foam ammunition at the animations, some of which were safe shooting situations and others risky (Appendix Figure G). Following presentation of eight randomly ordered images (four safe, four unsafe), youths were instructed to store their gun.

We considered four hunting simulation outcomes: (1) selection of one or more hunter orange–colored clothing articles; (2) number of dangerous shots taken during animated scenarios; (3) proper firearm storage, defined as gun unloaded and placed in safe with muzzle downward; and (4) total percentage of time engaged in unsafe actions through the simulation, defined as placing finger on trigger when shooting was not imminent, pointing muzzle toward self or others, and other clearly unsafe firearm behaviors.

Two outcomes were considered from the fence-climbing simulation: (1) safe climbing, scored objectively in a binary manner, and (2) percentage of time engaged unsafely, scored identically to the hunting simulation.

The second simulation replicated a shooting range. Youths were presented with a realistic-looking and -feeling dry-fire handgun and situated with a shooting bench and target. The researcher had an identical handgun, bench, and target and was positioned adjacently. Targets registered hits using laser, allowing participants to witness success and keep score. During a 5.5-minute shooting period, we presented five risk-inducing situations: (1) researcher went downrange to change target, (2) car alarm blared, (3) researcher shouted excitedly about the youth shooting well, (4) researcher received smartphone call, and (5) researcher requested help addressing a malfunctioning gun. At the end, youths were instructed to store the gun. We considered two outcomes: (1) percentage of time youths engaged unsafely and (2) safe storage, defined as unloading clip and locking both clip and firearm in storage case.

We coded outcomes through live and videotaped coding, with validity confirmed through independent coder interrater reliability on at least 10% of data with all $\kappa>0.87$ (categorical data) and all $\rho>0.93$ (continuous).

Analysis

In separate intention-to-treat analyses, we evaluated participants' knowledge, behavioral intention, and simulated behavior outcomes using linear mixed models, which accounted for correlation of measurement within study participants across time points. We used general linear mixed models for continuous variables, logistic mixed models for binary outcomes, and Poisson mixed models using empirical variance estimation for count outcomes. All models included intervention group and timepoint as categorical variables and interactions of time by group. To increase efficiency, we included two a priori identified covariates, youth age and sex.[12,13] The mixed models allowed use of all observed data, including data from participants with incomplete outcome measurement at follow-up, with missing-at-random assumption.[14] We conducted multiple imputation using chained equations as a sensitivity analysis.[15] We conducted analyses by using SAS version 9.4 (SAS Institute, Cary, NC) and R version 4.2.3 (R Foundation for Statistical Computing, Vienna, Austria), with two-sided tests and $\alpha = 0.05$.

Results

Supplementary Tables A and B show demographic and outcome data, respectively. Table 1 shows mixed model analysis results. Following training, youths randomized to ShootSafe

TABLE 1— Least-Squares Means of Primary and Secondary Outcome Measures and Between-Group Differences for ShootSafe Hunting Safety Intervention Group vs Nutrition Control Group: Birmingham, AL, 2022–2024

Outcome and Time Point	ShootSafe, Least-Squares Mean (SE) or %	Control, Least-Squares Mean (SE) or %	Between-Group Comparison	
			Measure (95% CI)	P
Knowledge assessment				
Questionnaire[a]				
Baseline	6.21 (0.23)	5.85 (0.22)	...	...
Postintervention	8.09 (0.23)	6.24 (0.22)	1.85 (1.22, 2.48)	<.001
4-mo follow-up	7.71 (0.23)	6.13 (0.22)	1.59 (0.95, 2.24)	<.001
Photographs[a]				
Baseline	8.77 (0.15)	9.04 (0.15)	...	...
Postintervention	9.93 (0.15)	9.60 (0.15)	0.33 (−0.09, 0.76)	.12
4-mo follow-up	10.11 (0.16)	9.70 (0.16)	0.42 (−0.02, 0.85)	.06
Behavioral intention				
Photographs[a]				
Baseline	9.17 (0.17)	9.37 (0.17)	...	...
Postintervention	9.96 (0.17)	9.62 (0.18)	0.34 (−0.14, 0.83)	.17
4-mo follow-up	9.77 (0.18)	9.19 (0.18)	0.58 (0.08, 1.07)	.023

Continued

TABLE 1— Continued

Outcome and Time Point	ShootSafe, Least-Squares Mean (SE) or %	Control, Least-Squares Mean (SE) or %	Between-Group Comparison: Measure (95% CI)	Between-Group Comparison: P
Storyboard[a]				
Baseline	8.06 (0.19)	7.99 (0.19)	. . .	. . .
Postintervention	9.12 (0.19)	7.99 (0.20)	1.12 (0.58, 1.67)	<.001
4-mo follow-up	8.87 (0.20)	8.01 (0.30)	0.86 (0.30, 1.41)	.003
Behavior: hunting scenario				
Safe clothing choice[b]				
Baseline	59.8	48.9	. . .	. . .
Postintervention	94.3	57.7	12.19 (4.09, 36.37)	<.001
4-mo follow-up	72.1	49.6	2.62 (1.24, 5.53)	.011
Unsafe shots taken[c]				
Baseline	5.19 (0.41)	5.00 (0.39)	. . .	. . .
Postintervention	3.27 (0.38)	5.69 (0.55)	0.58 (0.43, 0.78)	<.001
4-mo follow-up	3.00 (0.42)	4.87 (0.53)	0.62 (0.44, 0.87)	.007
Percentage of time unsafe[a]				
Baseline	6.69 (0.91)	3.39 (0.92)	. . .	. . .
Postintervention	4.70 (0.96)	5.17 (0.98)	−0.47 (−3.16, 2.23)	.73
4-mo follow-up	5.84 (0.95)	6.06 (0.96)	−0.22 (−2.87, 2.44)	.87
Safe storage[b]				
Baseline	42.1	33.2	. . .	. . .
Postintervention	62.1	51.2	1.56 (0.73, 3.32)	.25
4-mo follow-up	63.0	51.0	1.63 (0.76, 3.51)	.21
Behavior: fence scenario				
Cross fence safely[b]				
Baseline	16.6	13.0	. . .	. . .
Postintervention	51.8	33.1	2.17 (1.00, 4.69)	.049
4-mo follow-up	49.4	36.1	1.72 (0.78, 3.79)	.18
Percentage of time unsafe[a]				
Baseline	19.69 (2.40)	14.87 (2.46)	. . .	. . .
Postintervention	8.89 (2.46)	6.21 (2.52)	2.67 (−4.27, 9.61)	.45
4-mo follow-up	11.53 (2.60)	12.70 (2.57)	−1.16 (−8.36, 6.04)	.75
Behavior: range scenario				
Percentage of time unsafe[a]				
Baseline	7.46 (0.75)	7.59 (0.75)	. . .	. . .
Postintervention	6.25 (0.75)	7.80 (0.77)	−1.56 (−3.67, 0.56)	.15
4-mo follow-up	4.92 (0.77)	6.14 (0.78)	−1.22 (−3.37, 0.93)	.27
Safe storage[b]				
Baseline	62.3	60.8	. . .	. . .
Postintervention	64.9	60.4	1.21 (0.53, 2.79)	.65
4-mo follow-up	60.4	56.5	1.17 (0.52, 2.67)	.7

Note. CI = confidence interval. All analyses adjust for group, time, group–time interaction, youth age, and youth sex.

[a]Mean difference.

[b]Odds ratio.

[c]Mean ratio.

generally had higher firearm safety knowledge and safer behavioral intentions than youths randomized to vHappy. They also showed generally safer behavior in the hunting simulation. Although the direction of association was generally as hypothesized, groups did not differ significantly for behavioral assessments of safe storage, percentage of time unsafe, or fence-crossing safety. Figure 1 and Appendix Figure H illustrate results graphically. Sensitivity analyses concorded closely with primary analyses (Appendix Table C).

Youth impressions about ShootSafe were positive: 72% responded they enjoyed the website, 81% felt they learned to be safer with guns, and 94% reported they might or would recommend ShootSafe to same-age peers.

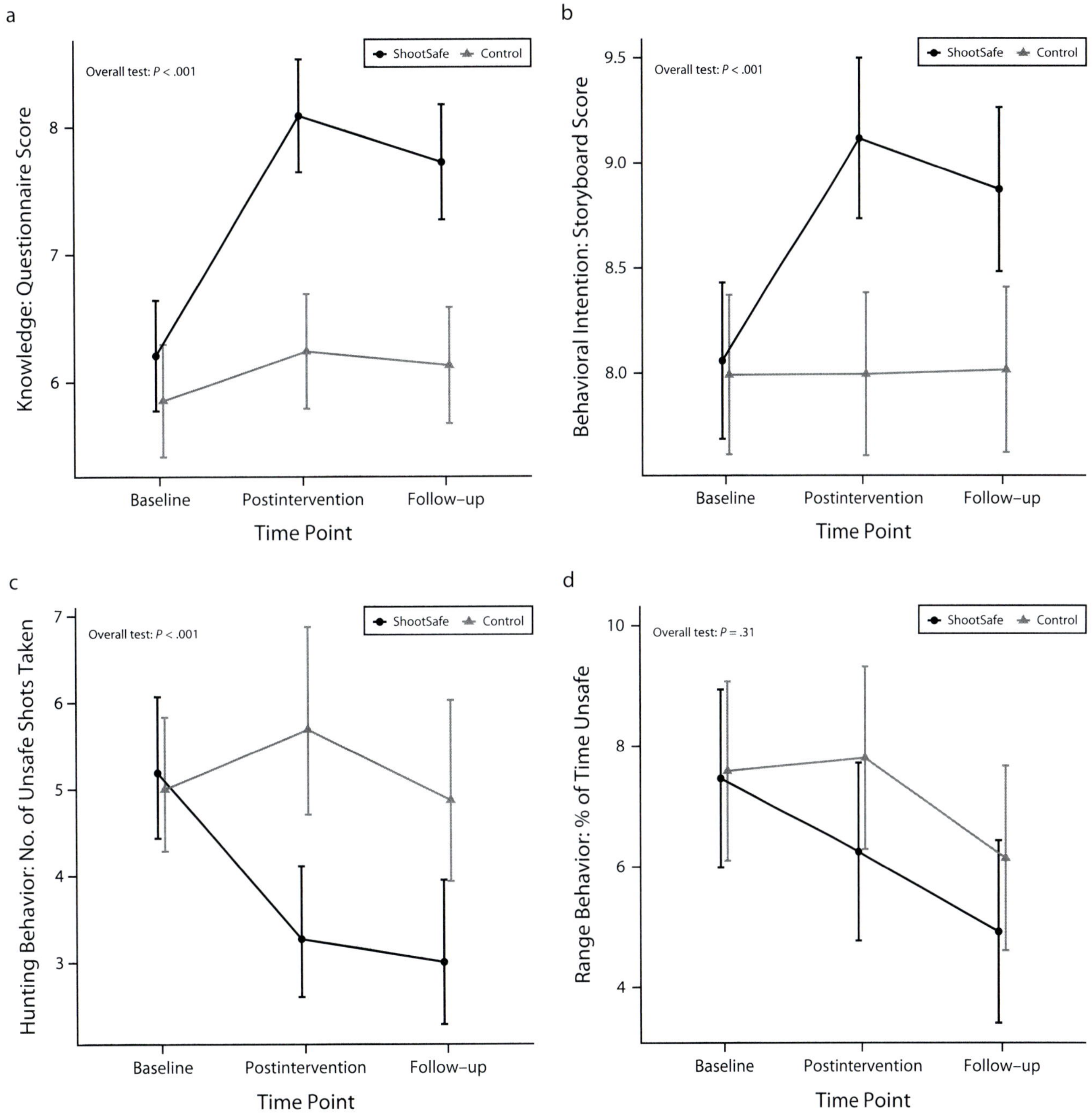

FIGURE 1— **Change Over Time for ShootSafe Hunting Safety Intervention Group vs Nutrition Control Group for (a) Knowledge Score, (b) Behavioral Score, (c) Hunting Behavior, and (d) Range Behavior: Birmingham, AL, 2022–2024**

AJPH December 2025, Vol. 115, No. 12

Adverse Effects

No adverse effects were seen.

SUSTAINABILITY

ShootSafe can be transmitted to any Internet-enabled device, including smartphones, and engaged in sequentially at the user's preferred pace (e.g., one chapter at a time; single sitting). Partnership with industry, nonprofits, or government may facilitate broad dissemination at no or low user cost.

PUBLIC HEALTH SIGNIFICANCE

Results suggest effectiveness, supporting widespread dissemination of ShootSafe or similar programs to train American youths aged 10 years and older in safe recreational firearms use, storage, and transport. Quality adult supervision is still recommended, but given youth firearm use practices, safety training is also essential. AJPH

ABOUT THE AUTHORS

David C. Schwebel was with the Department of Psychology, University of Alabama at Birmingham at the time of this study. D. Leann Long is with the Department of Biostatistics and Data Science, Wake Forest University School of Medicine, Winston-Salem, NC. Anna Johnston is with the Department of Psychology, University of Alabama at Birmingham. Yefei He, Joan Severson, and Katelyn Trullinger were with Digital Artefacts, Iowa City, IA, at the time of this study. Casie H. Morgan was with the Department of Psychology, University of Alabama with the Birmingham for part of this study and the Department of Psychiatry and Behavioral Sciences, Medical University of South Carolina for part of this study. Gregory Taylor is an independent contractor based in Los Angeles, CA.

CORRESPONDENCE

Correspondence should be sent to David C. Schwebel, University of Iowa Office of Research, 2660 University Capitol Centre, Iowa City, IA 52242 (e-mail: david-schwebel@uiowa.edu). Reprints can be ordered at https://www.ajph.org by clicking the "Reprints" link.

PUBLICATION INFORMATION

Full Citation: Schwebel DC, Long DL, Johnston A, et al. Evaluation of ShootSafe, an interactive, sequential website to teach youths firearms safety: a randomized clinical trial. *Am J Public Health*. 2025;115(12):1971–1977.

Acceptance Date: August 11, 2025.

DOI: https://doi.org/10.2105/AJPH.2025.308267

ORCID iDs:

David C. Schwebel https://orcid.org/0000-0002-2141-8970

D. Leann Long https://orcid.org/0000-0001-8614-7190

Anna Johnston https://orcid.org/0000-0002-2891-6569

Yefei He https://orcid.org/0009-0004-6239-7573

Casie H. Morgan https://orcid.org/0000-0002-1515-6548

Gregory Taylor https://orcid.org/0009-0004-1376-9270

CONTRIBUTORS

D. C. Schwebel contributed to conceptualization, methodology, writing the original draft, visualization, supervision, project administration, and funding acquisition. D. L. Long contributed to conceptualization, methodology, formal analysis, data curation, writing the original draft, article review and editing, visualization, and funding acquisition. A. Johnston contributed to conceptualization, methodology, investigation, data curation, article review and editing, visualization, supervision, and project administration. Y. He contributed to software, resources, and article review and editing. C. H. Morgan contributed to methodology, investigation, article review and editing, and supervision. J. Severson contributed to conceptualization, software, resources, visualization, and funding acquisition. G. Taylor contributed to conceptualization, resources, article review and editing, and visualization. K. Trullinger contributed to conceptualization, software, resources, and visualization. The fourth through eighth authors contributed similarly to the work and are listed alphabetically. All authors contributed to the conceptualization or design of the work or the acquisition, analysis, or interpretation of data for the work; drafted the work or revised it critically for important intellectual content; and approved the final version to be published.

ACKNOWLEDGMENTS

This publication was supported by the Centers for Disease Control and Prevention (CDC) of the US Department of Health and Human Services (HHS) as part of a financial assistance award totaling $1 950 000, with 100% funded by CDC/HHS. C. H. Morgan's work on article preparation was supported in part by a grant from the National Institute on Mental Health (T32MH018869, MPI: Danielson, Kilpatrick).

We thank the following individuals for their support of this project: Amanda Benson, Skylar Morriss, Jarius Rembert, Yixin Wang, and the full UAB Youth Safety team; Digital Artefacts team; Spring Creek Prop Farm, including Chris Story and Len Ward; advisory board members Marisa Futral (in memoriam), Dylan Baumgardner, Bo Garrett, Stephanie Mallory, and Steve McCormack; and actors and experts in ShootSafe videos.

Note. The contents are those of the author(s) and do not necessarily represent the official views of, nor an endorsement by, CDC/HHS or the US government.

CONFLICTS OF INTEREST

The authors have no conflicts of interest to report.

HUMAN PARTICIPANT PROTECTION

This research was reviewed and approved by the University of Alabama at Birmingham institutional review board. Adult participants provided informed consent, and child participants provided informed assent.

REFERENCES

1. Blakemore SJ, Choudhury S. Development of the adolescent brain: implications for executive function and social cognition. *J Child Psychol Psychiatry*. 2006;47(3-4):296–312. https://doi.org/10.1111/j.1469-7610.2006.01611.x
2. Inhelder B, Piaget J. *The Growth of Logical Thinking From Childhood to Adolescence: An Essay on the Construction of Formal Operational Structures*. Parsons A, Milgram S, trans. New York, NY: Basic Books; 1958.
3. Stewart M, Meinke DK, Snyders JK, Howerton K. Shooting habits of youth recreational firearm users. *Int J Audiol*. 2014;53(suppl 2):S26–S34. https://doi.org/10.3109/14992027.2013.857437
4. Morris TH. Experiential learning—a systematic review and revision of Kolb's model. *Interact Learn Environ*. 2020;28(8):1064–1077. https://doi.org/10.1080/10494820.2019.1570279
5. Schwebel DC, Long DL, Gowey M, Severson J, He Y, Trullinger K. Study protocol: developing and evaluating an interactive web platform to teach children hunting, shooting and firearms safety: a randomized controlled trial. *BMC Public Health*. 2021;21(1):308.
6. Roberts BK, Nofi CP, Cornell E, Kapoor S, Harrison L, Sathya C. Trends and disparities in firearm deaths among children. *Pediatrics*. 2023, Sep 1;152(3): e2023061296. https://doi.org/10.1542/peds.2023-061296
7. Centers for Disease Control and Prevention. Welcome to WISQARS. Available at: https://www.cdc.gov/injury/wisqars. Accessed January 18, 2025.
8. Holly C, Porter S, Kamienski M, Lim A. School-based and community-based gun safety educational strategies for injury prevention. *Health Promot Pract*. 2019;20(1):38–47. https://doi.org/10.1177/1524839918774571
9. Lee LK, Fleegler EW, Goyal MK, et al.; Council on Injury Violence and Poison Prevention. Firearm-

related injuries and deaths in children and youth: injury prevention and harm reduction. *Pediatrics.* 2022;150(6):e2022060070. https://doi.org/10.1542/peds.2022-060070

10. Ngo QM, Sigel E, Moon A, et al.; FACTS Consortium. State of the science: a scoping review of primary prevention of firearm injuries among children and adolescents. *J Behav Med.* 2019; 42(4):811–829. https://doi.org/10.1007/s10865-019-00043-2
11. Miller M, Hemenway D. Unsupervised firearm handling by California adolescents. *Inj Prev.* 2004;10(3):163–168. https://doi.org/10.1136/ip.2004.005447
12. Canner PL. Covariate adjustment of treatment effects in clinical trials. *Control Clin Trials.* 1991; 12(3):359–366. https://doi.org/10.1016/0197-2456(91)90016-f
13. Lingsma H, Roozenbeek B, Steyerberg E. Covariate adjustment increases statistical power in randomized controlled trials. *J Clin Epidemiol.* 2010;63(12):1391. https://doi.org/10.1016/j.jclinepi.2010.05.003
14. Molenberghs G, Thijs H, Jansen I, et al. Analyzing incomplete longitudinal clinical trial data. *Biostatistics.* 2004;5(3):445–464. https://doi.org/10.1093/biostatistics/kxh001
15. Li P, Stuart EA, Allison DB. Multiple imputation: a flexible tool for handling missing data. *JAMA.* 2015;314(18):1966–1967. https://doi.org/10.1001/jama.2015.15281

Building EXCITEment for Vaccines in Rural Communities

Michelle S. Rodgers, PhD, Laura H. Downey, DrPH, Tia M. Gregory, MS, Erica Weintraub Austin, PhD, Dawn E. Burton, PhD, Laura Clark, PhD, Ruth Hursman, RN, MSN, BCEN, Paula Peters, PhD, Kathryn A. Stofer, PhD, Jacqueline Wilkins, PhD, and Erica L. DeWald, BS

The Cooperative Extension System (CES) consists of 112 land-grant universities in the United States, including historically Black universities and Tribal colleges. In 2021, CES formed the Extension Collaborative on Immunization Teaching and Engagement (EXCITE) to increase confidence in and access to adult immunizations. From April 2021 to May 2023, EXCITE conducted 111 immunization education projects involving 76 land-grant universities. EXCITE reached more than 18 million individuals, and more than 48 000 COVID-19 and other adult-recommended vaccines were provided in partnership with local health organizations. (*Am J Public Health*. 2025;115(12):1978–1981. https://doi.org/10.2105/AJPH.2025.308258)

AJPH December 2025, Vol. 115, No. 12

When the first COVID-19 vaccines became widely available to the public in April 2021, demand and uptake varied across the United States. Vaccination coverage lagged in rural areas,[1] even though rural communities, on average, experienced disproportionate rates of COVID-19-related hospitalizations and mortality relative to urban and suburban areas.[2]

INTERVENTION AND IMPLEMENTATION

Key trusted messengers in rural communities are land-grant universities (LGUs), which offer science-based outreach programs through the Cooperative Extension System (CES) on topics ranging from nutrition and health to agriculture, youth development, and community vitality. Across 112 LGUs, including historically Black and Tribal colleges and universities, CES employs more than 32 000 professionals. CES has a presence in every county and parish in the United States.[3]

Through its nonprofit arm the Extension Foundation, CES formed the Extension Collaborative on Immunization Teaching and Engagement (EXCITE) to address vaccine confidence and demand in rural communities by (1) decreasing vaccine hesitancy among rural and medically underserved audiences, (2) increasing the accessibility of vaccination clinics among priority populations, (3) increasing connections and communication between priority populations and health care systems, and (4) helping both federal and local partners implement public health programs to reduce health disparities.[3]

Extension professionals use a variety of engagement approaches and communication technologies to disseminate science-based information. They also have relationships with a culturally, geographically, and economically diverse clientele as well as a network of state and local community partners. What they did not have, however, was a centralized leadership structure for a national initiative such as EXCITE.

The EXCITE national program team was established to provide overall leadership in operationalizing and managing the project. This team was composed of professionals at LGUs with expertise in administration, market research, project implementation, coaching, and evaluation. In addition, professionals with the Extension Foundation acted as the "solutions team," providing expertise in innovation and technology solutions, team building, marketing and communications, grant and contract management, and information technology.

Leaders at the US Department of Agriculture's National Institute of Food and Agriculture as well as the Centers for Disease Control and Prevention (CDC) were also valued leadership team members.

PLACE, TIME, AND PERSONS

The leadership team designed EXCITE in two phases of activity over the first three years of work. The first phase, the Rapid COVID-19 Campaign, was a one-year COVID-19 immunization awareness campaign designed to quickly disseminate tailored messaging to communities. The second phase, Adult Immunization Education Pilot Projects, funded two-year pilot projects to tailor vaccine messaging for specific populations, evaluate their success, and then reimplement the projects.

Each EXCITE project was developed by LGUs using a rapid community assessment of local needs documented through a vulnerability index. EXCITE projects focused on reaching rural and medically underserved communities and addressing health disparities. The priority populations served are summarized in Table 1. Many projects served more than one priority population. In addition to the priority populations shown in Table 1, 13 projects worked with communities on 17 Native American reservations.

PURPOSE

The Rapid COVID-19 Campaign was initiated in June 2021 to dispel myths about the COVID-19 vaccine and increase immunization rates among rural and medically underserved populations. All 112 LGUs were eligible to apply; 72 institutions chose to participate and were awarded funding in a noncompetitive process.

Information disseminated by CES was based on the CDC "Vaccinate with Confidence" messaging campaign.[4] Extension Foundation professionals quickly disseminated messages about the COVID-19 vaccine to priority populations, which were selected according to local community assessment tools developed by both the CDC and the Extension Foundation. Each LGU provided a COVID-19 vulnerability index for its select priority population indicating that the project focused on rural and medically underserved communities. The selected populations were verified with input from public health departments and medical providers as those with the greatest vaccine hesitancy. CES professionals then adopted, adapted, or developed tailored messages for the populations identified through the needs assessment process and in coordination with state public health departments. CES used various channels, including social media, faith communities, pop-up immunization clinics, and written or verbal messages, to share COVID-19 vaccine education materials.

The second phase, Adult Immunization Education Pilot Projects, was a two-year project beginning in May 2022 to reach further into key demographics with even more precise, effective messaging about the COVID-19 vaccine and other adult immunizations such as influenza and tetanus. Thirty-nine LGUs, 35 of which participated in the Rapid COVID-19 Campaign, were competitively selected with criteria to ensure diversity in methodology, partnership models, and target populations. Some LGUs within states chose to partner with other LGUs to expand their reach. All chosen pilot projects promoted immunization education, community uptake, and availability of vaccination clinics.

The first year of the pilot projects included the creation of campaigns informed by local market research to understand priority population views and perspectives and to inform future iterations of the intervention. The second year of the projects included worksite education, train-the-trainer sessions, media campaigns, development of community leaders as messengers, and use of volunteers for local program delivery.

EVALUATION AND ADVERSE EFFECTS

Seventy-six LGUs (67%) were involved in the first two phases of EXCITE. They were geographically dispersed across the country, with the largest percentage of involvement in the northeastern, southern, and central states. American Samoa was also involved in the Rapid COVID-19 Campaign (Figure 1).

During this time, EXCITE reached more than 18 million people through 174 467 engagement activities. EXCITE Rapid COVID-19 Campaign teams and Education Pilot teams reported mass media and social media as the engagement activities that reached the most individuals.

TABLE 1— Number of Extension Collaborative on Immunization Teaching and Engagement (EXCITE) Projects, by Priority Population: United States, 2021–2023

Priority Population	Number of Projects
Hispanic, Latino, and Spanish origin (including migrant farmworkers)	48
Black or African American	44
American Indian or Alaska Native	23
Asian	16
Native Hawaiian or other Pacific Islander	11

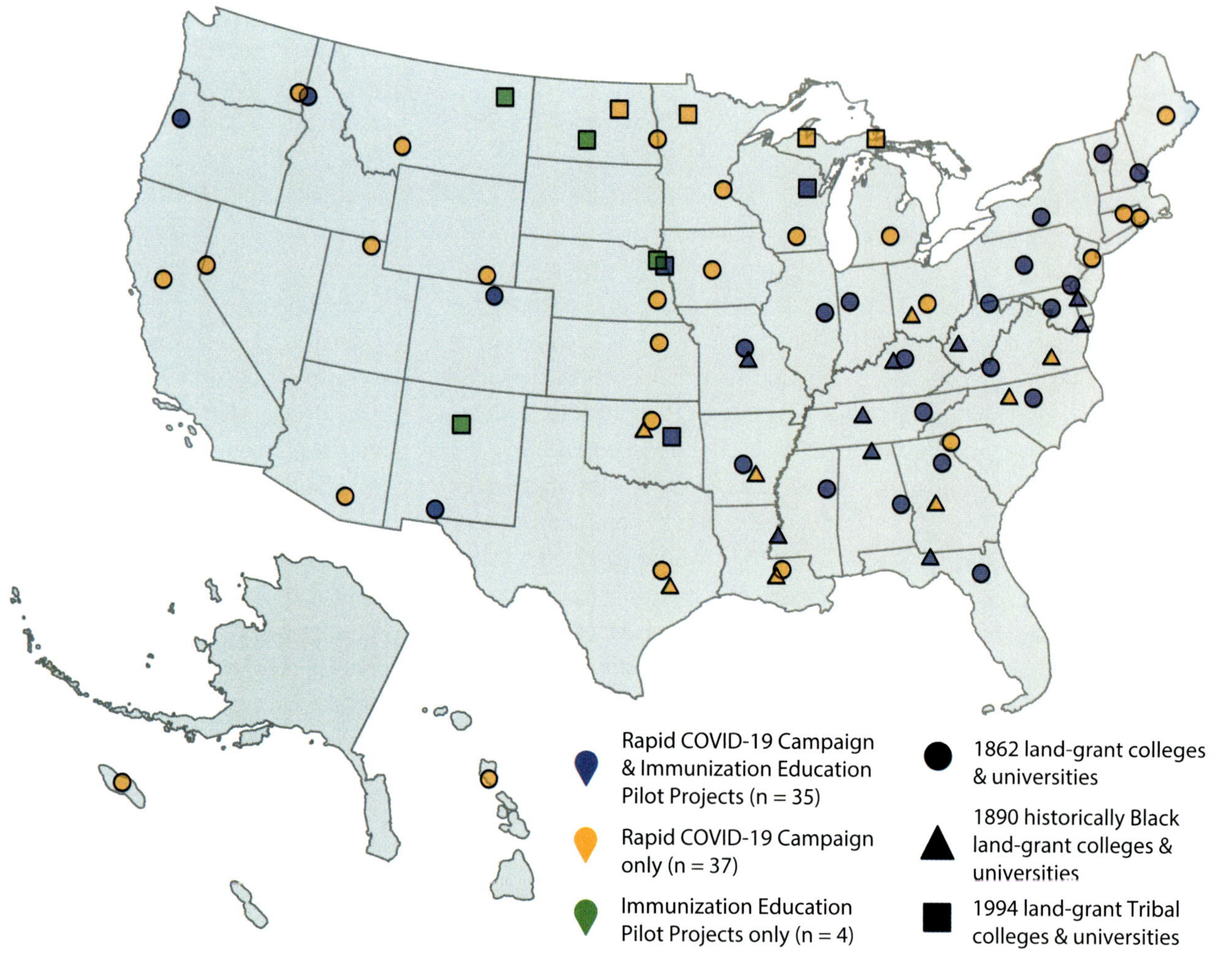

FIGURE 1— **Land-Grant Institutions Participating in the Extension Collaborative on Immunization Teaching and Engagement (EXCITE), by Project: United States, 2021–2023**

EXCITE teams also reported hosting 1034 vaccination clinics in collaboration with partners, directly administering 48 194 vaccines at these events.

In addition to measuring engagement activities, number and reach, assets developed or adopted, and campaign success, funded pilot projects used questions adapted from the CDC Vaccine Confidence Survey Question Bank to determine whether EXCITE was changing perceptions of and access to vaccines. By the conclusion of the pilot projects, teams had accomplished the goal of decreasing vaccine hesitancy among rural and medically underserved audiences.

In the final report, teams noted the following observed outcomes:

- Nine teams reported improved vaccination trust among their priority populations.
- Twelve teams reported improved vaccination rates.
- Nineteen teams reported improved perceived importance of vaccines for preventive health and disease prevention among their priority populations.
- Six teams reported improved social norms emphasizing the importance of vaccinations.

EXCITE's work would not have been possible without partners. By the end of May 2023, Rapid COVID-19 Campaign teams had worked with 410 partners and pilot project teams had collaborated with 234 partners.

SUSTAINABILITY

Although EXCITE met its goals, there were challenges involved. The pandemic itself affected staff time and availability as well as the ability to hire additional personnel. Staff also had to navigate moving all educational efforts to virtual platforms during the first year. In addition, our work had to begin with educating our own staff on the benefits of vaccination.

In the second year, staff turnover and retirements affected both the program teams and established partnerships. Personnel were also challenged by the need to rapidly provide up-to-date information, in multiple languages, as the pandemic progressed. Many rural communities require translated materials, including in Spanish, Haitian Creole, and Hmong, among other languages. EXCITE project teams also had to ensure that the materials developed reflected cultural differences. The program now maintains these materials in an asset library for ongoing immunization education efforts.

Despite the challenges, staff shared that EXCITE was both professionally and personally fulfilling. EXCITE continues beyond the pandemic by piloting the integration of immunization education into ongoing programs such as the Expanded Food and Nutrition Education Program and other family and consumer science programs (e.g., Dining with Diabetes).

PUBLIC HEALTH SIGNIFICANCE

Vaccination coverage among adults is low for most vaccines,[1] leaving many American adults unprotected from vaccine-preventable diseases. Adult vaccination rates, particularly in rural areas, remain stagnant despite widespread public health efforts.[1] The CDC and other public health agencies continue to seek evidence-based approaches to build the public's confidence in vaccines and eliminate barriers to immunizations. Public health agencies often turn to community-based organizations as trusted messengers to educate the public on the importance of vaccines in protecting individual and public health.

Lessons learned during the COVID-19 pandemic confirmed the importance of forming lasting, long-term relationships rather than short-term partnerships and the need to use multiple communication channels to achieve outcomes and sustain educational efforts.[5] The number and diversity of engagement activities underscore the long-standing role of CES as a trusted partner in rural and agricultural communities. Public health partners should strongly consider incorporating CES as a collaborating community-based organization, especially in attempts to reach rural audiences. AJPH

ABOUT THE AUTHORS

Michelle S. Rodgers, Ruth Hursman, and Erica DeWald are with the Extension Foundation, Kansas City, MO. The following authors are part of their respective Cooperative Extension programs. Laura H. Downey is with Auburn University, Auburn, AL. Tia M. Gregory is with Mississippi State University, Mississippi State, MS. Erica Weintraub Austin is with the Washington State University, Pullman. Dawn E. Burton is with Prairie View A&M University, Prairie View, TX. Laura Clark is with University of Tennessee, Knoxville. Paula Peters was with Kansas State University, Manhattan at the time of the study. Kathryn A. Stofer is with the University of Florida, Gainesville. Jacqueline Wilkins is with The Ohio State University, Columbus.

CORRESPONDENCE

Correspondence should be sent to Erica L. DeWald, One Kansas City Place, 1200 Main Street, Suite 3800, Kansas City, MO 64105-2122 (e-mail: ericadewald@extension.org). Reprints can be ordered at https://www.ajph.org by clicking the "Reprints" link.

PUBLICATION INFORMATION

Full Citation: Rodgers MS, Downey LH, Gregory TM, et al. Building EXCITEment for vaccines in rural communities. *Am J Public Health*. 2025;115(12): 1978–1981.

Acceptance Date: July 23, 2025.

DOI: https://doi.org/10.2105/AJPH.2025.308258

ORCID iDs:
Michelle S. Rodgers https://orcid.org/0009-0006-5174-0203

Tia M. Gregory https://orcid.org/0009-0007-4250-736X

Laura Clark https://orcid.org/0009-0006-2150-1738

Kathryn A. Stofer https://orcid.org/0000-0002-3659-490X

Erica L. DeWald https://orcid.org/0000-0002-8027-046X

CONTRIBUTORS

All of the authors were critical in the conception, development, and execution of this work.

ACKNOWLEDGMENTS

The Extension Collaborative on Immunization Teaching and Engagement (EXCITE) is made possible through an interagency agreement between the National Institute of Food and Agriculture and the Centers for Disease Control and Prevention and a cooperative agreement with the Extension Foundation in partnership with the Extension Committee on Policy Health Program Action Team. The Extension Foundation is a nonprofit organization that provides grant administration and fiscal oversight in support of the Cooperative Extension System.

We extend a special thank you to Julie Zajac, Alexandra M. Piasecki, R. Brent Elrod, and Edwin Lewis for their inspiration and support.

CONFLICTS OF INTEREST

The authors have no conflicts of interest.

HUMAN PARTICIPANT PROTECTION

No protocol approval was needed because no human participants were included.

REFERENCES

1. Andress L, Fitch C. Rural health inequities and the role of Cooperative Extension. Available at: https://open.clemson.edu/cgi/viewcontent.cgi?article=2018&context=joe. Accessed July 29, 2025.
2. Buys DR, Rennekamp R. Cooperative Extension as a force for healthy, rural communities: historical perspectives and future directions. *Am J Public Health*. 2020;110(9):1300–1303. https://doi.org/10.2105/AJPH.2020.305767
3. Extension Collaborative on Immunization Teaching and Engagement. EXCITE home page. Available at: https://excite.extension.org. Accessed July 29, 2025.
4. Centers for Disease Control and Prevention. Vaccinate with Confidence. Available at: https://www.cdc.gov/vaccines/partners/vaccinate-with-confidence.html. Accessed June 16, 2025.
5. Fiebelkorn AP, Adelsberg S, Anthony R, et al. The role of funded partnerships in working towards decreasing COVID-19 vaccination disparities, United States, March 2021–December 2022. *Vaccine*. 2024;42(suppl 3):125551. https://doi.org/10.1016/j.vaccine.2023.12.061

"I Didn't Have to Struggle": Caregivers' Perspectives on the Synergistic Interplay of WIC and SNAP on Family Health

Cristina M. Gago, PhD, MPH, Matthew M. Lee, PhD, MS, Nour M. Hammad, MSc, RD, Jhordan O. Wynne, PhD, MPH, Mary Kathryn Poole, PhD, MPH, Meghan Zimmer, MPH, Rebecca S. Mozaffarian, MS, MPH, Rachel Colchamiro, MPH, RD, CLC, Kelley May, MPH, Eric B. Rimm, ScD, and Erica L. Kenney, ScD, MPH

We explored how increased Special Supplemental Nutrition Program for Women, Infants, and Children (WIC) and Supplemental Nutrition Assistance Program (SNAP) benefits interacted for dually enrolled households. Twenty-five parents dually enrolled in WIC and SNAP in the spring of 2020 shared perceptions of expanded benefits and reduced administrative requirements via semistructured interviews. Specifically, parents shared that benefit increases minimized monthly cycles of limited or uncertain access to food, barriers to WIC redemption led many to prioritize SNAP benefits, reduced administrative requirements facilitated staying enrolled in both programs, and administrative flexibilities and benefit increases supported WIC and SNAP utilization. (*Am J Public Health*. 2025;115(12):1982–1987. https://doi.org/10.2105/AJPH.2025.308259)

AJPH December 2025, Vol. 115, No. 12

During the COVID-19 pandemic, when millions reported not having enough to eat and social distancing hindered access to services, Congress allowed the US Department of Agriculture to temporarily decrease administrative requirements and increase benefits for the Special Supplemental Nutrition Program for Women, Infants, and Children (WIC) and the Supplemental Nutrition Assistance Program (SNAP; Appendix B Table A, available as a supplement to the online version of this article at https://ajph.org). Changes to WIC allowed parents to recertify remotely and increased the cash value benefit for fruit and vegetable purchases from $9 to, currently, $26 per month per child. Simultaneously, SNAP extended the time between households' recertification applications, waived application interviews, permitted online shopping, and increased benefits (Appendix B, Figure A).

While growing literature has examined the impact of these changes on households enrolled in either WIC[1–4] or SNAP[5–7] alone,[8] few have examined the interplay across programs, despite one in three WIC-enrolled families participating in SNAP concurrently.[9] Better understanding of household experiences using both programs is critical for improving utilization.

STUDY OBJECTIVE

This qualitative study aimed to improve understanding of how expanded benefits and reduced administrative burden in WIC and SNAP simultaneously influenced eligible households' retention and utilization decisions.

RESEARCH QUESTION

How did expanded benefits and reduced administrative burden in WIC and SNAP influence dually eligible households' participation and utilization decisions?

PARTICIPANTS, SAMPLE, LOCATION, SETTING, AND YEAR OF STUDY

Parents with children who self-reported being enrolled in both WIC and SNAP in March 2020, were at least 18 years old, lived in Massachusetts, and spoke English or Spanish were eligible (December

2023–March 2024). All participants (n = 25) identified as female (Table A). Most were aged older than 30 years (54.2%), spoke English at home (62.5%), and identified as Puerto Rican (62.5%). Half reported sometimes worrying food would run out in the past year.

METHODS

This qualitative study was conducted in partnership with Massachusetts WIC.

Recruitment and Data Collection

Local WIC programs and community organizations shared information about the study via e-mail and text messages, social media, and physical flyer distribution. Interested participants contacted the study team via phone, e-mail, or QR code to complete an online eligibility screener. Researchers followed up with those deemed eligible to schedule an interview. After providing written informed consent, participants completed a brief demographic survey and a 45-minute semistructured Zoom interview. Interviews were led by trained qualitative researchers and audio recorded. Reporting aligns with the Standards for Reporting Qualitative Research.

Conceptual Framework and Interview Design

Our interview guide and analytic approach were grounded in the Getting to Equity Framework.[10] The framework posits four interrelated constructs as drivers of nutritional inequities, including increasing access to healthy food, reducing deterrents, improving resources, and building capacity. The study team developed a semistructured interview guide exploring these four constructs in relation to WIC and SNAP participation experiences, pandemic-related program changes, and the interaction between WIC and SNAP administrative burdens and benefits (Appendix A, available as a supplement to the online version of this article at https://www.ajph.org). We piloted the guide with two WIC participants and subsequently revised.

Analysis

Audio was transcribed verbatim by Sonix software (San Francisco, CA) and transcripts were analyzed by four trained researchers (C. M. G., M. M. L., N. M. H., and J. O. W.; see Appendix B, available as a supplement to the online version of this article at https://ajph.org, for positionality) in Dedoose 9.0.17 (Sociocultural Research Consultants LLC, Los Angeles, CA).[11] C. M. G. developed a preliminary codebook based on the Getting to Equity Framework,[10] predefined topics from the interview guide, and emergent topics from transcript review. Via deductive thematic analysis,[12] the researchers applied codes to the same five transcripts—meeting to iteratively revise the codebook, review code applications, and discuss discrepancies until reaching consensus. Once coding was deemed consistent, a team of analysts (C. M. G., M. M. L., N. M. H., and J. O. W.) coded the remaining transcripts independently. Researchers then reviewed the coded excerpts and met to generate, refine, and finalize themes through discussion.

KEY FINDINGS

Two key findings were identified. First, expanded WIC and SNAP benefits promoted dual program utilization; however, pandemic circumstances forced greater reliance on SNAP. Second, reduced administrative requirements for WIC and SNAP supported dual program retention, but differences in the quality of interactions with WIC and SNAP staff impacted participants' experiences of these changes.

Expanded Benefits Promoted Utilization

Increases to WIC and SNAP benefits served distinct, though synergistic, missions. Participants viewed the purposes of WIC and SNAP to be distinct. For example, they reported that WIC's cash value benefit increase aligned with WIC's goal to promote nutrition—allowing them to buy greater quantity, quality, and variety of fruits and vegetables (Box 1). Meanwhile, participants reported that SNAP's temporary emergency allotments and permanent Thrifty Food Plan adjustment improved access to flexible economic resources for poverty alleviation. Benefit increases interacted to facilitate benefit redemption across programs; for example, parents reported that increases in WIC's cash value benefit allowed them to save and stretch SNAP dollars further. However, the end of SNAP emergency allotments brought a return to monthly cycles of limited or uncertain food access.

Pandemic supply chain issues and fear of illness hindered access to WIC-approved foods, forcing greater reliance on SNAP. Parents identified three hindrances to WIC benefit uptake at the pandemic's start: low in-store inventory, transit barriers, and inability to shop in store for fear of COVID-19 exposure. Low inventory meant parents often could not fully redeem WIC benefits, even after traveling to multiple stores. Fear of illness led many to avoid stores,

BOX 1— Illustrative Quotes for Key Finding 1 From Analysis of Qualitative Interviews With 25 Parents Enrolled in WIC and SNAP in Massachusetts

Key finding 1: Expanded WIC and SNAP benefits promoted dual program utilization; however, pandemic circumstances hindered access to WIC-approved foods, forcing greater reliance on SNAP.

Subtheme 1.1: Increases to WIC and SNAP benefits served their distinct, though synergistic, missions.

- [WIC distinct role] "You could literally buy any fruits or vegetables, whether it's frozen fresh, canned, whatever it is. Uh, well, it made me try different stuff that I've never tried before, like zucchini and let's say, red bell peppers." –Participant B
- [SNAP distinct role] "[With the SNAP increases,] I didn't have to struggle and worry about my kids having food. And I didn't have to, like, cut back meals for myself to make sure my kids ate." –Participant P
- [Synergy] "I could buy the same things off my WIC . . . [and] it helps me out because it can make my food stamps last longer" –Participant D
- [Synergy] "When I noticed that, you know, I was, um, paying the fruits and vegetables more with the WIC than the SNAP, I, um, was pretty happy about it. Um, because, you know, that opened up a lot more space to buy other things that my daughters needed." –Participant G
- [Synergy] "I follow the WIC's guidelines even though I don't have to with the SNAP benefits—um, just to maintain the healthy overall aspect of what we're eating as a family in general." –Participant E
- [Positive affect] "It makes me happy that I even though I work, I don't make as much, but I get to provide for my kids what they want." –Participant B
- [SNAP rollback] "Because your regular benefits like run out like super quick within the first two weeks, and then after that it's like you're on your own. So having that was like, okay, I got something else to fall back on now, and I don't have to spend as much money on groceries right now." –Participant O
- [Other expenses] "I was able to pay my phone bills on time, pay my gas and electricity on time. Um, before it was like, we were like, juggling. If, you know, we'll pay this and then we'll pay this one later on." –Participant G

Subtheme 1.2: Pandemic circumstances (e.g., supply chain issues and fear of illness) hindered access to WIC approved foods, forcing greater reliance on SNAP.

- [Low inventory] "I had to go to multiple stores [to use WIC benefits]. It was repetitive because sometimes the shelves weren't stocked. So, then I would have to go somewhere else and see if they had it." –Participant C
- [Transit barriers] "I just feel like if it [WIC] was online for people that don't have transportation, it would just make it that much easier for them to have those benefits for their family instead of wasting them because they couldn't get to the store." –Participant E
- [Fear of COVID-19] "So during the pandemic, um, when everybody was freaking out about germs . . . no one knew what you know, COVID could really do to you or how it was really spread and all that, that fun jazz. Um, I placed a lot of Walmart orders, okay. And, uh, would, would drive up and they would bring the groceries to you, and, um, I did, uh, as fast as possible." –Participant J
- [SNAP online] So either, you know, Instacart, which I only use maybe like two times when I was really in a pinch because you have to pay for the fee and then the delivery and then you have to tip them. But the Walmart pickup was just literally a lifesaver during COVID, so that was amazing that they did that, because I think that also helped a lot of people use it and access it. –Participant Q
- [Rising prices] "Because everything is so expensive that you even know if you're getting more [SNAP] benefits, it doesn't really matter because you're still buying the same." –Participant R

Subtheme 1.3: Amid SNAP benefit increases, most continued to redeem the WIC benefits fully, while some redeemed WIC benefits more selectively.

- [Cash value benefit redemption] "Regardless of me using my SNAP I still use my WIC because . . . [they] give you $25 for fruit and vegetables." –Participant D
- [WIC redemption] "I will definitely still use the WIC benefits completely . . . and then with the SNAP I will just get whatever extra I wanted." –Participant F
- [WIC redemption] "I always still, no matter what I got for SNAP, I was still very smart and use[d] my WIC. I made sure whatever I could use on WIC, I used." –Participant A
- [Forfeiting WIC benefits] "I'm not going to grab it on my WIC, because I'm not going to go drag all my kids into the grocery store just to get the milk. . . . What do I care about $3–4 [for] milk on my food stamps?" –Participant Q

Note. SNAP = Supplemental Nutrition Assistance Program; WIC = Special Supplemental Nutrition Program for Women, Infants, and Children. Bracketed terms are intended to briefly summarize the topic of each illustrative quote.

even if it meant forfeiting WIC benefits. Alternatively, SNAP benefit increases and flexibilities gave families the resources to stock up on staples through a single monthly trip.

Amid SNAP benefit increases, some WIC participants redeemed WIC benefits more selectively. While grocery access changes drove initial reductions in WIC redemption, most parents still needed and intended to use WIC benefits fully—citing rising food prices and continued monthly cycles of limited or uncertain access to adequate food. However, some parents did note that SNAP benefit increases resulted in their redeeming WIC benefits less, even after initial grocery stocking issues were resolved, especially after the introduction of SNAP online shopping in Massachusetts in June 2020. Leveraging SNAP's flexibility and convenience, some reported using SNAP dollars on WIC items (and forfeiting WIC benefits) to save additional trips to WIC-approved stores. However, even those who reported under-redeeming components of their WIC food package still fully redeemed WIC's cash value benefit.

Reduced Requirements Supported Retention

WIC's transition to remote appointments was consistently described as the most important administrative change across both programs, ultimately facilitating retention in WIC (Box 2). This was especially true among parents with difficulty traveling to in-person appointments. While most parents reported no change in the quality of services, some felt in-person appointments were more thorough for monitoring growth; these parents advocated hybrid service options. Regarding SNAP, some parents reported that their recertification experiences did not change despite the administrative policy waivers, though some families noted that the extended certification periods protected against financial shocks.

Participants described broken communication with SNAP agency staff, including dropped calls and long wait times when attempting to reach caseworkers. Such interactions perpetuated feelings of shame and stigma. In contrast, open communication and positive relationships offered by WIC facilitated redemption and retention.

EVALUATION, TRANSFERABILITY, AND ADVERSE EFFECTS

In this study of the interactions between WIC and SNAP among dually enrolled households, parents reported that WIC and SNAP play distinct, though complementary, roles in enhancing food access.[8] WIC supports nutritional health and SNAP supports poverty alleviation. Despite intending to use both WIC and SNAP benefits fully, parents faced barriers to WIC access,[13] which prompted many to use SNAP's more flexible benefits to buy WIC items or alternatives. WIC's cash value benefit, which most closely resembles SNAP benefits in terms of maximizing autonomy, was the most highly valued and redeemed component of WIC's food package.[1–3]

Participation in WIC and SNAP for economically disadvantaged households is critical for reducing food insecurity, related health risks, and health care costs. It is also essential for preventing the widening of health inequities, given the intersection of food security with low income and structural racism. Our findings suggest that the pandemic-era streamlining of WIC and SNAP and increased benefit amounts should continue and be expanded—for example, through introducing WIC–SNAP

BOX 2— Illustrative Quotes for Key Finding 2 From Analysis of Qualitative Interviews With 25 Parents Enrolled in WIC and SNAP in Massachusetts

Key finding 2: Reduced administrative requirements for WIC and SNAP supported dual program retention, but differences in the quality of interactions with WIC and SNAP staff impacted participants' experiences of these changes.

Subtheme 2.1: Reduced administrative requirements for WIC supported long-term retention and those for SNAP protected against financial shock.

- [WIC remote] "I didn't have a car, so it was hard for me to get to the appointment to the office I had was a little bit far from where I live, so it was always a little situation when I was to go to the office. Um, then when they did this change where it was through the phone and stuff, like I still didn't have a car. That was amazing at that point because it makes it easy for me and then whatever. If they would need any paper for any reason, I would send it to through text message. And I wouldn't even have to show up to the, um, office at that point." –Participant F
- [WIC remote] "I don't have to worry about driving there. I don't have to worry about, um, you know, a fussy kiddo that doesn't want to be there. I don't have to worry about germs right now." –Participant J
- [SNAP extended certification] "If your income went up or it went down, either way, you were still getting the max benefit. You didn't have to do anything. Um, so that was very, very nice. It was very helpful." –Participant I
- [SNAP extended certification] "Honestly, to me it didn't really make much of a difference because I still tried to . . . get the paperwork for like recertification . . . as quickly as possible." –Participant H

Subtheme 2.2: Differences in quality of interactions with WIC and SNAP staff impacted participant understanding of programmatic changes during the pandemic.

- [SNAP communication] "I don't talk to my caseworker because my caseworker is never available. I've already went through probably five of them now." –Participant A
- [SNAP communication] "I was a little confused about why my food stamps got reduced, and I called, and it said, like a week for them to, like, call me back and like, like explaining what was going on. And sometimes they don't even, like, call you back." –Participant H
- [SNAP communication] "I wouldn't say because of miscommunication, but when they increase the amount that they were giving, I was surprised when I received my monthly benefit and I was like, wait, this is too much. What have they done? [And] it like caused stress because it was like, what's going on here?" –Participant E
- [SNAP communication] "You just always feel like you're walking into this entity, like the jailhouse. . . . You're walking through metal detectors. It just doesn't feel welcoming. And you always just feel so ashamed." –Participant A
- [WIC communication] "Someone always answers the phone and directs you to who you have to speak to, or they answer your question and if they don't have an answer for you, they'll get back to you" –Participant E
- [WIC communication] "They're pretty good with, like, giving us a call back and if not, like, answering the actual phone. Yeah. Um, we speak with nutritionists. Um, they're on the site, so I've never really had a problem with that. Um, and usually our benefits are, like, recharged right there the same day that they say it's going to be recharged. I never had a problem with that." –Participant G

Note. SNAP = Supplemental Nutrition Assistance Program; WIC = Special Supplemental Nutrition Program for Women, Infants, and Children. Bracketed terms are intended to briefly summarize the topic of each illustrative quote.

dual-approved online shopping, adding more WIC food package flexibilities, and maintaining remote benefit services. Participants' description of the critical role of respectful, open communication with WIC agency staff also highlights the need to design policies to support this.

However, most pandemic-era relief programs have ended, resulting in significant increases in food insecurity nationwide (affecting 10.2% in 2021, 12.8% in 2022, and 13.5% in 2023[14]), aligning with the United States' largest one-year increase in poverty (doubling from 5.2% in 2021 to 12.4% in 2022).[15] Despite this, Congress passed legislation to restrict access to SNAP, increase administrative burdens, and reduce benefit amounts over time.[16]

Study transferability may be limited; most data were collected from participants recruited from one local WIC program in Massachusetts. However, findings align with those from other states[5,7] and federal policies examined hold implications for states across the nation.

SCALABILITY

Scalability was not applicable.

PUBLIC HEALTH SIGNIFICANCE

Findings support that permanent reinstatement of pandemic-era administrative flexibilities (e.g., H.R. 2424 - MODERN WIC Act of 2023) and benefit increases may support long-term retention and redemption among low-income parents eligible for WIC and SNAP. Furthermore, continuing to improve WIC- and SNAP-approved retail access and maintaining the current WIC cash-value benefit allowance of $26 per month long-term will support equitable redemption of benefits. *AJPH*

ABOUT THE AUTHORS

Cristina M. Gago is with the Department of Community Health Sciences, Boston University School of Public Health, Boston, MA. Matthew M. Lee is with the Department of Social and Behavioral Sciences, Harvard T. H. Chan School of Public Health, Boston. Nour M. Hammad, Jhordan O. Wynne, Mary Kathryn Poole, Meghan Zimmer, and Rebecca S. Mozaffarian are with the Department of Nutrition, Harvard T. H. Chan School of Public Health. Rachel Colchamiro and Kelley May are with the Massachusetts Department of Public Health, Boston. Eric B. Rimm is with the Department of Nutrition and the Department of Epidemiology, Harvard T. H. Chan School of Public Health, and the Channing Division of Network Medicine, Brigham and Women's Hospital, Harvard Medical School, Boston. Erica L. Kenney is with the Department of Nutrition and the Department of Social and Behavioral Sciences, Harvard T. H. Chan School of Public Health.

CORRESPONDENCE

Correspondence should be sent to Cristina Gago, PhD, MPH, Department of Community Health Sciences, Boston University School of Public Health, 801 Massachusetts Ave, #428, Boston, MA 02118 (e-mail: gago@bu.edu). Reprints can be ordered at https://www.ajph.org by clicking the "Reprints" link.

PUBLICATION INFORMATION

Full Citation: Gago CM, Lee MM, Hammad NM, et al. "I didn't have to struggle": caregivers' perspectives on the synergistic interplay of WIC and SNAP on family health. *Am J Public Health*. 2025;115(12):1982–1987.

Acceptance Date: July 23, 2025.

DOI: https://doi.org/10.2105/AJPH.2025.308259

ORCID iDs:

Cristina M. Gago https://orcid.org/0000-0003-3159-705X

Matthew M. Lee https://orcid.org/0000-0002-1510-3753

Nour M. Hammad https://orcid.org/0000-0001-9578-7261

Jhordan O. Wynne https://orcid.org/0000-0002-4651-3392

Mary Kathryn Poole https://orcid.org/0000-0003-3466-8650

Meghan Zimmer https://orcid.org/0000-0001-6811-8847

Rebecca S. Mozaffarian https://orcid.org/0000-0003-0118-2574

Eric B. Rimm https://orcid.org/0000-0002-1402-7250

Erica L. Kenney https://orcid.org/0000-0003-1437-3724

CONTRIBUTORS

C. M. Gago contributed to study design, data acquisition, analysis, interpretation, and drafting of the article. M. M. Lee and M. K. Poole contributed to data acquisition, analysis, interpretation, and critical revision of the article. N. M. Hammad and J. O. Wynne contributed to analysis, interpretation, and critical revision of the article. M. Zimmer contributed to interpretation and critical revision of the article. R. S. Mozaffarian contributed to data acquisition and critical revision of the article. R. Colchamiro, K. May, E. B. Rimm, and E. L. Kenney contributed to study design and critical revision of the article. All authors gave final approval of the version to be published.

ACKNOWLEDGMENTS

This research was supported by Healthy Eating Research (grant 283-5114), a national program of the Robert Wood Johnson Foundation. M. Zimmer was supported by a training grant (T32-DK-007703) of the National Institute of Diabetes and Digestive and Kidney Diseases. M. M. Lee and M. K. Poole were supported by a training grant (5T32HL098048-14) of the National Heart, Lung, and Blood Institute.

We thank Areli Caballero-González, MPH, for her assistance conducting interviews.

Note. The funder had no role in the design, analysis, or interpretation of the research and had no restrictions regarding publication.

CONFLICTS OF INTEREST

The authors reported no conflicts of interest.

HUMAN PARTICIPANT PROTECTION

Study procedures were approved by the Harvard T. H. Chan School of Public Health institutional review board. All participants provided informed consent.

REFERENCES

1. Halverson MM, Karpyn A. WIC participants' perceptions of the cash-value benefit increase during the COVID-19 pandemic. *Nutrients.* 2022;14(17):3509. https://doi.org/10.3390/nu14173509
2. Gago C, Colchamiro R, May K, Rimm EB, Kenney EL. Caregivers' perceived impact of WIC's temporary cash-value benefit (CVB) increases on fruit and vegetable purchasing, consumption, and access in Massachusetts. *Nutrients.* 2022;14(23):4947. https://doi.org/10.3390/nu14234947
3. Duffy EW, Vest DA, Davis CR, et al. "I think that's the most beneficial change that WIC has made in a really long time": perceptions and awareness of an increase in the WIC cash value benefit. *Int J Environ Res Public Health.* 2022;19(14):8671. https://doi.org/10.3390/ijerph19148671
4. Tsai M, Au L, Ritchie L, Anderson C, Martinez C, Whaley S. Larger WIC cash value benefit for vegetables and fruit is associated with lower

food insecurity and improved participant satisfaction in WIC families with children. *Current Developments in Nutrition*. 2022;6:231. https://doi.org/10.1093/cdn/nzac048.045

5. Restrepo BJ. The protective effect of SNAP during economic downturns: evidence from the COVID-19 pandemic. *Applied Eco Perspectives Pol.* 2023;45(4):2141–2160. https://doi.org/10.1002/aepp.13345
6. Molitor F, Doerr C, Kehl S. Unemployment, SNAP enrollment, and food insecurity before and after California's COVID-19 shutdown. *J Nutr Educ Behav*. 2021;53(12):1055–1059. https://doi.org/10.1016/j.jneb.2021.09.001
7. Jackson KE, Chiang AY, Hamad R. The association of increased SNAP benefits during COVID-19 with food insufficiency and anxiety among US adults: a quasi-experimental study. *Public Health Nutr*. 2024;27(1):e186. https://doi.org/10.1017/S1368980024001447
8. Crespo-Bellido M, Headrick G, López MÁ, et al. A systematic review: the impact of COVID-19 policy flexibilities on SNAP and WIC programmatic outcomes. *Adv Nutr*. 2025;16(2):100361. https://doi.org/10.1016/j.advnut.2024.100361
9. Hall L, Neuberger Z. Eligible low-income children missing out on crucial WIC benefits during pandemic. Center on Budget and Policy Priorities. July 12, 2021. Available at: https://www.cbpp.org/research/food-assistance/eligible-low-income-children-missing-out-on-crucial-wic-benefits-during. Accessed November 12, 2024.
10. Kumanyika S, Getting to equity in obesity prevention: a new framework. *NAM Perspectives*. 2017;7(1). https://doi.org/10.31478/201701c
11. Dedoose Version, cloud application for managing, analyzing, and presenting qualitative and mixed method research data. 2021. Available at: https://www.dedoose.com. Accessed May 22, 2025.
12. Braun V, Clarke V. Thematic analysis. In: Cooper H, Camic PM, Long DL, Panter AT, Rindskopf D, Sher KJ, eds. *APA Handbook of Research Methods in Psychology, Vol 2: Research Designs: Quantitative, Qualitative, Neuropsychological, and Biological*. Washington, DC: American Psychological Association; 2012:57–71. https://doi.org/10.1037/13620-004
13. Barnes CY. "It takes a while to get used to": the costs of redeeming public benefits. *J Public Adm Res Theory*. 2021;31(2):295–310. https://doi.org/10.1093/jopart/muaa042
14. Economic Research Service. Food Security in the US—Interactive Charts and Highlights. US Department of Agriculture. Available at: https://www.ers.usda.gov/topics/food-nutrition-assistance/food-security-in-the-us/interactive-charts-and-highlights. Accessed May 22, 2025.
15. Padilla CM, Thomson D. Nearly 1 million more children were in poverty in 2023 than 2022, despite economic growth. ChildTrends. September 10, 2024. Available at: https://www.childtrends.org/publications/more-children-in-poverty-in-2023-than-2022-economic-growth. Accessed February 24, 2025.
16. Arrington JC. One Big Beautiful Bill Act. HR 1, 119th Cong (July 4, 2025). Available at: https://www.congress.gov/bill/119th-congress/house-bill/1/text. Accessed July 17, 2025.

Integrating Primary Care and Public Health: Promising Pathways to Building Infrastructure and Delivering Services

Katherine M. Anderson, MPH, Luisa N. Borrell, DDS, PhD, and Lorna Thorpe, PhD

ABOUT THE AUTHORS

Katherine M. Anderson is a doctoral candidate in the Department of Behavioral, Social, and Health Education Sciences, Emory University Rollins School of Public Health, Atlanta, GA, and a past student editor of AJPH. *Luisa N. Borrell is a distinguished professor in the Department of Epidemiology and Biostatistics, City University of New York Graduate School of Public Health and Health Policy, New York, and an* AJPH *associate editor. Lorna Thorpe is a professor in the Department of Population Health, New York University Grossman School of Medicine, New York, and an* AJPH *associate editor.*

See also Primary Care and Public Health in the Community, pp. 1992–2019.

Forty-six years after the World Health Organization's 1978 *Alma-Ata Declaration on Primary Health Care*,[1] the call to better integrate primary care and the public health entity still reverberates. As described in the 2012 Centers for Disease Control and Prevention and Health Resources and Services Administration–funded report *Primary Care and Public Health: Exploring Integration to Improve Population Health*,[2] "Integration of primary care and public health could enhance the capacity of both sectors to carry out their respective missions"[2(p1)] and form partnerships "to catalyze a collaborative, intersectoral movement toward improved population health."[2(p1)] The need for such integration has only grown in the face of recent population-level health challenges, including the COVID-19 pandemic, climate change, international conflict, social media health-related misinformation, and efforts to address social determinants of health.

Compounding this, both sectors are facing crises induced by actualized reductions in, and ongoing threats to, federal funding for health programming and services that have been shown to reduce the burden of disease and save lives domestically and internationally.[3–6] In recent months, community health centers have been unable to access federal funds, disease outbreak responses (e.g., to measles) were halted, rural outreach programs were scaled back, and many other services have been paused or canceled because of funding cuts.[7,8] In this context, the integration of the public health sector and primary care may be not only an opportunity but also a survival tactic for both fields to continue to serve the health and well-being of individuals and populations.

Continued on page 1989...

HISTORY CORNER

13 YEARS AGO

A Call for Action on Primary Care and Public Health Integration

The fields of primary care and public health in the United States have for the last century generally functioned independently of each other. This is not optimal; our current health challenges require improved efforts to work together in an integrated fashion to address the root causes of illness and prevent additional cases of disease, and to make the default choice a healthy one. . . .On March 28, 2012, the Institute of Medicine (IOM) released the report, "Primary Care and Public Health: Exploring Integration to Improve Population Health.". . . [T]he IOM committee developed a set of principles that they deem essential for successful integration of primary care and public health: 1. a shared goal of population health improvement; 2. community engagement in defining and addressing population health needs; 3. aligned leadership; 4. sustainability, including shared infrastructure; and 5. sharing and collaborative use of data and analysis. The IOM report notes that integration can start with any of these principles and that starting is more important than waiting until all are in place.

From *AJPH*, June 2012, p. S307

PUBLIC HEALTH–PRIMARY CARE INTEGRATION MODEL

Those gathered at Alma-Ata defined and committed to building a health care policy approach that not only focuses on providing primary care—"first-contact, accessible, continued, comprehensive, and coordinated patient-focused care"[9(pXIII)]—but also considers environmental and social determinants of health, health as an inherent right of all people, equity as a primary value of health care, and integration and collaboration with communities to facilitate health for all.[10]

Terming this *primary health care*, the World Health Organization defines it as a "whole-of-society approach" to improve health equity and well-being, with three major components: primary care and public health as the core of integrated health services, collaborative policy and action across sectors, and empowered communities and individuals.[9] By definition, the integration of primary care and public health can involve a wide variety of sectors and encompass many different strategies. This special section highlights compelling examples of integration, and the breadth of articles spans a range of topics, including public health workforce development, nutritional incentives for communities and individuals at risk for chronic disease, integration of preventive care in inpatient treatment settings, hypertension control, and rural health service delivery.

TRANSFORMING PRIMARY HEALTH CARE FOR BETTER HEALTH

Mills (p. 2002) discusses the development of infrastructure to increase access to primary care in rural counties, particularly those without a local health department, in "Integration of Health Care, Public Health, and Communities: A New Model for Rural Public Health." The author describes hub-and-spokes style infrastructure developed by MaineHealth through community partnerships and public health integration, suggesting that the model might increase rural health capacity and improve health in other rural health contexts nationwide. Furthermore, the author identifies evidence of sustainability, highlighting future considerations for infrastructure development.

Allaudeen et al. (p. 1997), in their article "Advancing Equity in Preventive Care: Leveraging Hospital Admissions for Vulnerable Populations," describe the implementation and outcomes of a program to reach individuals receiving inpatient care with preventive services they may otherwise not access. Using hospital admissions data, the authors identified overdue preventive care for admitted patients, including cancer screenings, laboratory monitoring tests, and vaccinations, allowing preventive services to be provided during onsite care. Notably, the authors found that patients who experienced housing instability or had not engaged in primary care for more than a year were most likely to benefit from this program.

Focusing on primary care infrastructure, Soltani et al. (p. 1992), in their article "Improving Hypertension Control in Southern Arizona: A Collaboration Between Community Health Centers and Local Health Departments," describe a partnership between federally qualified health centers and local health departments in Arizona: the Southern Arizona Hypertension Control Collaborative. This addresses undiagnosed and

Continued on page 1990...

HISTORY CORNER

23 YEARS AGO

Community-Oriented Primary Care: New Relevance in a Changing World

In 1940, two young South African physicians, Sidney and Emily Kark, went to live and work in an impoverished, rural, Zulu tribal reserve called Pholela in the province of Natal. . . .Their responsibilities, as they embraced them, entailed not only treating illness presented to them, but also taking a census of the local population and performing basic epidemiologic surveys to establish a baseline of illness in the community as a starting point for planned interventions. . . .The melding of population health principles with the practice of clinical medicine in community-based settings has been a feature of some health delivery settings throughout the world for the past half century. Under the increasingly recognized heading of community-oriented primary care, this constellation of activities has provided collaborative programs of intervention and prevention in service delivery not always achieved by primary care practices. COPC [community-oriented primary care] has provided an important stimulant for teaching and an exemplar of best practices for community health delivery.

From *AJPH*, November 2002, p. 1748

untreated hypertension in three counties. The authors describe augmented primary care infrastructure to facilitate identification and treatment of hypertension, and they share their experience using multisectoral expertise to improve clinical care, increase community awareness of hypertension, enhance connections to care, and coordinate public health strategic activities moving forward.

In their analytic essay "Retooling the Workforce for Collaboration: Centering Collective Efficacy in Public Health and Primary Care Leadership Development," Martelino and Bekemeier (p. 2006) propose a framework for collective leadership development that integrates both public health and primary care professionals. Noting that sector leaders' collaborative engagement is vital for successful integration, the authors advocate the development of communication, relational, and effective skills to promote collective efficacy and performance across sectors. The authors offer a practice-informed model to guide the future integration of workforce members from both disciplines to facilitate the successful implementation of collaborative work.

Finally, Byker Shanks et al. (p. 2015) present enrollment data for a national produce prescription program in "Characteristics of the People and Communities Served by GusNIP Produce Prescriptions: United States, 2020–2024." This article discusses a food is medicine intervention that aims to increase access to and consumption of fruits and vegetables among those at risk for chronic diseases. The authors analyze the national distribution of enrollment to identify whether the program is reaching those most in need of support, concluding that, indeed, those using the program are experiencing food insecurity and have insufficient fruit and vegetable intake. Finally, they assess areas for potential expansion, particularly in a changing political and funding landscape.

Taken together, this collection of articles underscores the importance of integrating primary care and public health from structural- to individual-level approaches through traditional and innovative ways to improve population health. Such integration is more important than ever, given the recent budget cuts directly affecting preventive programs, especially those focused on chronic diseases throughout local and national agencies. AJPH

CORRESPONDENCE

Correspondence should be sent to Katherine M. Anderson, Emory University Rollins School of Public Health, 1518 Clifton Rd NE, Atlanta, GA 30322 (email: kmande9@emory.edu). Reprints can be ordered at https://www.ajph.org by clicking the "Reprints" link.

PUBLICATION INFORMATION

Full Citation: Anderson KM, Borrell LN, Thorpe L. Integrating primary care and public health: promising pathways to building infrastructure and delivering services. *Am J Public Health*. 2025;115(12):1988–1991.

Acceptance Date: September 14, 2025.

DOI: https://doi.org/10.2105/AJPH.2025.308297

ORCID iD:
Katherine M. Anderson https://orcid.org/0000-0001-9675-3653

CONTRIBUTORS

K. M. Anderson conceptualized, drafted, and edited the editorial. L. N. Borrell and L. Thorpe edited and reviewed the editorial.

CONFLICTS OF INTEREST

The authors have no conflicts of interest to report.

REFERENCES

1. International Conference on Primary Health Care. Declaration of Alma-Ata. September 1978. Available at: https://www.who.int/docs/default-source/documents/almaata-declaration-en.pdf. Accessed October 4, 2025.
2. Institute of Medicine. *Primary Care and Public Health: Exploring Integration to Improve Population*

Continued on page 1991...

HISTORY CORNER

46 YEARS AGO

Physicians' Patient Referrals to a Nurse Practitioner in a Primary Care Medical Clinic

At present, public interest in controlling the costs of medical care has reached a stage where legislative limits have been proposed. In addition, consumer dissatisfaction with depersonalized and crisis-oriented health care is well documented. One of the ways in which the health professions have responded to these concerns is by introducing the concept of the nurse practitioner (NP). NPs are currently being educated to manage common ailments and to monitor the chronic but stabilized medical conditions of patients referred to them by physicians. The rationale behind utilization of NPs is that their services would enable physicians to concentrate their efforts on patients with more complicated medical problems. . . .Our study has shown that physicians in one particular clinic use the services of an NP to a much lesser extent than would be expected from an inspection of their attitudes towards the NP role. . . .[P]hysicians were reluctant to consider hiring an NP or to have a member of their own family treated by an NP. . . . Accordingly, one step toward improving this situation could be provided by increased socialization opportunities for physicians and NPs, e.g., in educational and clinical contexts.

From *AJPH*, January 1979, pp. 73–74

Health. Washington, DC: National Academies Press; 2012.

3. Amon J, Sharfstein JM. The domestic consequences of defunding global health. *JAMA Health Forum.* 2025;6(5):e252462–e252462. https://doi.org/10.1001/jamahealthforum.2025.2462
4. Martinez-Alvarez M, Amouzou A, Barros AJD, et al. Broken promises: the USA foreign aid freeze threatens women's, children's, and adolescents' health. *Lancet.* 2025;405(10488):1448–1450. https://doi.org/10.1016/S0140-6736(25)00558-6
5. Coria AL, Wahl B, Thacker N, Vreeman R, Zühlke L. USAID's role in saving children's lives: past legacy and future directions. *Pediatrics.* 2025;156(2): e2025071260. https://doi.org/10.1542/peds.2025-071260
6. Bleich SN, Leung CW, Hamad R. Implications of recent federal actions on food assistance programs. *JAMA Health Forum.* 2025;6(4):e251567. https://doi.org/10.1001/jamahealthforum.2025.1567
7. Association of Schools & Programs of Public Health. Broken lifelines: the economic consequences of defunding academic public health. May 2025. Available at: https://aspph-webassets.s3.us-east-1.amazonaws.com/Economic+Impact+Report.pdf. Accessed October 4, 2025.
8. Ungar L, Smith MR. Trump administration's deep cuts to public health leave system reeling. May 31, 2025. Available at: https://www.pbs.org/newshour/health/trump-administrations-deep-cuts-to-public-health-leave-system-reeling. Accessed October 4, 2025.
9. World Health Organization; United Nations Children's Fund. *Operational Framework for Primary Health Care: Transforming Vision Into Action.* 2020. Available at: https://iris.who.int/bitstream/handle/10665/337641/9789240017832-eng.pdf?sequence=1. Accessed October 4, 2025.
10. Hone T, Macinko J, Millett C. Revisiting Alma-Ata: what is the role of primary health care in achieving the sustainable development goals? *Lancet.* 2018;392(10156):1461–1472. https://doi.org/10.1016/S0140-6736(18)31829-4

Improving Hypertension Control in Southern Arizona: A Collaboration Between Community Health Centers and Local Health Departments

Lisa Soltani, MD, MPH, Andrew Saal, MD, MPH, and Theresa Cullen, MD, MS

See also Primary Care and Public Health in the Community, pp. 1988–2019.

Federally qualified health centers and local health departments in three Southern Arizona counties formed a partnership in 2023 to address unrecognized and undertreated high blood pressure in the region. By augmenting primary care infrastructure with the surveillance, communication, and policy functions of local health departments, the partnership seeks to improve population health outcomes by sharing clinical best practices, increasing community awareness, enhancing connections to primary care, and coordinating public health department strategic activities. (*Am J Public Health*. 2025;115(12): 1992–1996. https://doi.org/10.2105/AJPH.2025.308196)

AJPH December 2025, Vol. 115, No. 12

In September 2023, a group of clinicians and quality improvement staff from six federally qualified health centers (FQHCs) in Southern Arizona and their corresponding local health departments (LHDs) formed a loose coalition, which became known as the Southern Arizona Hypertension Control Collaborative (SAHCC). Interest in the endeavor evolved from health centers' involvement in the National Hypertension Control Initiative, a Health Resources and Services Administration (HRSA) grant–funded effort focused on improving hypertension control nationally. Team members hoped to leverage successes from the initiative along with public health approaches to benefit a larger, regional population. These efforts became the impetus for the formation of the SAHCC, which now meets on a quarterly basis.

INTERVENTION AND IMPLEMENTATION

Drawing on the "waterfall" strategy for chronic disease management (improved prevention, screening, diagnosis, and treatment while reducing the impacts of disease complications), SAHCC has explored and implemented a range of both clinic- and community-based activities to improve clinical care, increase community awareness, enhance patient connection to primary care, and coordinate public health strategic activities (Box 1).

Activities undertaken by SAHCC parallel the framework outlined in the 2017 National Association of County and City Health Officials toolkit that promotes collaborations between LHDs and community health centers.[1] FQHC members began the dialogue by sharing the most successful practices they had adopted through their participation in the National Hypertension Control Initiative. Discussions then evolved to identify areas where collaboration and coordination could have a synergistic impact for the community at large.

PLACE, TIME, AND PERSONS

SAHCC includes six Arizona FQHCs (Chiricahua, Desert Senita, El Rio, Marana, Mariposa, and United Community Health Centers), three county health departments (Cochise, Pima, and Santa Cruz), the Arizona American Heart Association (AHA), and representatives of area hospitals. The target populations are adult residents of Cochise, Pima, and Santa Cruz counties, including health center patients as well as individuals without a medical home who are

BOX 1— Selected Activities of the Southern Arizona Hypertension Control Collaborative

Improve Clinical Care Activities	Increase Community Awareness Activities	Enhance Connection to Primary Care Activities	Coordinate Public Health Strategic Activities
FQHCs share clinical best practices. Present at the state's primary care association for FQHCs. Arrange peer-to-peer physician champion presentations for staff meetings at sister FQHCs. Share workflow aids such as policies and standing orders that support hypertension screening and control across organizations.	Develop joint activities for Heart Health Month (February) and Hypertension Awareness Month (May). Coordinate ongoing social media campaigns. Organize community talks and clinician champion interviews on local media and for advocacy organizations serving affected populations. Host public screening events, including blood pressure kiosks and public library monitor-lending programs.	Create telephone hotlines for health department staff to connect people with elevated blood pressures to medical homes. Meet with local hospitals to improve the transition of patients with uncontrolled hypertension from emergency department and hospital settings to primary care medical homes. Train community health workers in screening for hypertension and connection to primary care.	Assessment: Geo-locate high-risk areas to enhance screening and linkages to primary care. Policy: Develop programs that improve screening opportunities internally as well as with community partners. Build opportunities for community health workers to increase their scale, skills, and scope in community cardiovascular health. Assurance: Build collaborations among partners to share resources and broaden participation in regional health boards and partner agencies.

Note. FQHC = federally qualified health center.

at increased risk for high blood pressure (BP). The combined population of the three counties is approximately 939 000 adults, of whom 26% to 30% have hypertension. The six health centers combined serve 52 000 individuals living with hypertension.

PURPOSE

Cardiovascular disease is the leading cause of mortality for adults in Arizona[2] and in the nation at large.[3] Systolic BP is the number-one risk factor for years of life lost in the United States.[4] Poor population outcomes from hypertension stem from a combination of unrecognized disease, lack of access to care, and suboptimal treatment intensification. SAHCC fosters dialogue and collaboration between FQHC hypertension champions and LHDs and seeks to (1) share clinical best practices in the care of patients with hypertension, (2) improve community awareness of environmental and lifestyle contributors, (3) screen for unrecognized hypertensive disease and connect those individuals to care, and (4) coordinate public health strategic activities.

EVALUATION

There were four outcomes of interest.

Outcome 1: Improve Clinical Care

Provider–champions at the FQHCs served as resources for one another, sharing treatment protocols, standing orders, and speakers' resources. In the first year of collaboration, five of the six participating FQHCs achieved improved rates of BP control as defined by the HRSA measure of hypertension control (< 140/90). Recognizing that the HRSA goal for BP control has not been updated in many years, the partners agreed to work toward AHA Target: BP goals and recognition.

Outcome 2: Increase Community Awareness

SAHCC members have engaged in a wide array of activities, independently and in collaboration, to increase public consciousness of the importance of screening, identifying, and effectively treating hypertension. Many new projects were planned for February Heart Health and May Hypertension Awareness months. These activities included coordinated social media campaigns, educational publications in local newspapers, local interview-style talk shows, health fairs, community "heart health" classes, "know your numbers" billboard and bus ad campaigns, health department webpages on hypertension and lifestyle resources, a public library lending program for BP monitors, and BP kiosks in several public buildings. During the May hypertension awareness campaign, more than 700 unique users accessed the new health department webpages on cardiovascular health, 337 county library patrons borrowed home BP monitors, more than 1000 viewers accessed "Talks with a Doc" webchats, and rural health fairs screened more than 220 people in remote areas.

Outcome 3: Enhance Connections to Care

The collaborative aims to enhance primary care access for individuals identified with elevated BP in community settings. One county established a direct hotline between health department staff members and a local FQHC to expedite patient entry into care. As the program matures, "patients assisted with navigation to primary care" is being developed as a metric for community health worker activity.

Outcome 4: Coordinate Public Health Activities

The three core functions of public health departments are assessment, policy development, and assurance. To improve the assessment of the burden of hypertensive disease in the region, health department epidemiologists used geo-mapping software to crosswalk several large data sets (Figures 1 and 2). The resultant map overlays 2021 Centers for Disease Control and Prevention (CDC) Behavioral Risk Factor Surveillance System survey data describing the percentage of respondents aware they have high BP but not taking medication, FQHC and LHD locations, and the CDC Social Vulnerability Index. Interactive functionality

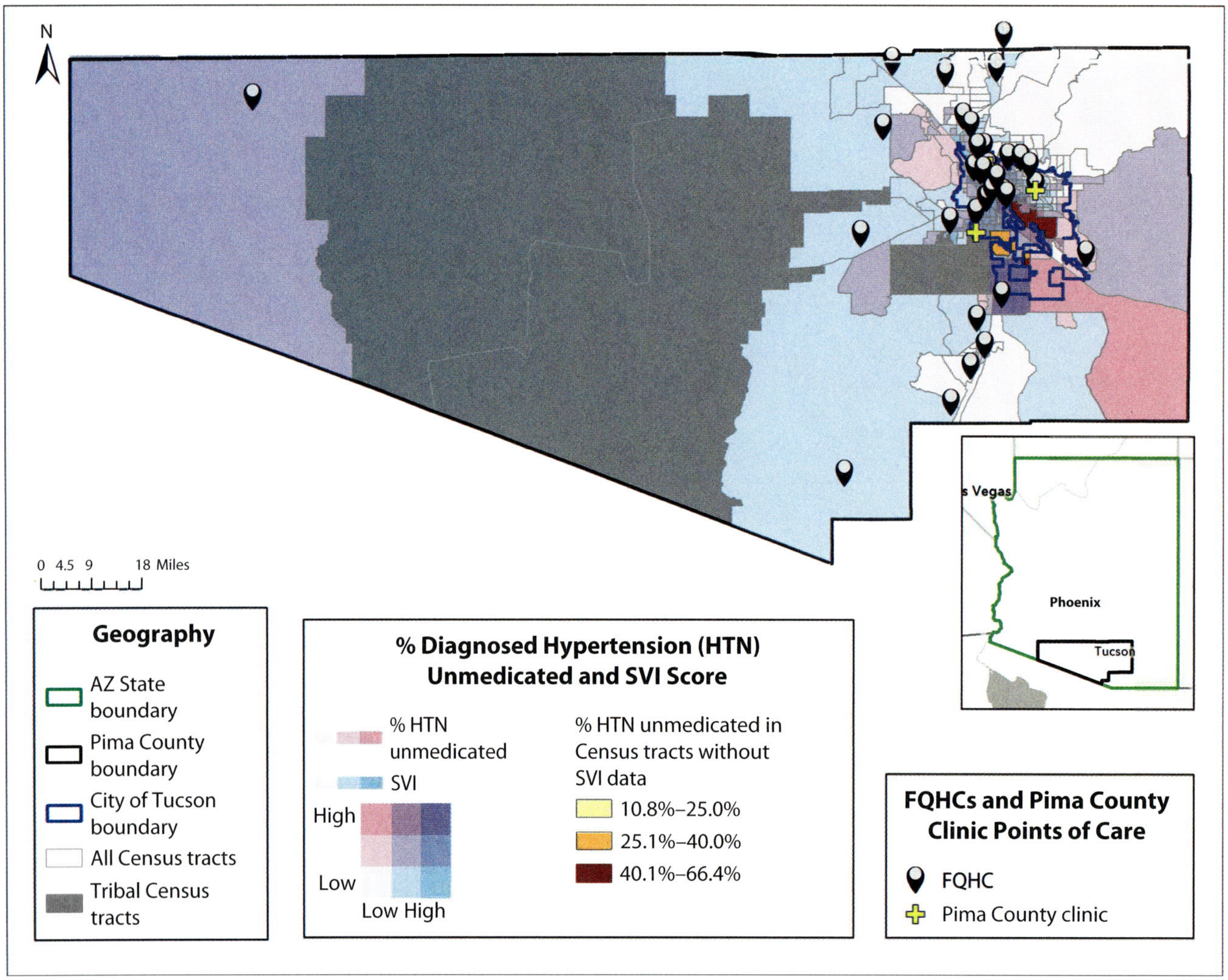

FIGURE 1— Map of Pima County, Arizona, Showing Self-Reported Rates of Having Hypertension and Not Being on Medication, Overlapped With the Social Vulnerability Index (SVI) Score for Each Census Tract: 2021

Note. FQHC = federally qualified health center. Please see Figure 2 for a close-up of the Tucson Metro area. Map layers include the percentage of adults with hypertension who are not currently taking medication,[5] census tracts with increased socioeconomic needs (Centers for Disease Control and Prevention/Agency for Toxic Substances and Disease Registry Social Vulnerability Index),[6] and 27 geolocated FQHCs and Pima County clinic locations.[7] Additional layers can include patient demographics and self-reported rates of hypertension and medication adherence. Out of respect for tribal data sovereignty, census tracts on tribal lands (gray areas) have been excluded from this analysis.

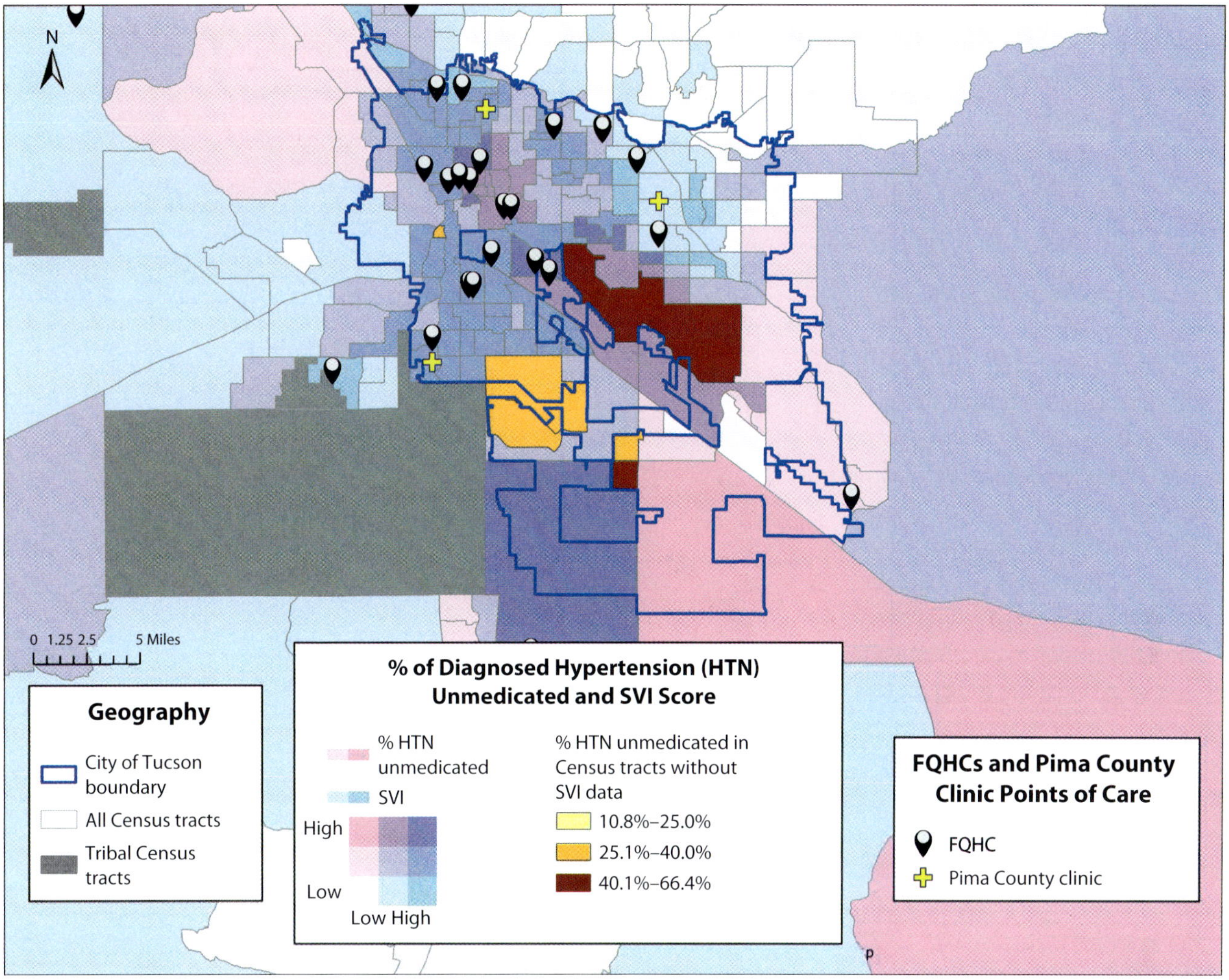

FIGURE 2— **Map of Pima County With a Close-Up of the Tucson Metro Area, Showing Self-Reported Rates of Having Hypertension and Not Being on Medication, Overlapped With the Social Vulnerability Index (SVI) Score for Each Census Tract: 2021**

Note. FQHC = federally qualified health center. Map layers include the percentage of adults with hypertension who are not currently taking medication,[5] census tracts with increased socioeconomic needs (Centers for Disease Control and Prevention/Agency for Toxic Substances and Disease Registry Social Vulnerability Index),[6] and 27 geolocated FQHC and Pima County clinic locations.[7] Additional layers can include patient demographics and self-reported rates of hypertension and medication adherence. Out of respect for tribal data sovereignty, census tracts on tribal lands (gray areas) have been excluded from this analysis.

of the map tool enables a drill down for each FQHC that indicates the number of patients with hypertension, the level of control, and demographic information. The bivariate map defines census tracts of concern where vulnerable populations experience lower hypertension care. These findings have been subsequently supported in a novel CDC report that estimates county-level hypertension prevalence and control.[8] Team members hope to use data to better deploy resources to achieve improved hypertension awareness and control in key census tracts.

Policy development engages stakeholders in public health issues. Through increased exposure, several FQHC clinicians now serve on the Pima County Board of Health and other regional committees in developing regional action plans as well as helping to craft public health communications. In addition, the health department's initiative to increase the regional workforce of community health workers has incorporated a standard curriculum on BP screening and linkage to care, as well as partnering with the AHA to provide training workshops in English and Spanish.

Lastly, in the category of assurance, LHDs have incorporated more opportunities for screening, including adding BP protocols to county immunization and family planning clinics as well as supplying loaner monitors and vitals kiosks in public spaces.

SUSTAINABILITY

FQHCs are patient-centered medical homes capable of delivering comprehensive care and aim to become the health care of choice for all. LHDs increasingly have the role of providing situational awareness of evolving health threats paired with the strategic goal of building healthier communities. Timely sharing of data and iterative improvements in care delivery galvanize these partners to respond more effectively to the changing landscape of disease and wellness in the shared community. Quarterly virtual meetings, along with asynchronous updates from team members and focused efforts for national commemorative heart-health months, have led to a sustainable model for ongoing partnership.

PUBLIC HEALTH SIGNIFICANCE

Collaboration between FQHCs and LHDs can leverage the unique skill set of each to improve regional hypertension control. Enhanced relationships between health departments and community health centers create a generational opportunity that amplifies each agency's resources. Working together can foster sustainable improvements in the health of individuals and in the larger communities they serve. AJPH

ABOUT THE AUTHORS

Lisa Soltani is with the El Rio Community Health Center in Tucson, AZ. Andrew Saal and Theresa Cullen are with the Pima County Health Department, Tucson.

CORRESPONDENCE

Correspondence should be sent to Andrew Saal, MD, MPH, 3950 S Country Club Rd, Suite 100, Tucson, AZ 85714 (e-mail: andrew.saal@pima.gov). Reprints can be ordered at https://www.ajph.org by clicking the "Reprints" link.

PUBLICATION INFORMATION

Full Citation: Soltani L, Saal A, Cullen T. Improving hypertension control in Southern Arizona: a collaboration between community health centers and local health departments. *Am J Public Health*. 2025;115(12):1992–1996.

Acceptance Date: May 8, 2025.

DOI: https://doi.org/10.2105/AJPH.2025.308196

ORCID iDs:

Lisa Soltani https://orcid.org/0009-0002-1486-9818

Andrew Saal https://orcid.org/0009-0008-7300-1246

Theresa Cullen https://orcid.org/0000-0002-8730-5688

CONTRIBUTORS

All authors contributed equally to the work.

ACKNOWLEDGMENTS

The authors would like to acknowledge the providers, staff, and patrons of the federally qualified health centers of Southern Arizona (Chiricahua, Desert Senita, El Rio, Marana, Mariposa, and United Community Health Centers) and the Cochise, Pima, and Santa Cruz County Health Departments, as well as Matthew Jager (science editor). Thank you especially to Erin Woods, MPH, and Haley Oura, MPH, for their data mapping and visualization skills.

CONFLICTS OF INTEREST

The authors report no conflicts of interest.

HUMAN PARTICIPANT PROTECTION

The study did not involve human participants.

REFERENCES

1. National Association of County and City Health Officials. Local Health Department–Community Health Center Collaboration Toolkit. 2017. Available at: https://www.naccho.org/uploads/downloadable-resources/Programs/Public-Health-Infrastructure/NACCHO-LHD-CHC-collaboration-toolkit.pdf. Accessed November 7, 2024.
2. Arizona Department of Health Services. *Arizona State Health Assessment: 2022 Annual Update.* Available at: https://www.azdhs.gov/documents/operations/strategic-initiatives/arizona-state-health-assessment-2022.pdf. Accessed November 15, 2024.
3. Ahmad FB, Cisewski JA, Anderson RN, et al. Mortality in the United States—provisional data, 2023. *MMWR Morb Mortal Wkly Rep.* 2024;73(31):677–681. https://doi.org/10.15585/mmwr.mm7331a1.
4. Martin SS, Aday AW, Allen NB, American Heart Association Council on Epidemiology and Prevention Statistics Committee and Stroke Statistics Committee, et al. 2025 heart disease and stroke statistics: a report of US and global data from the American Heart Association. *Circulation.* 2025;151(8):e41–e660. https://doi.org/10.1161/CIR.0000000000001303.
5. Centers for Disease Control and Prevention. Behavioral Risk Factor Surveillance System Survey Data. Atlanta, GA: US Department of Health and Human Services; 2021.
6. Centers for Disease Control and Prevention/Agency for Toxic Substances and Disease Registry/Geospatial Research, Analysis, and Services Program. CDC/ATSDR Social Vulnerability Index 2022 Database for Arizona. Available at: https://www.atsdr.cdc.gov/placeandhealth/svi/data_documentation_download.html. Accessed March 14, 2025.
7. Health Resources and Services Administration. Uniform Data System. Rockville, MD: US Department of Health and Human Services; 2023.
8. Weng X, Vaughan AS, He S, et al. County-level hypertension prevalence and control in the United States: a ZIP 3-county crosswalk using electronic health record data. *Prev Chronic Dis.* 2024;21:E95. https://doi.org/10.5888/pcd21.240185.

Advancing Equity in Preventive Care: Leveraging Hospital Admissions for Vulnerable Populations

Nazima Allaudeen, MD, David B. Huberman, PhD, and Elizabeth Le, MD

See also Primary Care and Public Health in the Community, pp. 1988–2019.

To supplement traditional preventive care models, we leveraged hospital admission to address overdue vaccinations, cancer screening, and laboratory tests. A total of 28.7% of patients had at least one overdue preventive care item; 70.9% of these patients received at least one preventive care intervention during their hospitalization. Patients experiencing housing instability or with more than a year since their last primary care appointment were more likely to benefit. This intervention demonstrates hospitalization as an opportunity to address inequities in preventive care. (*Am J Public Health.* 2025;115(12):1997–2001. https://doi.org/10.2105/AJPH.2025.308218)

AJPH December 2025, Vol. 115, No. 12

Preventive care is a crucial but underutilized component of optimal population health management. Improving preventive care in the United States could save more than 100 000 lives and $3.7 billion annually.[1,2] Of eligible patients, 69.0% have received pneumococcal vaccine, 24.1% zoster vaccine, and 30.0% hepatitis B vaccine.[3] Cancer screening rates are similarly low, with 12.5% of eligible patients screened for lung cancer and 71.6% for colorectal cancer.[4,5] Gaps in preventive care are even larger in racially minoritized subgroups and those experiencing housing instability, substance use, or severe mental illness.[6–11] The need overwhelms primary care's ability to address alone, with an estimated 8.6 hours per day required to deliver recommended preventive care across a typical patient panel.[12]

Hospital admission offers an opportunity for patients to obtain overdue preventive care. Targeted projects to improve pneumonia vaccination and mammography[13,14] and pandemic initiatives for COVID-19 vaccination[15,16] have demonstrated feasibility in addressing specific preventive care elements during hospitalization. To our knowledge, no previous interventions have addressed preventive care comprehensively for hospitalized patients.

INTERVENTION AND IMPLEMENTATION

We developed a protocol to evaluate inpatients for overdue preventive care and leverage the admission to complete any appropriate items. The Veterans Affairs (VA) electronic health record (EHR) utilizes an automated clinical reminder system, which applies guideline-directed preventive care recommendations to patient characteristics (see Appendix A, available as a supplement to the online version of this article at https://www.ajph.org, for technical definitions). Because this system includes only information within our own medical center, patients outside our catchment were excluded.

A physician lead screened inpatients on medicine, orthopedic, neurosurgery, and podiatry services for clinical reminders in three domains: vaccines, cancer screening, and laboratory tests. Vaccines included COVID-19, zoster, pneumonia, hepatitis A, and hepatitis B. Cancer screening included low-dose computed tomography for lung cancer, ultrasound for hepatocellular cancer, and fecal immunochemical test for colorectal cancer. Laboratory tests included lipid panel, hemoglobin A1C, and hepatitis B and C screening.

For patients with any overdue care in these three domains, the chart was reviewed. Patients with limited life expectancy were excluded. For vaccinations, the EHR was reviewed for contraindications such as infection, fever, or active symptoms. The state immunization registry was reviewed to ascertain any vaccinations received outside VA. Any remaining patients were deemed appropriate to offer preventive care. The physician (1) entered orders for the inpatient care (vaccines, radiologic tests, and laboratory tests), (2) informed the inpatient team through secure messaging, (3) followed up on the laboratory and radiographic results, and (4) ordered remaining care for outpatient when applicable (e.g., to complete remaining doses of a vaccination series).

The primary measure was the percentage of patients offered preventive care. For the subset offered overdue preventive care, a secondary outcome was whether the patient completed the care. We compared demographic and psychosocial characteristics between patients who were offered overdue preventive care and patients without overdue preventive care. Race and ethnicity are self-reported fields in the EHR. Severe mental illness, substance use, and housing instability were defined by *International Classification of Diseases, 10th Revision* (Geneva, Switzerland: World Health Organization; 2015) codes on either the EHR problem list or discharge diagnoses.[17] Patients who used VA housing assistance services within the last five years were also included as having housing instability. Last primary care appointment included completed appointments within our VA health care system.

We conducted univariable and multivariable logistic regression analyses to assess the effects of the selected characteristics on patients offered overdue care versus patients without overdue care. For the subset of patients offered overdue preventive care, we performed univariable and multivariable logistic regressions to determine the impact of these characteristics on those who completed the care and those who did not. For all regressions, we calculated parameter estimates and associated 95% confidence intervals and *P* values for each characteristic. We considered a *P* value of less than .05 to be statistically significant. We performed all analyses with R statistical software, version 4.2.1.[18]

PLACE, TIME, AND PERSONS

VA Palo Alto Health Care System is a level 1a facility (VA's highest complexity level) affiliated with Stanford University, serving approximately 67 000 veterans across seven outpatient locations. The acute care hospital contains approximately 80 medical–surgical floor beds, 15 intermediate intensive care unit beds, and 15 intensive care unit beds. The intervention period was April 24, 2023, to April 23, 2024. The preintervention baseline was January 1, 2022, to December 31, 2022.

PURPOSE

The goal of our intervention was to increase preventive care during hospital admission.

EVALUATION AND ADVERSE EFFECTS

Over the one-year intervention period, 2171 patients were screened. The top medical admission source was the emergency department (85.5%). The 520 patients who were outside our medical center catchment were excluded. Of the remaining 1651 patients, 474 (28.7%) patients were offered at least one preventive care intervention (Figure 1). Of these patients, 336 (70.9%) patients received at least one preventive care intervention during their admission. Compared with the baseline period, the number of inpatient vaccinations increased by 117.9% (112 vs 244), and lung cancer screening increased by 233.3% (12 vs 40).

Characteristics of patients with and without overdue preventive care are shown in Table 1. Patients with overdue preventive care were more likely to be Black (15.2% vs 9.3%; $P = .008$), have a diagnosis of severe mental illness (39.7% vs 30.0%; $P = .001$) or substance use (27.2% vs 10.8%, $P < .001$), or experience housing instability (24.3% vs 9.3%; $P < .001$). Patients with overdue care were more likely to have more than three years since their last primary care visit (17.1% vs 7.8%; $P < .001$). In the multivariable analysis, age, housing instability, and time since last primary care visit remained significant. Mean age for patients with overdue care was lower (68.3 vs 76.8 years), likely in part attributable to some interventions having recommended maximum age cutoffs. Of the 474 patients offered overdue care, the majority of patients in all subgroups completed the care (Appendix A).

Like previous studies, we demonstrated that patients can successfully receive preventive care during hospital admission.[13–16] However, this study shows the feasibility of addressing preventive care more comprehensively with vaccines, cancer screening, and laboratory tests. Vaccinations more than doubled and lung cancer screening more than tripled with these efforts. Overdue preventive care was common among inpatients, with nearly one third of patients having relevant overdue care, underscoring the potential impact of leveraging hospital admission to deliver missed care.

As with other hospitals, during the pandemic, our site instituted a nursing protocol to offer COVID-19 vaccines to inpatients, representing 80.4% of vaccines in our baseline period. While

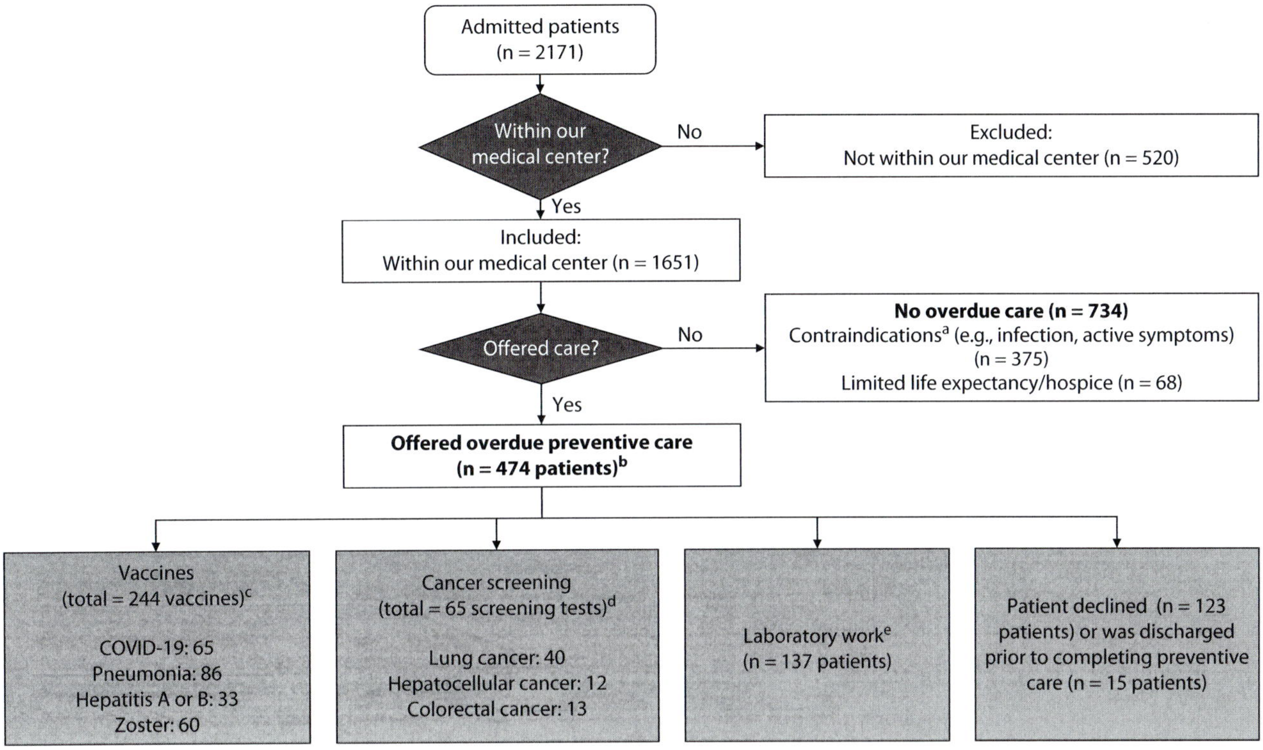

FIGURE 1— Patient Flow for Inclusion and Completed Preventive Care: Veterans Affairs, Palo Alto, CA, 2023–2024

[a]Contraindications applied only to vaccines.
[b]Patients may have been offered > 1 preventive care intervention.
[c]A total of 191 patients received a total of 244 vaccines.
[d]A total of 64 patients completed a total of 65 cancer screening tests.
[e]Laboratory work included lipid panel, hemoglobin A1C, hepatitis B antibody, and hepatitis C antibody.

these crucial outreach efforts increased access to COVID-19 vaccination early in the pandemic, these protocols were not sustained, nor did they address other preventive care. They did, however, serve as a model to reach vulnerable patients who may not otherwise access this care.

Patients who were Black or experiencing severe mental illness, substance use, or housing instability were more likely to have overdue preventive care and therefore benefit from our intervention. By bringing care to where the patient is in space and time, inpatient preventive care bypasses myriad potential barriers to outpatient care. Issues with transportation, time off work, or caregiver obligations are overcome by maximizing the hospital care encounter.[19] Furthermore, bypassing the steps of scheduling the care can increase completion rates. For example, one study showed that 59.3% of patients referred for low-dose computed tomography never connected with the lung cancer screening program.[20] Additional barriers of engagement, mistrust, fatalism, and patient knowledge, which may be more common among racially minoritized groups, were not directly addressed in our study.[21–23] However, our overall completion rate of 70.9% suggests that factors of convenience and being in the care of a trusted inpatient team can overcome these barriers nonetheless.

Patients with overdue care were less likely to have had a recent primary care visit. This finding is consistent with previous studies demonstrating that patients receiving primary care were more likely to receive cancer screening, vaccinations, and laboratory tests for diabetes and cholesterol.[24] While some patients may have barriers to primary care, they may still engage with hospital care, offering an opportunity to maximize the inpatient care encounter. Our study highlights that traditional care models miss some patients, and additional pathways to preventive care during admission can help close the gap.

Our study has several limitations. First, this study's participants were enrolled in VA health care, mitigating potential barriers of lack of insurance and direct patient costs. However, other payer sources allow for reimbursement of preventive care delivered during hospitalization. Second, VA is a

TABLE 1— Characteristics of Patients With and Without Overdue Preventive Care: Veterans Affairs, Palo Alto, CA, 2023–2024

Characteristics	Overdue Preventive Care (n = 474), Mean ±SD or No. (%)	No Overdue Preventive Care (n = 734), Mean ±SD or No. (%)	b (95% CI) or Categorical *P*	
			Univariable	Multivariable
Age, y			<.001	<.001
b (95% CI)	68.3 ±12	76.8 ±10.4	−0.07 (−0.08, −0.06)	−0.06 (−0.08, −0.05)
Race			.008	.18
White	315 (66.5)	496 (67.6)	0 (Ref)	0 (Ref)
Black	72 (15.2)	68 (9.3)	0.51 (0.15, 0.87)	0.28 (−0.11, 0.68)
Asian	17 (3.6)	34 (4.6)	−0.24 (−0.86, 0.35)	−0.24 (−0.92, 0.41)
Other	70 (14.8)	136 (18.5)	−0.21 (−0.54, 0.11)	−0.27 (−0.68, 0.13)
Ethnicity			.5	.97
Hispanic	61 (12.9)	84 (11.4)	0 (Ref)	0 (Ref)
Not Hispanic	368 (77.6)	567 (77.2)	−0.11 (−0.47, 0.25)	−0.05 (−0.45, 0.35)
Unknown	45 (9.5)	83 (11.3)	−0.29 (−0.79, 0.20)	−0.02 (−0.60, 0.55)
Marital status			.021	.46
Married	173 (36.5)	325 (44.3)	0 (Ref)	0 (Ref)
Never married	94 (19.8)	118 (16.1)	0.40 (0.08, 0.73)	−0.21 (−0.60, 0.16)
Other	207 (43.7)	291 (39.6)	0.29 (0.03, 0.55)	0.004 (−0.29, 0.29)
Severe mental illness				
Yes	188 (39.7)	220 (30.0)	0 (Ref)	0 (Ref)
No	286 (60.3)	514 (70.0)	−0.43 (−0.67, −0.19)	−0.06 (−0.34, 0.21)
Substance use				
Yes	129 (27.2)	79 (10.8)	0 (Ref)	0 (Ref)
No	345 (72.8)	655 (89.2)	−1.13 (−1.44, −0.83)	−0.36 (−0.73, 0.01)
Gender				
Male	454 (95.8)	698 (95.1)	0 (Ref)	0 (Ref)
Female	20 (4.2)	36 (4.9)	−0.16 (−0.73, 0.39)	−0.60 (−1.25, 0.02)
Housing instability				
Yes	120 (25.3)	71 (9.7)	0 (Ref)	0 (Ref)
No	354 (74.7)	663 (90.3)	−1.15 (−1.48, −0.84)	−0.49 (−0.87, −0.10)
Years since last primary care appointment			<.001	<.001
<1	324 (68.4)	613 (83.5)	0 (Ref)	0 (Ref)
1–3	69 (14.6)	64 (8.7)	0.71 (0.35, 1.08)	0.52 (0.12, 0.92)
>3 or never	81 (17.1)	57 (7.8)	0.99 (0.63, 1.36)	0.92 (0.52, 1.33)

Note. CI = confidence interval. Univariable logistic regression was conducted for each listed characteristic, and a multivariable logistic regression was conducted with all listed characteristics included. For categorical characteristics, overall *P* values were obtained using likelihood ratio tests comparing the fully specified models and similar models without the respective characteristic being tested.

comprehensive health care system with a shared EHR, easing transparency of preventive care needs. However, many other EHRs and state immunization registries provide similar guidance. Rates of severe mental illness, substance use, and housing instability may be higher in our VA population than other settings. Lastly, the prepost study design lacked a control group.

SUSTAINABILITY

Providing high value preventive care remains an enduring goal of health care. Unfortunately, barriers to receiving preventive care are pervasive. This intervention leverages existing hospital infrastructure and resources to overcome these barriers.

PUBLIC HEALTH SIGNIFICANCE

Preventive care can be successfully delivered to inpatients to meet the needs of underserved patients. Supplementing traditional models by offering preventive care during admission can reduce health inequities and meet the needs of a diverse population. AJPH

ABOUT THE AUTHORS

Nazima Allaudeen, David B. Huberman, and Elizabeth Le are with Veterans Affairs Palo Alto Health Care System, Palo Alto, CA.

Note. Views expressed are those of the authors and not necessarily those of the Department of Veterans Affairs.

CORRESPONDENCE

Correspondence should be sent to Nazima Allaudeen, MD, 3801 Miranda Ave, MC 111, Palo Alto, CA 94304 (e-mail: nazima.allaudeen@va.gov). Reprints can be ordered at https://www.ajph.org by clicking the "Reprints" link.

PUBLICATION INFORMATION

Full Citation: Allaudeen N, Huberman DB, Le E. Advancing equity in preventive care: leveraging hospital admissions for vulnerable populations. *Am J Public Health*. 2025;115(12):1997–2001.

Acceptance Date: June 11, 2025.

DOI: https://doi.org/10.2105/AJPH.2025.308218

ORCID iD:

Nazima Allaudeen https://orcid.org/0000-0002-4941-8729

CONTRIBUTORS

All authors contributed substantially to this work, including design of the project, data analysis, interpretation of the data, and drafting, revising, and final approval of the article. All authors agree to be accountable for all aspects of the work.

CONFLICTS OF INTEREST

The authors declare no conflict of interest.

HUMAN PARTICIPATION PROTECTION

The Stanford institutional review board determined this study to be quality improvement and exempt from human participant review.

REFERENCES

1. Partnership for Prevention. Preventive Care: A National Profile on Use, Disparities, and Health Benefits. August 2007. Available at: https://search.issuelab.org/resource/preventive-care-a-national-profile-on-use-disparities-and-health-benefits.html. Accessed August 2, 2024.
2. Maciosek MV, Coffield AB, Flottemesch TJ, Edwards NM, Solberg LI. Greater use of preventive services in US health care could save lives at little or no cost. *Health Aff (Millwood).* 2010;29(9):1656–1660. https://doi.org/10.1377/hlthaff.2008.0701
3. Lu PJ, Hung MC, Srivastav A, et al. Surveillance of vaccination coverage among adult populations—United States, 2018. *MMWR Surveill Summ.* 2021;70(3):1–26. https://doi.org/10.15585/mmwr.ss7003a1
4. Richards TB, Soman A, Thomas CC, et al. Screening for lung cancer—10 states, 2017. *MMWR Morb Mortal Wkly Rep.* 2020;69(8):201–206. https://doi.org/10.15585/mmwr.mm6908a1
5. QuickStats: age-adjusted percentage of adults aged 50–75 years who received the recommended colorectal cancer screening, by sex and family income—National Health Interview Survey, United States, 2021. *MMWR Morb Mortal Wkly Rep.* 2023;72(25):699. https://doi.org/10.15585/mmwr.mm7225a7
6. Alba C, Zheng Z, Wadhera RK. Changes in health care access and preventive health screenings by race and ethnicity. *JAMA Health Forum.* 2024;5(2):e235058. https://doi.org/10.1001/jamahealthforum.2023.5058
7. Gierisch JM, Beadles C, Shapiro A, et al. Health Disparities in Quality Indicators of Healthcare Among Adults With Mental Illness. Washington, DC: Department of Veterans Affairs; October 2014.
8. Shepherd-Banigan M, Drake C, Dietch JR, et al. Primary Care Engagement Among Veterans With Experiences of Homelessness and Serious Mental Illness: An Evidence Map. Washington, DC: Department of Veterans Affairs; April 2021.
9. Saleh S, Mohammed A, Davila J, Paranji N, Niu B. Disparities in hepatocellular cancer screening in cirrhotic patients with psychiatric disorders. *Cureus.* 2022;14(3):e23516. https://doi.org/10.7759/cureus.23516
10. Ladhani S, Ohri A, Wong RJ. Disparities in hepatocellular carcinoma surveillance: dissecting the roles of patient, provider, and health system factors. *J Clin Gastroenterol.* 2020;54(3):218–226. https://doi.org/10.1097/MCG.0000000000001313
11. Montgomery MP, Meehan AA, Cooper A, et al. Notes from the field: COVID-19 vaccination coverage among persons experiencing homelessness—six US jurisdictions, December 2020–August 2021. *MMWR Morb Mortal Wkly Rep.* 2021;70(48):1676–1678. https://doi.org/10.15585/mmwr.mm7048a4
12. Privett N, Guerrier S. Estimation of the time needed to deliver the 2020 USPSTF preventive care recommendations in primary care. *Am J Public Health.* 2021;111(1):145–149. https://doi.org/10.2105/AJPH.2020.305967
13. Jolin J, van Aalst R, Volpp B, Taylor T, Cohen E. Using an inpatient quality improvement curriculum for internal medicine residents to improve pneumococcal conjugate vaccine administration rates. *Jt Comm J Qual Patient Saf.* 2018;44(6):328–333. https://doi.org/10.1016/j.jcjq.2017.12.005
14. Khaliq W, Siferd C, Kantsiper ME, Jacobs L, Howell EE, Wright SM. Capturing the rest: inpatient mammography for nonadherent hospitalized women. *Am J Prev Med.* 2021;61(5):709–715. https://doi.org/10.1016/j.amepre.2021.04.026
15. Smith TE, Rodgers IT, Silverman DJ, et al. COVID-19 case rates after surveillance and vaccinations in a statewide psychiatric hospital system. *Am J Public Health.* 2021;111(10):1780–1783. https://doi.org/10.2105/AJPH.2021.306444
16. Martinot M, Mohseni-Zadeh M, Marion L, Roncalez D. COVID-19 vaccine: missed opportunities and hospital vaccine implementation. *Clin Microbiol Infect.* 2022;28(8):1174–1175. https://doi.org/10.1016/j.cmi.2022.03.036
17. US Department of Veterans Affairs. Serious mental illness. Available at: https://www.va.gov/PREVENTS/docs/PRE013_FactSheets_SeriousMentalillness_508.pdf. Accessed July 16, 2024.
18. The R Foundation: The R project for statistical computing. Available at: https://www.R-project.org. Accessed October 24, 2024.
19. Kobayashi KJ, Karson AS. Bringing care to underserved and vulnerable patient populations: meeting patients where they are. *Med Care.* 2022;60(1):1–2. https://doi.org/10.1097/MLR.0000000000001671
20. Navuluri N, Morrison S, Green CL, et al. Racial disparities in lung cancer screening among veterans, 2013 to 2021. *JAMA Netw Open.* 2023;6(6):e2318795. https://doi.org/10.1001/jamanetworkopen.2023.18795
21. Lin JJ, Mhango G, Wall MM, et al. Cultural factors associated with racial disparities in lung cancer care. *Ann Am Thorac Soc.* 2014;11(4):489–495. https://doi.org/10.1513/AnnalsATS.201402-055OC
22. Navuluri N, Lanford T, Shapiro A, et al. Barriers and facilitators impacting lung cancer screening uptake among Black veterans: a qualitative study. *J Natl Compr Canc Netw.* 2024;22(4):231–236. https://doi.org/10.6004/jnccn.2023.7098
23. Thompson HS, Manning M, Mitchell J, et al. Factors associated with racial/ethnic group-based medical mistrust and perspectives on COVID-19 vaccine trial participation and vaccine uptake in the US. *JAMA Netw Open.* 2021;4(5):e2111629. https://doi.org/10.1001/jamanetworkopen.2021.11629
24. Levine DM, Landon BE, Linder JA. Quality and experience of outpatient care in the United States for adults with or without primary care [errata in *JAMA Intern Med.* 2019;179(6):854. https://doi.org/10.1001/jamainternmed.2019.1010; *JAMA Intern Med.* 2019;179(5):733. https://doi.org/10.1001/jamainternmed.2019.0618.]. *JAMA Intern Med.* 2019;179(3):363–372. https://doi.org/10.1001/jamainternmed.2018.6716

Integration of Health Care, Public Health, and Communities: A New Model for Rural Public Health

Dora Anne Mills, MD, MPH

See also Primary Care and Public Health in the Community, pp. 1988–2019.

Rural public health has been hit with a triple set of challenges: overstretched health care, poor health status, and limited public health capacities. MaineHealth, a nonprofit integrated 10-hospital health system, serves a mostly rural area with no local public health departments in its rural communities. By integrating primary care with public health and partnering with communities, MaineHealth has developed an infrastructure to successfully address these challenges. We believe this approach is worthy of consideration in other rural areas. (*Am J Public Health*. 2025;115(12):2002–2005. https://doi.org/10.2105/AJPH.2025.308233)

AJPH December 2025, Vol. 115, No. 12

By leveraging the resources of the health care system and by building partnerships, MaineHealth has developed a hub-and-spokes model for community health called the Center for Health Improvement (CHI) that has successfully addressed some rural disparities and built capacity for nonregulatory functions of public health. In this unique way, CHI is able to impact some challenges faced by rural public health.[1]

INTERVENTION AND IMPLEMENTATION

MaineHealth CHI's hub is an organizational hub of resources that includes

- health data and analytics,
- a grants office,
- operational and management resources for program planning and strategy,
- program evaluation, and
- system-wide and statewide programs that work with other providers, state and federal government agencies, statewide nonprofits, businesses, and other partners across the system and state.

CHI's spokes are community health departments in each local hospital's service area that serve all of the residents of that area. The departments (spokes) consist of a community health director and other public health professionals who oversee partnerships with primary care clinicians, local government agencies, schools, and community-based organizations (CBOs; e.g., community action programs). These partnerships are guided by a multisector community coalition that forms a council that is convened by the community health director or a community member. With resources from the CHI hub, the local community health department teams facilitate community health needs assessments (CHNAs), foster partnerships, apply for grants (that include subawards to CBOs), and oversee strategies to address health issues that are prioritized by the CHNA.

The CHI team has developed well-defined roles and responsibilities of the hub and spokes derived from the 10 essential public health services framework, competencies for the community health departments derived from national public health competencies, and standards for the community health departments that include a multisector community council that guides the local departments' work. (Figure A, available as a supplement to the online version of this article at https://ajph.org).

PLACE, TIME, AND PERSONS

MaineHealth's headquarters and tertiary care hospital are in the city of Portland, Maine, though the vast majority of its service area is rural, and all of its community hospitals are in rural areas. MaineHealth employs about 2000 providers in 200 primary care and specialty practice sites as well as in its 10 hospitals and serves 85% of Maine.

Maine's median household income is the 35th lowest, the cost of living is higher than the national average, it is the oldest state in the nation (highest median age and highest proportion of people aged older than 64 years), and it is the most rural state in the country.[2–6] Like the rest of New England and much of the country, there are no local accredited public health departments headquartered in rural areas.[7]

CHI was created in 1997 and has further developed over time to serve various needs, including evolving to a hub-and-spokes model. Since 2019, when the MaineHealth system unified under one 501(c)(3), the model has been more fully defined, and CHI officially became a system-wide department in 2022.

PURPOSE

MaineHealth's motivation is driven by its vision, "working together so our communities are the healthiest in America." Three additional factors are behind the formation of CHI. First, coverage of many nonregulatory public health services by the state's public health agency is unrealistic because staffing is sparse in rural areas because of the lack of a sufficient government infrastructure, yet nonprofit hospitals with primary care practices scattered across rural areas provide an alternative infrastructure to leverage. Second, few municipal or county government agencies or CBOs in rural Maine have the resources to take responsibility for public health services, including applying for and managing government public health grants. Third, primary care providers are overstretched serving patients' health care needs to directly provide many nonclinical public health services.

EVALUATION AND ADVERSE EFFECTS

Box 1 provides several examples of how the CHI hub-and-spokes infrastructure has improved health in rural communities. There are several themes.

First, the local community health departments (spokes) provide public health leadership and assure community and primary care partnerships, including by either convening or participating in a multisector coalition that forms a council. These partnerships have been critical in addressing public health needs. For instance, during the COVID-19 mass vaccination campaign, these partnerships helped identify and provide effective community education and vaccination strategies.

In addition, using the hub's data analyses on patients' SDOH (social determinants of health) screening, showing a tripling of the screen-positive rates for those with a behavioral health diagnosis and a doubling for those who are non-English speakers, the local community health departments leveraged their partnerships to codevelop appropriate strategies. Examples include CHI's local food pantries providing satellites in addiction medicine clinics and working with ethnic CBOs to determine culturally appropriate foods and operations for food pantries in locations with large immigrant communities.

Second, CHI's hub provides centralized resources that would be otherwise challenging to replicate in rural areas. For example, MaineHealth's centralized information technology department builds connections between primary care and CHI's public health programs (e.g., the nicotine treatment program and the National Diabetes Prevention Program). And CHI's centrally located epidemiologists provide analyses on SDOH screening and other programs.

Third, CHI's work at the nexus between public health and health care in both the hub and spokes has been a critical asset. For instance, CHI's Healthy Aging and Maternal Child Health teams, both located centrally in the hub, provide trainings to clinical sites to achieve the age-friendly designation and on the Maternal Opioid Misuse Model. Local community health departments are also educated on these models, to help reinforce the importance of them in community and local clinical settings as well as to reinforce two-way linkages between these settings with SDOH and other community-based resources. In addition, our Access to Care team works across CHI with clinical sites (MaineHealth and others), CBOs, government agencies, and schools to address health coverage issues.

Box 1 illustrates just a few of our programs and their results. We believe this hub-and-spokes work also influences the overall health of our communities, which ranks highly. For instance, in the 2025 County Health Rankings, MaineHealth's nine counties served directly by CHI have *z* scores that average in the top two healthiest groups out of 10 groupings of peer counties nationally.[13] And comparing states through America's Health Rankings' 2024 report, Maine ranked first among those states with similar median household incomes (±$5,000 of Maine's income of $73,463).[14]

SUSTAINABILITY

We believe this hub-and-spokes model is a sustainable one. MaineHealth invests approximately $16 million annually in CHI, much of which counts toward the community benefits required

BOX 1— Some Examples of Center for Health Improvement (CHI) Initiatives: Maine, 2017–2025

Initiative	Function	Results
Connecting primary care with CHI's public health programs	Electronic health records send automatic notices to primary care providers regarding patient eligibility for CHI's National Diabetes Prevention Program (NDPP) and nicotine treatment programs.	Starting in 2020, NDPP sustained enrollment increased 10 times, from 15 to 160 patients per month. CHI's NDPP program is recognized as a Centers for Disease Control and Prevention Full Plus program, which means it reaches high completion and health outcome goals. Starting in 2017, referrals to CHI's statewide nicotine treatment program (Maine QuitLink) from MaineHealth patients saw a sustained increase of 500%, with 6000 additional patients referred annually with an average of 800 of them successfully treated. CHI's program has a 40% quit rate, much higher than 3%–5% without assistance.[8]
Social determinants of health (SDOH)	Led by CHI, MaineHealth screens 80% of patients, with a 16% overall screen-positive rate for at least one of five health-related social needs.	Screen-positive patients referred to a CHI community health worker in 2024–2025 experience a 90% decrease in 60-day unplanned readmissions. Sharing screening data with community-based organizations (CBOs) starting in 2024 has resulted in partnerships to address underlying SDOH (e.g., legislation to reduce deposits required by power companies for those without a credit rating).
COVID-19 vaccination	CHI, CBOs, primary care, and pharmacy led 2020–2021 community COVID-19 vaccination clinics.	More Mainers received their vaccination from MaineHealth than any other organization during 2020–2021. Maine reached the highest in the nation vaccination rates, with higher rates among racial and ethnic minorities compared with non-Hispanic Whites.[9]
Maternal substance use disorder	Via a federal Maternal Opioid Misuse (MOM) grant, CHI implemented integrated obstetrical and opioid treatment and addressed SDOH.[10]	Starting in 2021, women with an opioid use disorder and Medicaid participating in MOM versus those not participating in MOM showed sustained improved birth outcomes with a 44% reduction in low birth weight and 24% reduction in preterm birth.
Age-friendly designation	CHI is working with primary care and hospital sites to meet the age-friendly designation.	Eleven primary care practices and one hospital have met this designation so far. National studies show this designation contributes toward improvements in health outcomes, patient satisfaction, and lowering costs.[11,12]
Access to care	CHI helps enroll patients and others into public health programs (SNAP, WIC), and health insurance and pharmaceutical access programs; addresses transportation, housing, and other SDOH needs; and provides case management.	In fiscal year 2024, a total of 29 846 individuals were assisted through access to care services: • There were 13 625 encounters through the patient assistance line to help with health care coverage and to address transportation, housing, and other SDOH; • 8652 Medicaid applications were submitted; • 914 asylum seekers were connected with health care and social services; • 3685 patients were provided with low-cost or free medications; and • 7880 prescription assistance applications were completed.

Note. SNAP = Supplemental Nutrition Assistance Program; WIC = Special Supplemental Nutrition Program for Women, Infants, and Children.

of all nonprofit hospitals. These dollars in turn help leverage an additional $19 million in external funding, mostly federal and state public health dollars. Seventeen percent of these external dollars are subawarded to CBOs. Currently, about 300 employees work for CHI, with about half based in local community health departments and the rest in the central hub. Most have a public health education background.

Lessons Learned

Key strategies of CHI include

- developing and maintaining partnerships that include a multisector coalition at the local community level;
- hiring public health professionals to lead the local community health departments (spokes);
- engaging clinicians, which is likely easier because CHI is housed within a health system, even when engaging external clinicians such as those working in federally qualified health centers (FQHCs); and
- building foundational resources in the hub (e.g., data analytics, grant writing, and grants management).

While some have encouraged us to help develop county or municipal public health departments, we feel this is unrealistic in many rural areas, because government capacity there is extremely limited, without the ability to apply for and manage federal or state grants. Community action programs, schools, and FQHCs are other common infrastructures in rural areas. However, nonprofit hospitals are distinguished by having the requirements to conduct CHNAs as well as to provide community benefits. Of note, CHNAs across Maine are co-led with the community action programs.

Challenges include sustainability, which is always a challenge for any local public health organization. However, with the requirement for nonprofit hospitals to conduct a CHNA and provide community benefits, and with the ability for the organization to seek numerous grants, CHI has existed and grown for more than 25 years. Challenges may increase with the reduction in government grant opportunities and if the federal requirements for CHNAs or community benefits are rescinded.

Also, assuring CHI's work is primarily serving the rural communities that make up the vast majority of its service area is sometimes a challenge because the health system's headquarters is in an urban community. The local (rural) community health directors, local multisector councils, the triennial CHNA with resulting plans, and a CHI leadership team that includes each local community health director help ensure CHI's work is addressing the needs of its service area.

PUBLIC HEALTH SIGNIFICANCE

Rural communities are often home to primary care networks that are members of a nonprofit hospital-based system or a FQHC system. Centralized resources of both types of systems have the potential to support local teams to work in the nexus between public health and health care, in partnership with communities. Community benefits and CHNA requirements can be leveraged in the case of nonprofit hospital-based systems. In rural areas of the country with overstretched health care, poor health status, and limited public health capacities, we believe this hub-and-spokes model can be replicated to improve health and nonregulatory public health capacity. AJPH

ABOUT THE AUTHOR

Dora Anne Mills is with MaineHealth, Portland, ME.

CORRESPONDENCE

Correspondence should be sent to Dora Anne Mills, MD, MPH, Chief Health Improvement Officer, MaineHealth, 110 Free St, Portland, ME 04101 (e-mail: doraanne.mills@mainehealth.org). Reprints can be ordered at https://ajph.org by clicking the "Reprints" link.

PUBLICATION INFORMATION

Full Citation: Mills DA. Integration of health care, public health, and communities: a new model for rural public health. *Am J Public Health.* 2025;115(12): 2002–2005.

Acceptance Date: June 20, 2025.

DOI: https://doi.org/10.2105/AJPH.2025.308233

ORCID iD:
Dora Anne Mills https://orcid.org/0009-0004-8523-7505

ACKNOWLEDGMENTS

The work reflected in this article is that of the more than 300 team members of MaineHealth's Center for Health Improvement and its many MaineHealth, clinical, community, and governmental partners. The author is deeply grateful to all of them.

CONFLICTS OF INTEREST

The author reports no conflicts of interest.

HUMAN PARTICIPANT PROTECTION

This analysis did not involve human participants, so no institutional review board approval was necessary.

REFERENCES

1. Rural Health Information Hub. Rural health disparities. November 12, 2024. Available at: https://www.ruralhealthinfo.org/topics/rural-health-disparities#disparities-and-inequities. Accessed November 15, 2024.
2. National Institute on Minority Health and Health Disparities. Median household income. HDPulse: An ecosystem of minority health and health disparities resources. Available at: https://hdpulse.nimhd.nih.gov/data-portal/social/table?age=001&age_options=ageall_1&demo=00011&demo_options=income_3&race=00&race_options=race_7&sex=0&sex_options=sexboth_1&socialtopic=030&socialtopic_options=social_6&statefips=00&statefips_options=area_states. Accessed November 10, 2024.
3. Missouri Economic Research and Information Center. Cost of Living Data Series. Available at: https://meric.mo.gov/data/cost-living-data-series. Accessed November 10, 2024.
4. America's Health Rankings. Analysis of CDC WONDER, single-race population estimates. United Health Foundation. Available at: https://www.americashealthrankings.org/explore/measures/pct_65plus. Accessed November 10, 2024.
5. US Census Bureau. "Median Age by Sex" American Community Survey. ACS 5-Year Estimates Detailed Tables, Table B01002. 2020. Available at: https://data.census.gov/table/ACSDT5Y2020.B01002?q=American+Community+survey&g=050XX00US26065$1500000&y=2020&d=ACS+5-Year+Estimates+Detailed+Tables. Accessed November 11, 2024.
6. America's Health Rankings. Analysis of US Census Bureau, American Community Survey. United Health Foundation. Available at: https://www.americashealthrankings.org/explore/measures/pct_rural_b. Accessed November 10, 2024.
7. Public Health Accreditation Board. Accreditation activity. Available at: https://phaboard.org/accreditation-recognition/accreditation-activity. Accessed November 13, 2024.
8. Truth Initiative. Quitting tobacco: facts and stats. April 22, 2024. Available at: https://truthinitiative.org/research-resources/quitting-smoking-vaping/quitting-tobacco-facts-and-stats. Accessed September 11, 2025.
9. Mills DA, Boomsma J. Lessons learned from Maine's nation-leading vaccination efforts. *Health Affairs Forefront.* July 27, 2021. Available at: https://www.healthaffairs.org/do/10.1377/hblog20210722.638604/full. Accessed November 10, 2024.
10. Hirai AH, Ko JY, Owens PL, Stocks C, Patrick SW. Neonatal abstinence syndrome and maternal opioid-related diagnoses in the US, 2010–2017. *JAMA.* 2021;325(2):146–155. https://doi.org/10.1001/jama.2020.24991
11. American Hospital Association. Creating value with age-friendly health systems. *Value Initiative Issue Brief.* August 2020. Available at: https://www.aha.org/system/files/media/file/2020/08/value-initiative-issue-brief-10-creating-value-with-age-friendly-health-systems.pdf. Accessed May 10, 2025.
12. Mate K, Fulmer T, Pelton L, et al. Evidence for the 4Ms: interactions and outcomes across the care continuum. *J Aging Health.* 2021;33(7-8):469–481. https://doi.org/10.1177/0898264321991658
13. University of Wisconsin Population Health Institute. County Health Rankings & Roadmaps. March 2025. Available at: https://www.countyhealthrankings.org. Accessed May 10, 2025.
14. America's Health Rankings. 2024 Annual Report. January 2025. Available at: https://www.americashealthrankings.org/learn/reports/2024-annual-report. Accessed May 10, 2025.

Retooling the Workforce for Collaboration: Centering Collective Efficacy in Public Health and Primary Care Leadership Development

Janelle Zamora Martelino, RN, PhD, MN, and Betty Bekemeier, RN, PhD, MPH

See also Primary Care and Public Health in the Community, pp. 1988–2019.

Enhanced integration of public health and primary care sectors is necessary to advance population health equity. Integration requires engagement from leaders adept at working collaboratively, yet barriers persist. While leadership development has been a promising means to address interpersonal obstacles, traditional approaches typically focus on teaching discipline-based cognitive skills while underplaying communication, relational, and affective skills that leaders need to excel in increasingly networked and collaborative organizations.

Building on previous efforts to foster collaborative leadership in public health, we propose a framework to support the intentional development of collective leadership among public health and primary care professionals. The framework emphasizes collaborative leader behaviors, collective efficacy, and collective performance, and it acknowledges the critical interactions among team members with diverse expertise. It also conceptualizes leadership as a dynamic, shared process among members rather than focusing on a defined person.

We offer recommendations for incorporating this framework into intersectoral leadership development programs to strengthen the collective abilities of the workforce and accelerate integration across sectors.
(*Am J Public Health*. 2025;115(12):2006–2014. https://doi.org/10.2105/AJPH.2025.308216)

AJPH December 2025, Vol. 115, No. 12

The World Health Organization[1] and the National Academy of Medicine[2,3] have issued calls to improve public health and primary care sector collaboration to advance population health outcomes. Amid recent public health challenges, like the COVID-19 pandemic, structural racism, and extreme weather events, multisectoral partnerships have become increasingly important, requiring engagement from knowledgeable leaders capable of working across sectors. However, barriers that inhibit integration persist, like inadequate understanding of specific roles, ineffective communication, and poor rapport between primary care and public health.[2,4,5] Leadership development has been offered as a promising way to address interpersonal obstacles and encourage more complete integration between public health and primary care.[3,4]

Leadership development programs often focus on improving participants' knowledge, technical skills, and perceived ability. While individual-level outcomes can be a starting point for leadership development, these programs are limited in that individual skills may not assist leaders in working interorganizationally or across sectors. Public health initiatives such as the National Public Health Leadership Institute began incorporating team-based approaches to leadership development as early as the mid-2000s, demonstrating positive outcomes in collaborative practice and cross-agency alignment.[6] More recently, emerging leadership development programs have continued to bridge public health and primary care, focusing on systems leadership, equity, and community collaboration. Programs such as the Northwest Public Health and Primary

Care Leadership Institute and the Region IV Public Health & Primary Care Leadership Institute bring together leaders from health departments, primary care, and community organizations to build shared capacity for collective action.

Evaluation of these programs improved alignment of goals, enhanced cross-sector partnerships, and stimulated implementation of community-level interventions.[7,8] These programs point to a broader shift toward collective approaches to leadership. To build on this momentum, a structured framework could help further support and accelerate the development, sustainability, and scaling of collective leadership capacity across sectors.

We propose a framework for conceptualizing collective leadership development among public health and primary care professionals, emphasizing improving collaborative leader self-efficacy and collective efficacy. Given the complexities of population health improvement, the framework described here acknowledges the critical interactions between the leader and team members with diverse skills and expertise while viewing leadership as a dynamic, shared process among members rather than focusing on a defined person.[9]

CURRENT CONCEPTS OF LEADER AND LEADERSHIP DEVELOPMENT

The concepts of leader development and leadership development are often confused. While the terms may appear synonymous and are used interchangeably, they are different but related concepts. Leader development is a process whereby a leader builds intrapersonal knowledge, skills, abilities, values, and identities that enhance the leader's effectiveness in setting direction, creating alignment, and maintaining commitment in groups of people who share common work.[10–12] Leadership development emphasizes the group-level processes that develop in the interaction between an individual leader and the social and organizational environment and include vital components like empathy, service orientation, collaboration and cooperation, and conflict management.[10] Leadership development seeks to enhance the collective capacity of organizational members to engage effectively in leadership roles and processes. Day clarifies that leadership development can be understood as an organizational strategy by

> helping people understand how to relate to others, coordinate their efforts, build commitments, and develop extended social networks by applying self-understanding to social and organizational imperatives.[10(p586)]

Leader development is an aspect of the broader concept of leadership development.

In science and practice, leadership has been traditionally viewed as an individual-level phenomenon, where a single leader provides direction and inspiration to a group of followers in a hierarchical organizational structure.[13,14] The behaviors of successful leaders are seen as observable and transferrable—skills that can be cultivated through education and experience.[15] This person-centered approach to leader development focuses on intrapersonal attributes that enhance a leader's effectiveness at establishing goals, synchronizing efforts, and ensuring engagement of teams who share common work.[11,12] Friedrich et al.[9] describe these competencies as baseline leadership skills, categorized into 3 domains: (1) conceptual skills, such as intelligence, creativity, and foresight, which are critical to effective problem-solving and decision-making; (2) interpersonal skills, including communication, emotion regulation, political skill, and perspective taking, which support engagement and delegation; and (3) technical skills, referring to procedural knowledge and domain-specific expertise that informs problem-solving. Traditional leadership development thus centers around individual behaviors and leader–follower dynamics, typically within vertical organizational hierarchies—a perspective that continues to dominate popular and professional approaches to leadership development.

While this approach to leader development is necessary, leadership in practice is rarely a solitary endeavor. The complexities of population health require multiple individuals and entities to engage in actions requiring leadership and collaboration, depending on the context and situation. Traditional notions of developing individual leaders and their interactions with followers could be interpreted as misaligned with interprofessional collaboration and practice principles. In interprofessional collaboration, different health and social care professional groups work together to affect health outcomes positively and are involved in regular negotiation and interaction between professionals, and the contributions of various professionals are valued.[16] Traditional models of leadership and development may help to clarify the challenges of leading within organizational boundaries. However, working across organization and sector boundaries to address shared challenges presents different demands on leaders and requires new leadership paradigms.[17] Our current health environment necessitates a leadership approach that acknowledges multiperson interactions and the interorganizational context and elevates the importance of a collective mindset to achieve shared goals. A collective leadership approach is more congruent with the principles and values of interprofessional collaboration and practice.

We thus use the term "collaborative" to characterize the style in which the focal leader acts or behaves, emphasizing expressed power-sharing among groups. "Collective" is more of an orientation in this case, where the individual or group is mindful of how the group, or collective, works together to achieve goals.

COLLECTIVE LEADERSHIP

According to Friedrich et al., collective leadership is "a dynamic leadership process in which a defined leader, or set of leaders, selectively utilize skills and expertise within a network, effectively distributing elements of the leadership role as the situation or problem at hand requires."[9(p933)] This approach shifts focus away from individual leaders as the central figures, distinguishing between the person who leads and the broader construct of leadership. Leadership is understood to emerge at the collective level—a system of relationships—rather than solely from individuals or dyads. As Ospina notes, "individuals' decisions, interactions, and actions are embedded [at the collective level], which is where leadership emerges."[18(p281)] Leadership in this context is shaped by shared practices, informed by situational demands. Formal and informal networks of relationships provide leaders and team members access to distributed expertise, supporting activities such as information exchange, collaboration, and joint decision-making.[13] These responsibilities are fluid and shift across individuals over time. Ultimately, collective leadership cultivates the capacity for effective collaboration and achieving shared goals.[18]

BENEFITS OF COLLECTIVE LEADERSHIP

Collective leadership offers many benefits to organizations. Expecting an individual to be an exceptional leader in all situations is unrealistic. Collective leadership encourages other leaders and team members to view leadership as a joint endeavor[9] and can promote the rise of leaders on the basis of expertise. This leadership approach shares responsibility and accountability, allowing other team members to feel empowered, engaged, and a part of the decision-making process. Because decisions are made collectively, the expertise of leaders and team members is appropriately utilized, and they are more likely to buy into any changes. With this approach, team members feel valued, respected, listened to, and heard, and a sense of mutual and shared understanding is fostered.[19] In effective collective leadership, well-established relationships within the network enable the group to respond quickly to changing situations.[9]

FRAMEWORK FOR COLLECTIVE LEADERSHIP DEVELOPMENT

While there is increasing interest in collective leadership, the science and practice of collective leadership development are limited,[13] particularly in the field of interprofessional studies.[20] Given the existing challenges of working in complex population health environments, we believe that leader and leadership development in public health and primary care should adopt a collective leadership approach that highly regards the expertise of multiple leaders. Traditional models of leadership development should be moderated with an added focus on collaborative problem-solving, working in horizontal leadership structures, and incentivizing behavior in new ways.

Drawing upon the work of Bronfenbrenner,[21] Bandura,[22] Friedrich et al.,[9] and Hannah et al.,[23] we propose a framework for conceptualizing collective leadership development (Figure 1) with an emphasis on collaborative leader self-efficacy, collaborative leader behaviors, and collective efficacy. Collective efficacy is the shared belief in a group's capacity to achieve its goals.[24] Our framework is depicted in concentric circles based on Bronfenbrenner's[21] socioecological model. It provides a systems perspective that considers individual and environmental factors influencing an individual's behavior on different levels. Bandura's[25] theoretical model of self-efficacy is embedded within the individual level of leader development, illustrating the relationship between developmental activities, leader self-efficacy, and leader behavior and performance. Collective efficacy beliefs are thought to operate within the individual through similar processes as self-efficacy.[22] However, these individual perceptions of collective efficacy can evolve to form group perceptions of collective efficacy over time.[23] Collective behavior and performance are depicted in the interpersonal and organizational levels. Our framework values the interactions between the leader and team members with diverse skills and expertise[9] and acknowledges collective

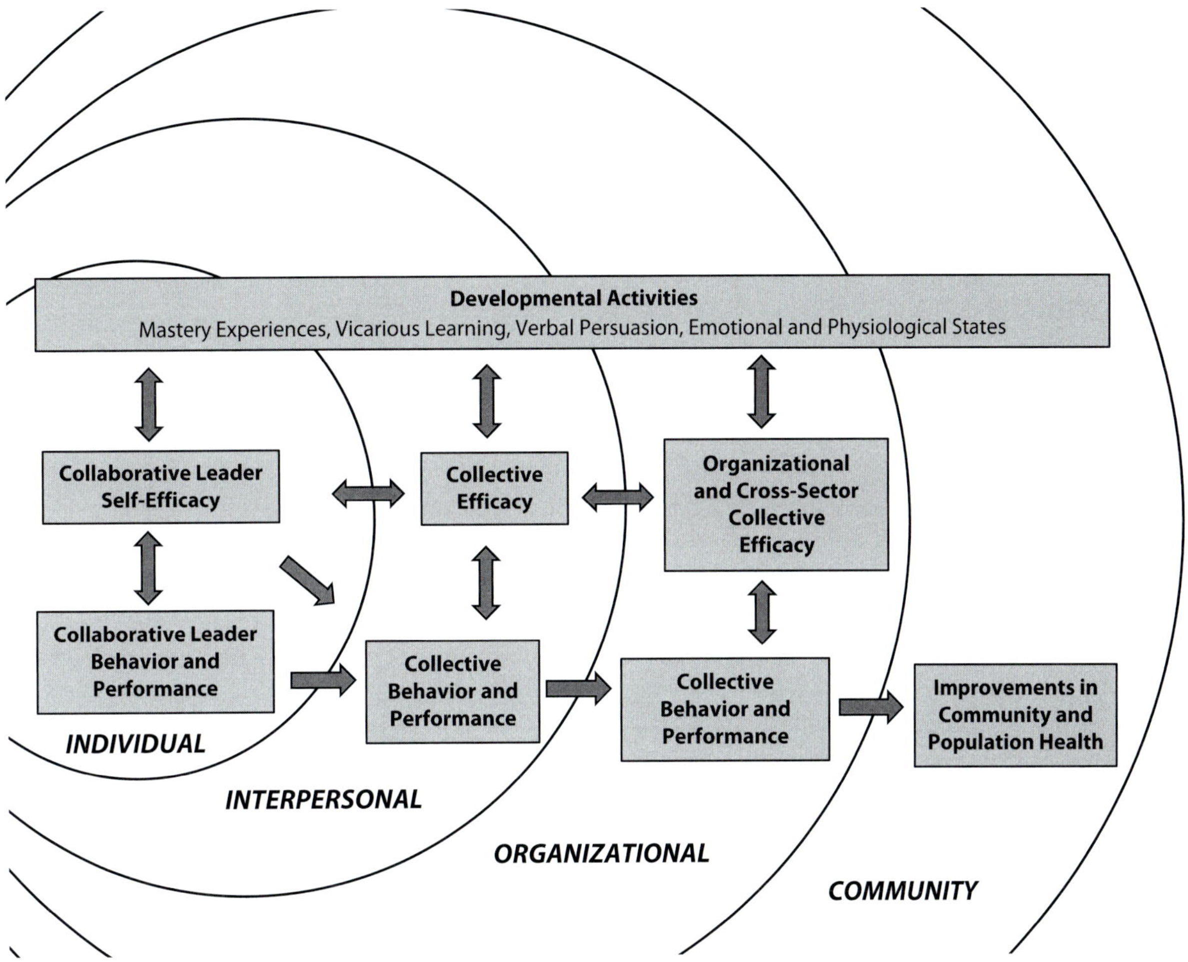

FIGURE 1— A Framework for Collective Leadership Development in Cross-Sector Interprofessional Collaboration

Note. Conceptualized by the authors, this framework is informed by Bronfenbrenner's socioecological model,[21] Bandura's theory of self-efficacy,[22] and existing scholarship on collective leadership (Friedrich et al.[9]; Hannah et al.[23])

leadership development as a shared process among members. By developing leaders in a collaborative leadership approach, the individual can model behaviors and practices to other team members that promote greater collective efficacy.

Key Constructs in Collective Leadership Development

Collaborative leader self-efficacy. Day et al.[26] posit that leader development is at the heart of successful leadership development. Without a good leader, successful leadership will be difficult to develop among teams. Internal self-confidence of the leader, termed "leader self-efficacy," has been attributed as a critical element of their effectiveness and development. According to Machida and Schaubroeck, leader self-efficacy is "a leader's confidence in their abilities, knowledge, and skills in areas needed to lead others effectively."[27(p460)] Empirical research demonstrates that leader self-efficacy is associated with positive work outcomes, leader performance, perception of leader effectiveness, motivation of others, and group performance.[23]

Given the benefits of leader self-efficacy, questions arise regarding how best to develop it. Based on Bandura's[25] work with self-efficacy, leader self-efficacy can be developed through (1) mastery experiences based on past leader accomplishments, as in successful practice at a skill or behavior; (2) modeling or vicarious learning through role models successfully performing similar tasks; (3) verbal persuasion or positive feedback and encouragement on leadership roles; and (4) emotional and physiological states—that is, the well-being of the individual. Participants from an existing public health and primary care leadership development program reported higher levels of leader self-efficacy several months after program completion, providing them the confidence to move into more formalized leadership roles (J. Martelino; interview data collected January 2023).

While the empirical literature does not appear to characterize leadership styles in leader self-efficacy, we argue that leader self-efficacy should be specified to indicate the leadership approach for development. For example, a proficient leader with an authoritarian style may find it challenging to operate in a collective leadership environment. Thus, collaborative leader self-efficacy is specified in the framework to align with the collective leadership approach. Adapting both Machida and Schaubroeck's[27] definition of leader self-efficacy and Ibarra and Hansen's[28] definition of a collaborative leader, we define collaborative leader self-efficacy as a leader's confidence in their abilities, knowledge, and skills to engage people and groups inside and outside of one's formal control and inspire them to work toward common goals.

Collaborative leader behaviors and performance. Leader self-efficacy is believed to help individuals manage their leader behavior via goal setting and influences effective leadership, motivation, and performance.[29] Based on Bandura's[24,25] social cognitive theory of motivation and behavior, individuals with high self-efficacy will outperform those with low self-efficacy. In collective leadership, leader performance is contingent upon the individual creating conditions that support the effective exchange of information and expertise among team members.[30] Accordingly, many essential collaborative leader behaviors (Box 1) are oriented toward fostering such exchanges. While traditional leader development programs often focus on building foundational leadership skills and behaviors,[14] programs with a collective leadership orientation should prioritize cultivating collaborative leadership behaviors. Recruiting midcareer leaders may be advantageous, as they are likely to have already developed core leadership competencies, and a focus on refining and advancing collaborative leader behaviors can be applied. Evidence from a cross-sector leadership development program demonstrated improvements in network awareness, bidirectional communication, and relationship building within participants' teams well after program completion (J. Martelino; interview data collected January 2023).

BOX 1— Examples of Collaborative Leader Skills and Behaviors

Skill or Behavior	Description
Bidirectional communication	Communication that involves an exchange between 2 parties, such as consultation, exchanging feedback, or information sharing, across levels
Unidirectional communication	Communication that is directed from one party to another, typically from leader to team member, that is motivating (e.g., direction-giving language to clarify expectations, meaning-making to communicate values of the group or organization, or empathetic language to demonstrate compassion and emotion)
Network awareness and development	Gaining familiarity with connections and available expertise in networks; developing relationships with others
Wielding influence	Being able to identify unproductive discussions and exert influence to move things forward
Delegation	Transferring tasks, responsibilities, or decision-making to other team members with clear expectations and regular monitoring
Empowerment of others	Distribution or sharing of leadership with those who have relevant knowledge or expertise via delegation of authority or information sharing
Consultation	Utilization of others' expertise by seeking problem clarification and monitoring of problems
Trust-building	Interpersonal exchange relationship that is developed between 2 members whereby members prove themselves responsible and trustworthy—for example, through accomplishment of tasks or serving as a confidante
Facilitating opportunities for contact among members	Creating conditions to connect and encourage collaboration among heterogenous team members to promote innovation
Giving members voice	Permitting team members to participate in problem-solving
Sense-giving	Ensuring team members possess a common understanding of the problem, their work related to the issue, and how to engage
Ensuring diverse representation in network	Engaging others from different backgrounds, experiences, disciplines, cultures, and generations for effective problem identification, implementation of solutions, and revision

Note. From Friedrich et al.,[9] Friedrich et al.,[14] and Ibarra and Hansen.[28]

Collective efficacy. Collective efficacy is defined as a group's shared belief in its ability to produce desired results.[22] It is assessed by the group's confidence in members' abilities to perform their individual duties and the group's belief in the collective's ability as a whole to produce desired results. It is important to note that collective efficacy beliefs first reside within the individual (e.g., "I believe that our group can accomplish our task.") but over time can emerge as group-level perceptions of collective efficacy (e.g., "We believe that our group can accomplish our task.").[22] In public health and primary care leadership development, collective efficacy can be enhanced by allowing leaders to better understand cross-sector roles, values, philosophies, and collaborative working styles and by developing mutual trust and respect. In unpublished data from a cross-sector leadership development program, participants reported enhanced levels of collective efficacy after the program (J. Martelino; interview data collected January 2023). Although evidence on collective efficacy in cross-sector leadership programs—particularly in public health and primary care—is limited, research from the education sector offers relevant parallels. Leadership development programs that promote shared leadership and relational trust have been shown to enhance collective efficacy.[31] Similar public health and primary care approaches may help build collective efficacy by strengthening collaboration and shared responsibility across sectors.

In the collective leadership approach, team-level processes and related theories are understood to play out at the interpersonal level.[9,30] Thus, an exchange exists between the individual leader, team members, and the broader network. While scant empirical findings exist, it is conceivable that high leader self-efficacy affects both the individual and collective efficacy of team members and their performance and reciprocally affects the leader's self-efficacy. High leader self-efficacy has been associated with higher leader performance and higher levels of group performance.[23] Therefore, it is proposed in our framework that collaborative behaviors exercised by the leader have a positive effect on the behaviors and performance of team members, not only at the interpersonal level but at the wider organizational or interorganizational network level as well. These collaborative behaviors exhibited by both leaders and team members during social interactions with the group would indicate to team members that they are successful at doing their part in achieving group tasks and that collective efficacy would increase.[23] Taggar and Seijts[32] have demonstrated that both leader and follower efficacies predict collective efficacy.

Collective leadership behaviors and performance. The collective leadership environment manifests when most leaders and members in a team, unit, or organization work collaboratively and consistently exercise collaborative leader behaviors (Box 1). Cullen et al.[33] argue that collective leadership development focuses on collective outcomes that are beyond the development of individual leaders' competencies to one that is on the collective's ability to produce direction, alignment, and commitment. Direction is the agreement on what the group is trying to accomplish, alignment is when activities are coordinated and integrated toward the shared goal, and commitment is when individuals prioritize the collective's success.

In collective leadership development, developmental activities are fostered across multiple levels to reinforce the collective mindset. Our framework assumes that this leadership development approach is cultivated on multiple levels. At the individual level, leadership is developed through participation in a formal leadership development program. At the interpersonal level, growth occurs in dyadic and group work within the program setting. At the organizational level, senior leaders, administrators, and executives play a key role in reinforcing leadership practices. Finally, at the community level, leadership is expressed through engagement with community members, patients, or recipients of a population health intervention or change. Cullen et al.[33] refer to the collective's shared beliefs and practices for understanding and producing direction, alignment, and commitment as leadership culture. Concerning collective performance, scholars have long suggested that organizational outcomes are a byproduct of improvements in learning and transfer, and there is empirical support for leadership development outcomes.[12] Some studies have demonstrated improved organizational performance through enhanced strategic thinking, change management, and systems leadership capacity,[34] resulting in increased retention and engagement of leaders and staff because of supportive and inclusive leadership practices.[35]

Community and population health improvements. Leadership development programs embedded in collective leadership principles have demonstrated the potential to generate improvements beyond individual skill-building, contributing to broader community-level outcomes. These programs emphasize collaborative capacity, systems thinking, and cross-sector engagement, enabling participants to start or strengthen initiatives addressing social determinants of health and structural inequities. For example, the multisector leadership program Culture of Health Leaders through the Robert Wood Johnson Foundation has demonstrated strengthened cross-sector collaboration and increased capacity to influence local and state systems.[36] While research conditions such as temporal design, control conditions, sample representation, and other contextual factors[37] may limit our ability to establish causal effects of distal outcomes from the leadership development program, the evidence we have thus far highlights its potential as a lever for advancing population health and health equity.

Factors of Collective Leadership Development

There are individual differences that can influence the development of collaborative leader capacity. An individual's cognitive ability is thought to affect recall, information processing for problem-solving, and interpretation and analysis of the collective's network. Leader experience with collaboration, both within organizations and in specific leader roles, and personality traits may also affect how collaborative behaviors are developed.[23]

Elements in the external environment can also facilitate or inhibit collaborative leader capacity. Because our leader development framework depends on the expertise of the collective network, network characteristics like size, density, and embeddedness of connections are thought to affect collaborative leader capacity.[14] Given these dependencies, communication is vital for collaboration within a collective leadership approach. Ongoing, open exchange among leaders and team members is required[30]; however, it is important to note that not all working environments have cultures that permit open communication. Finally, time is a factor in the development of collaborative leaders. Collective leadership is a demanding cognitive activity, and when there is inadequate time to foster relationships and work collaboratively and where stress is high, leaders may not practice those behaviors.[30]

FROM FRAMEWORK TO IMPLEMENTATION

The provision of public- and private-sector health promotion and social services requires leadership across organizations to work together to meet changing expectations and new priorities to advance population health equity. Enhanced integration of health and social services across sectors is necessary to reduce the burden of chronic disease and health inequities across populations.[38] It requires leaders who are adept at working collaboratively. Indeed, a recent review noted that the most effective leadership styles in the health care setting were more collaborative, multifaceted, and dynamic and that such behaviors were strongly associated with quality care outcomes and patient and employee satisfaction.[39] However, traditional approaches to developing leaders typically focus on teaching discipline-based cognitive skills and development while underplaying communication, relational, and affective skills that organizations need to operate in with increasingly networked and collaborative organizations.

We offer a framework to guide the evolution of collective leadership development programs to meet the needs of today's complex work environments. While public health leadership programs have increasingly incorporated collaborative approaches over the past 2 decades,[6] there remains a need for structured frameworks that can support the intentional development and scaling of collective leadership capacity across levels and sectors. Our proposed framework builds on these foundations and centers collaborative leader behaviors, collective efficacy, and collective performance to support the integration of public health and primary care. By focusing specifically on developmental activities that cultivate a view of leadership as a joint endeavor, team members share responsibility and accountability and increase members' engagement and feelings of empowerment (J. Martelino; interview data collected January 2023).

Key activities that promote teamwork should be prioritized, including conflict resolution, communication, and interpersonal skills; problem-solving through complex health and community issues; setting a joint vision and motivating others toward such a vision; and time and resource management.[40] While there is no consensus on the optimal duration of leadership development programs, it is generally accepted that programs spanning several months result in greater knowledge acquisition and allow participants to incorporate skills into practice.[11] An investment of time and space is necessary to develop long-term relationships across organizations to support interdependent, collective leadership development.[33] We recommend that cross-sector leadership development efforts be enhanced by incorporating this framework into programs to boost the collective abilities of the workforce. Integrating this approach would not replace programs that seek to build management and technical skills but rather complement them by elevating the importance of building collective efficacy within and across agencies.

The framework does not assume that all participants—particularly those from public health and primary care—enter the leadership development programs with the same baseline knowledge or experience related to cross-sector collaboration. We recognize that primary care leaders often operate in settings oriented toward individual patient care, while public health leaders more commonly work at population and systems levels. To address this variation, leadership development programs adopting this framework should include foundational activities early in the program that surface differing leadership perspectives, build a shared language, and explicitly develop competencies in collaborative problem-solving, mutual goal-setting, and interprofessional communication. These elements are intended to scaffold collective leadership development in a way that is responsive to participants' varied professional backgrounds and organizational contexts.

However, implementing this framework may present challenges. For example, deeply ingrained professional norms and organizational structures may resist collective leadership models. Leaders may also experience uncertainty around role boundaries, especially when leadership is not necessarily defined by formal authority but by influence, collaboration, and context. Finally, some leaders may question the practicality of collective leadership, particularly in high-pressure environments where top-down decision-making is common. Intentional program design and skilled facilitation will be essential to reinforcing collective leadership development over time.

The framework presented is grounded in the authors' experience designing and implementing a leadership development program focused on cultivating collective leadership among public health and primary care professionals. Although a full evaluation of the program is currently unpublished, insights gained through its design, facilitation, and iterative refinement directly informed the development of the framework. The recommendations reflect both practical experience and alignment with principles drawn from the literature on interprofessional collaboration, systems leadership, and collective efficacy. As such, the framework represents both a practice-informed and evidence-aligned model for guiding future collective leadership development efforts.

Collective leadership is gaining traction in health service delivery debates, though there is little consensus about how to conceptualize, define, or measure collective leadership.[13] This framework advances the science of collective leadership development by leveraging current research on the growth and development of individual leaders working in teams and extends it to leadership across networks and sectors. It acknowledges the multifaceted, interprofessional nature of health and health care delivery and expands the notion of collective efficacy into leadership development programs. This framework can also guide further research to explore optimal program duration to increase collective efficacy and connect program elements to more distal outcomes.

CONCLUSION

The complex public health challenges of our time require a workforce capable of operating in integrated environments that span public health and primary care. This collective leadership development framework conceptualizes leadership as a dynamic, shared process and acknowledges the critical interactions among team members with diverse skills and expertise. By emphasizing collaborative behaviors and building collective efficacy, this approach can help reengineer the public health and primary care workforce to lead more effectively across sectors and advance population health. AJPH

ABOUT THE AUTHORS

Janelle Z. Martelino was with the School of Nursing, University of Washington, Seattle, at the time of this study. Betty Bekemeier is with the Department of Child, Family and Population Health, School of Nursing, and the Northwest Center for Public Health Practice, School of Public Health, both at the University of Washington, Seattle.

CORRESPONDENCE

Correspondence should be sent to Janelle Z. Martelino, PhD, MN, RN, FACMPE, 30 211th St SW, Bothell, WA 98021 (e-mail: jzamora@uw.edu). Reprints can be ordered at https://www.ajph.org by clicking the "Reprints" link.

PUBLICATION INFORMATION

Full Citation: Martelino JZ, Bekemeier B. Retooling the workforce for collaboration: centering collective efficacy in public health and primary care leadership development. *Am J Public Health*. 2025;115(12): 2006–2014.

Acceptance Date: June 11, 2025.

DOI: https://doi.org/10.2105/AJPH.2025.308216

ORCID iDs:
Janelle Zamora Martelino https://orcid.org/0000-0002-1133-7608

Betty Bekemeier https://orcid.org/0000-0002-9034-2746

CONTRIBUTORS

J. Z. Martelino originated and provided the first draft of the article with contributions from B. Bekemeier. Both authors contributed to editing and revising the article and approved the final version.

ACKNOWLEDGMENTS

This work was supported by the National Institute for Occupational Safety and Health (NIOSH) under federal training grant T42OH008433.

Note. The content is solely the responsibility of the authors and does not necessarily represent the official views of NIOSH.

CONFLICTS OF INTEREST

The authors declare no potential conflicts of interest with respect to the research, authorship, or publication of this article.

HUMAN PARTICIPANT PROTECTION

No human participants were involved in the research reported in this article.

REFERENCES

1. Rechel B. *How to Enhance the Integration of Primary Care and Public Health? Approaches, Facilitating Factors and Policy Options.* Copenhagen, Denmark: World Health Organization; 2020.
2. Institute of Medicine. *Primary Care and Public Health: Exploring Integration to Improve Population Health.* Washington, DC: Institute of Medicine; 2012.
3. Global Forum on Innovation in Health Professional Education; Board on Global Health; Institute of Medicine. *Interprofessional Education for Collaboration: Learning How to Improve Health From Interprofessional Models Across the Continuum of Education to Practice: Workshop Summary.* Washington, DC: National Academies Press; 2013.
4. Valaitis RK, O'Mara L, Wong ST, et al. Strengthening primary health care through primary care and public health collaboration: the influence of intrapersonal and interpersonal factors. *Prim Health Care Res Dev.* 2018;19(4):378–391. https://doi.org/10.1017/S1463423617000895
5. Pratt R, Gyllstrom B, Gearin K, et al. Identifying barriers to collaboration between primary care and public health: experiences at the local level. *Public Health Rep.* 2018;133(3):311–317. https://doi.org/10.1177/0033354918764391
6. Umble K, Steffen D, Porter J, et al. The National Public Health Leadership Institute: evaluation of a team-based approach to developing collaborative public health leaders. *Am J Public Health.* 2005;95(4):641–644. https://doi.org/10.2105/AJPH.2004.047993
7. Karnik H, Barbiero J, Zemmel DJ, et al. Building adaptive leaders: a formative evaluation of the Region V Public Health Leadership Institute using ripple effect mapping and focus groups. *J Public Health Manag Pract.* 2025;31(4):591–599. https://doi.org/10.1097/PHH.0000000000002150
8. Brandert K, Alperin M, Lloyd LM, et al. Learning to lead: 3 models to support public health leadership development. *J Public Health Manag Pract.* 2022;28(suppl 5):S203–S211. https://doi.org/10.1097/PHH.0000000000001519
9. Friedrich TL, Vessey WB, Schuelke MJ, Ruark GA, Mumford MD. A framework for understanding collective leadership: the selective utilization of leader and team expertise within networks. *Leadersh Q.* 2009;20(6):933–958. https://doi.org/10.1016/j.leaqua.2009.09.008
10. Day DV. Leadership development. *Leadersh Q.* 2000;11(4):581–613. https://doi.org/10.1016/S1048-9843(00)00061-8
11. Day DV, Dragoni L. Leadership development: an outcome-oriented review based on time and levels of analyses. *Annu Rev Organ Psychol Organ Behav.* 2015;2(1):133–156. https://doi.org/10.1146/annurev-orgpsych-032414-111328
12. Lacerenza CN, Reyes DL, Marlow SL, Joseph DL, Salas E. Leadership training design, delivery, and implementation: a meta-analysis. *J Appl Psychol.* 2017;102(12):1686–1718. https://doi.org/10.1037/apl0000241
13. Yammarino FJ, Salas E, Serban A, Shirreffs K, Shuffler ML. Collectivistic leadership approaches: putting the "we" in leadership science and practice. *Ind Organ Psychol.* 2012;5(4):382–402. https://doi.org/10.1111/j.1754-9434.2012.01467.x
14. Friedrich TL, Griffith JA, Mumford MD. Collective leadership behaviors: evaluating the leader, team network, and problem situation characteristics that influence their use. *Leadersh Q.* 2016;27(2):312–333. https://doi.org/10.1016/j.leaqua.2016.02.004
15. Bradley EH, Nembhard IM, Taylor L, Brewster A, Banaszak-Holl J. Leadership and management: a framework for action. In: Burns LR, Bradley EH, Weiner BJ, eds. *Shortell & Kaluzney's Health Care Management: Organization Design and Behavior.* 7th ed. Boston, MA: Cengage; 2018:32–55.
16. Reeves S, Pelone F, Harrison R, Goldman J, Zwarenstein M. Interprofessional collaboration to improve professional practice and healthcare outcomes. *Cochrane Database Syst Rev.* 2017;6(6):CD000072. https://doi.org/10.1002/14651858.CD000072.pub3
17. Getha-Taylor H, Morse RS. Collaborative leadership development for local government officials: exploring competencies and program impact. *Public Adm Q.* 2013;37(1):71–102.
18. Ospina SM. Collective leadership and context in public administration: bridging public leadership research and leadership studies. *Public Adm Rev.* 2017;77(2):275–287. https://doi.org/10.1111/puar.12706
19. Sanders K, Webster J, Manley K, Cardiff S. Recognising and developing effective workplace cultures across health and social care that are also good places to work. In: Manley K, Wilson V, Øye C, eds. *International Practice Development in Health and Social Care.* Oxford, UK: John Wiley and Sons; 2021:205–219.
20. Brewer ML, Flavell HL, Trede F, Smith M. A scoping review to understand "leadership" in interprofessional education and practice. *J Interprof Care.* 2016;30(4):408–415. https://doi.org/10.3109/13561820.2016.1150260
21. Bronfenbrenner U. *The Ecology of Human Development: Experiments by Nature and Design.* Cambridge, MA: Harvard University Press; 1979.
22. Bandura A. Exercise of human agency through collective efficacy. *Curr Dir Psychol Sci.* 2000;9(3):75–78. https://doi.org/10.1111/1467-8721.00064
23. Hannah ST, Avolio BJ, Luthans F, Harms PD. Leadership efficacy: review and future directions. *Leadersh Q.* 2008;19(6):669–692. https://doi.org/10.1016/j.leaqua.2008.09.007
24. Bandura A. Social cognitive theory: an agentic perspective. *Annu Rev Psychol.* 2001;52:1–26. https://doi.org/10.1146/annurev.psych.52.1.1
25. Bandura A. *Self-Efficacy: The Exercise of Control.* New York, NY: W H Freeman/Times Books/Henry Holt & Co; 1997.
26. Day DV, Harrison MM, Halpin SM. *An Integrative Approach to Leader Development: Connecting Adult Development, Identity, and Expertise.* 1st ed. New York, NY: Routledge; 2008. https://doi.org/10.4324/9780203809525
27. Machida M, Schaubroeck J. The role of self-efficacy beliefs in leader development. *J Leadersh Organ Stud.* 2011;18(4):459–468. https://doi.org/10.1177/1548051811404419
28. Ibarra H, Hansen MT. Are you a collaborative leader? *Harvard Business Review.* July–August 2011. Available at: https://hbr.org/2011/07/are-you-a-collaborative-leader. Accessed March 20, 2022.
29. Murphy SE, Johnson SK. Leadership and leader developmental self-efficacy: their role in enhancing leader development efforts. *New Dir Stud Leadersh.* 2016;2016(149):73–84. https://doi.org/10.1002/yd.20163
30. Mumford MD, Friedrich TL, Vessey WB, Ruark GA. Collective leadership: thinking about issues vis-à-vis others. *Ind Organ Psychol.* 2012;5(4):408–411. https://doi.org/10.1111/j.1754-9434.2012.01469.x
31. Leithwood KA, Louis KS, Anderson S, Wahlstrom K. *Review of Research: How Leadership Influences Student Learning.* Minneapolis, MN: University of Minnesota; 2004.
32. Taggar S, Seijts GH. Leader and staff role-efficacy as antecedents of collective-efficacy and team performance. *Hum Perform.* 2003;16(2):131–156. https://doi.org/10.1207/S15327043HUP1602_2
33. Cullen KL, Palus CJ, Chrobot-Mason D, Appaneal C. Getting to "we": collective leadership development. *Ind Organ Psychol.* 2012;5(4):428–432. https://doi.org/10.1111/j.1754-9434.2012.01475.x
34. Day DV, Fleenor JW, Atwater LE, Sturm RE, McKee RA. Advances in leader and leadership development: a review of 25 years of research and theory. *Leadersh Q.* 2014;25(1):63–82. https://doi.org/10.1016/j.leaqua.2013.11.004
35. Cummings GG, Tate K, Lee S, et al. Leadership styles and outcome patterns for the nursing workforce and work environment: a systematic review. *Int J Nurs Stud.* 2018;85:19–60. https://doi.org/10.1016/j.ijnurstu.2018.04.016
36. Burke NS, Christopher GC, Hacker TS, Moy J, Williams A. Culture of health leaders: building a diverse network to advance health equity. In: Fernandez CSP, Corbie-Smith G, eds. *Leading Community Based Changes in the Culture of Health in the US—Experiences in Developing the Team and Impacting the Community.* London, UK: IntechOpen; 2021. https://doi.org/10.5772/intechopen.98452
37. Martin R, Hughes DJ, Epitropaki O, Thomas G. In pursuit of causality in leadership training research: a review and pragmatic recommendations. *Leadersh Q.* 2021;32(5):101375. https://doi.org/10.1016/j.leaqua.2019.101375
38. Integrated Health Services. Technical Series on Primary Health Care: Integrating Health Services Brief. Geneva, Switzerland: World Health Organization; 2018.
39. Sfantou D, Laliotis A, Patelarou A, Sifaki-Pistolla D, Matalliotakis M, Patelarou E. Importance of leadership style towards quality of care measures in healthcare settings: a systematic review. *Healthcare (Basel).* 2017;5(4):73. https://doi.org/10.3390/healthcare5040073
40. Bowman C, Paal P, Brandstötter C, Cordina M. Evidence of successful interprofessional education programs—models, barriers, facilitators and success: a systematic review of European studies. *J Health Organ Manag.* 2023;37(8):526–541. https://doi.org/10.1108/JHOM-04-2022-0115

Characteristics of the People and Communities Served by GusNIP Produce Prescriptions: United States, 2020–2024

Carmen Byker Shanks, PhD, Victoria A. Zigmont, PhD, MPH, Ruth Quattro, MPH, Christopher R. Long, PhD, Courtney A. Parks, PhD, MHK, Hollyanne Fricke, MPH, Elise Mitchell, MS, MPH, Bailey Houghtaling, PhD, MS, Hilary Seligman, MD, MAS, Sarah Stotz, PhD, MS, and Amy L. Yaroch, PhD

See also Primary Care and Public Health in the Community, pp. 1988–2014.

Objectives. To examine enrollment in Gus Schumacher Nutrition Incentive Program (GusNIP) produce prescriptions and identify opportunities to expand their reach.

Methods. We conducted descriptive analyses of cross-sectional baseline surveys of 21 635 participants (living in the Southern, West, North Central, or Northeast region of the United States) in GusNIP produce prescriptions between 2020 and 2024. We applied geographic information system mapping and inferential statistics to fruit and vegetable intake data.

Results. At enrollment, 43.2% of participants were aged 45 to 65 years, 77% were women, 32.7% were Hispanic, 24.4% were non-Hispanic Black/African American, and 26.2% were non-Hispanic White. Mean fruit and vegetable intake was 2.39 cups (SD = 0.78) daily, varying by region. Approximately two thirds of participants reported food insecurity (67.2%).

Conclusions. GusNIP produce prescriptions are reaching intended communities, including people with low fruit and vegetable intake, chronic disease risk, and food insecurity. Opportunities exist to broaden reach.

Public Health Implications. GusNIP produce prescriptions offer a national lens on Farm Bill–funded policy in action. As "food is medicine" interventions, including GusNIP produce prescriptions, evolve, it is important to understand who enrolls, who is not yet represented, and who could benefit most by extending reach to individuals and their communities. (*Am J Public Health*. 2025;115(12):2015–2019. https://doi.org/10.2105/AJPH.2025.308293)

AJPH December 2025, Vol. 115, No. 12

Consuming enough fruits and vegetables is vital for preventing and managing chronic diseases. Produce prescriptions are a "food is medicine" intervention designed to promote healthy food consumption among people experiencing or at risk for chronic disease and food insecurity. These interventions engage health care partners to prescribe free or reduced-cost fresh fruits and vegetables for eligible patients. There is mixed but growing evidence that produce prescriptions can increase fruit and vegetable intake, reduce household food insecurity, and improve chronic disease biomarkers and clinical measures.[1,2]

Since 2018, the US Department of Agriculture (USDA) has funded Gus Schumacher Nutrition Incentive Program (GusNIP) produce prescriptions in communities nationwide as well as the National Training, Technical Assistance, Evaluation, and Information Center to provide technical assistance and evaluation support.[3] GusNIP produce prescriptions aim to increase fresh fruit and vegetable intake, reduce food insecurity, increase health care utilization, and decrease costs associated with health care.[4] Participants are eligible if they receive benefits under the Food and Nutrition Act of 2008 (Pub L No. 88–525) or have medical assistance under state Medicaid and belong to a low-income household with or at risk for a diet-related health condition.

We examined who enrolls in GusNIP-funded produce prescriptions. We assessed characteristics of people and communities that enrolled from 2020 through 2024 to identify gaps where GusNIP produce prescriptions can expand. Because fruits and vegetables are the primary intervention, we mapped fruit and vegetable intake to identify opportunities in reach that may guide policy and resource allocation for greater GusNIP produce prescription impact.

METHODS

We used a cross-sectional design to analyze baseline enrollment data collected between 2020 and 2024 from participants in all 96 GusNIP-funded produce prescription projects that operated across 1992 health care, farm direct, brick-and-mortar, and clinic sites, where participants received and redeemed a "prescription" for fruits and vegetables.

We collected baseline surveys from 21 635 participants using sampling plans that aimed for 75 to 130 or more participants per GusNIP produce prescription project, based on grant amount, to ensure demographic and project-specific representativeness. Recruitment occurred in clinics, at food retail sites, via telephone, and via e-mail to reflect variation in demographics, project models, and geography. Follow-up surveys are beyond the scope of this enrollment-focused article.

At enrollment, participants received prescriptions from a health care provider for fruits and vegetables. GusNIP produce prescriptions differed across projects, varying by food retail sites (e.g., farmers market, supermarket), clinic types, prescription amount (≥ $20–$100 per month), prescription type (e.g., token, discount, produce box), and whether and what kind of nutrition education was offered to participants.

Adult participants (≥ 18 years) completed a baseline 27-item self-report survey when enrolling in a GusNIP produce prescription (details are reported elsewhere).[5] Most participants were offered a $10 stipend. We analyzed 23 survey items, including demographics, ZIP code (for spatial analysis), GusNIP produce prescription use, fruit and vegetable intake (assessed with the National Cancer Institute's 10-Item Dietary Screener Questionnaire fruit and vegetable module, which estimates intake in cups/day equivalents during the past 30 d),[6] food insecurity (assessed with the USDA Household Food Security Survey Module: Six-Item Short Form with 30-d lookback),[7] and perceived health.[8] Each question had the option to skip or decline. Data collected from GusNIP produce prescription implementors included grantee award number, eligibility criteria, National Institute of Food and Agriculture (NIFA) regions,[9] and geographic mapping variables: state, city, latitude, and longitude. Although some GusNIP produce prescriptions included having children in the household as eligibility criteria, we excluded nonadult survey participants from analysis.

Table A (available as a supplement to the online version of this article at http://www.ajph.org) summarizes enrollment criteria from grantee-reported annual data. Most GusNIP produce prescriptions served adults (86.5%) who screened positive for food insecurity (63.5%) or a diet-related disease (79.2%), including diabetes (97.4%), prediabetes (81.6%), hypertension (75.0%), and obesity (69.7%).

We used the National Cancer Institutes' scoring algorithm to convert the Dietary Screener Questionnaire frequency responses to cups per day for fruit intake alone, vegetable intake (not counting French fries) alone, and combined fruit and vegetable intake (not counting French fries).[6] We defined food insecurity by the number of affirmative responses: high (0), marginal (1), low (2–4), and very low (5–6).[7] We used frequencies and percentages for categorical variables and means and SDs for continuous variables. We used linear regression to compare differences in fruit and vegetable intake by cups per day across NIFA regions ($\alpha = 0.05$). We conducted analyses in Stata version 18 (StataCorp LP, College Station, TX).

We used proximity-based clustering to analyze patterns of fruit and vegetable intake in NIFA regions[9] using ArcGIS Online version 10.9.1 (Esri, Redlands, CA). We identified and mapped clusters of participant locations based on geographic proximity using self-reported ZIP codes, and we aggregated average fruit and vegetable intake (cups/day).

RESULTS

This analysis included 21 635 participants' self-reported baseline survey data. Almost half (43.2%) of participants were aged between 45 and 65 years; the mean was 51.6 (SD = 15.87) years. Most identified as a woman (77.0%). One third of participants identified as Hispanic (32.7%), 24.3% as non-Hispanic Black/African American, and 29.1% as non-Hispanic White. Most participants were from the Southern region (37.2%), followed by the West (35.4%), North Central (14.5%), and Northeast (13.4%) regions.

Most respondents (82.1%) were first-time GusNIP produce prescription participants. Some participants reenroll across program cycles, and the baseline survey is readministered. Participants consumed an average of 2.39 cups of fruits and vegetables per day during the past 30 days (SD = 0.78), including an average intake of 0.92 cups per day of fruits (SD = 0.49) and 1.48 cups per day of vegetables (SD = 0.45). In total, 67.2% experienced food insecurity during the previous 30 days. More than half (59.4%) perceived their current health status to be poor or fair (Table B, available as a supplement to the online version of this article at http://www.ajph.org).

Figure 1 depicts average daily fruit and vegetable intake (n = 16 927) across the 4 regions of the United States. When comparing differences in fruit and vegetable intake by NIFA region, the North Central (−0.15; 95% confidence interval [CI] = −0.19, −0.10), Southern (−0.09; 95% CI = −0.12, −0.05), and Western (−0.037; 95% CI = −0.072, −0.002) regions had lower average fruit and vegetable intake compared with the Northeast region ($P < .05$).

DISCUSSION

The data set used in this study, the largest cross-sectional baseline sample of GusNIP produce prescriptions, presented an unparalleled opportunity to examine who enrolls. GusNIP produce prescriptions are intended to reach populations with low income and high risk or prevalence of chronic disease. GusNIP produce prescriptions largely serve participants who screen positive for chronic disease (79.2%). Overall, 67.4% reported food insecurity and 59.4% reported poor or fair health. These data suggest that GusNIP produce prescriptions are reaching the intended audience.

Participants' mean baseline fruit and vegetable intake (2.39 cups/day) was similar to the US average (2.6 cups/day), which are both below the recommended 5 cups per day.[10] NIFA

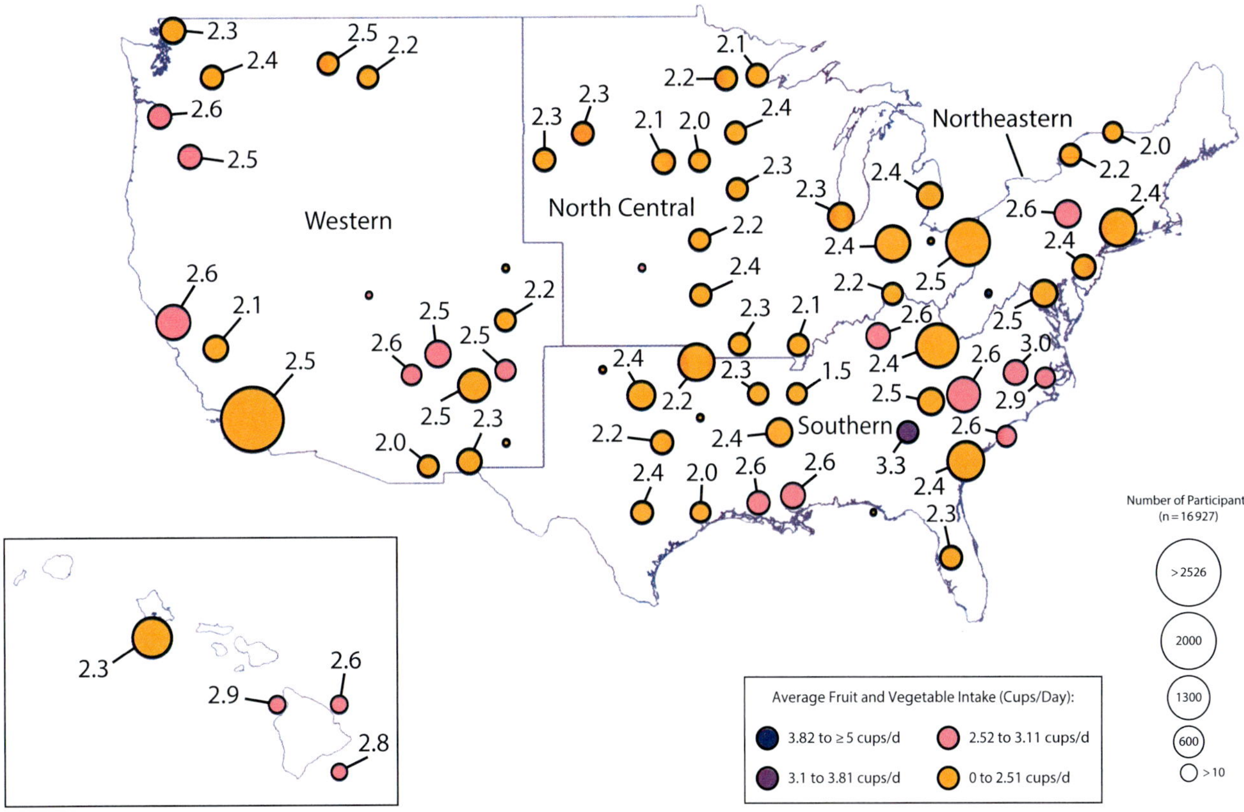

FIGURE 1— Average Daily Fruit and Vegetable Intake at Enrollment, by Participant Clusters and Across National Institute of Food and Agriculture Regions: Gus Schumacher Nutrition Incentive Program Produce Prescriptions; US Southern, West, North Central, and Northeast Regions, 2020–2024

Note. Data are from a sample of the Gus Schumacher Nutrition Incentive Program produce prescription participants who completed self-reported baseline surveys. Our analyses used unweighted data, and we included participants on the map who reported both fruit and vegetable intake and a ZIP code. US regions included North Central, Northeastern, Southern, and Western. We selected National Institute of Food and Agriculture regions to align with US Department of Agriculture program administration and support policy-relevant interpretation. Cutpoints (0–2.51, 2.52–3.11, 3.12–3.81, ≥ 3.82–5.0 cups/day) were data driven to reflect natural breaks in self-reported fruit and vegetable intake to emphasize observed variation and facilitate interpretation by geographic differences.

regional differences were statistically significant but small. Importantly, even modest, sustained differences in fruit and vegetable intake can yield clinical benefits, especially at the population level.[11] These patterns may reflect region-level factors, such as food availability, economics, agriculture, and cultural preferences. For example, variations in fruit and vegetable intake may indicate access and affordability challenges that GusNIP produce prescriptions could mitigate through broader enrollment outreach.

Although GusNIP produce prescriptions reach many households, enrollment remains uneven across certain characteristics. Only 5.5% of participants were aged 18 to 24 years, and men were enrolled at lower rates than women; both groups are important for chronic disease prevention through healthy dietary habits, regardless of enrollment reasons. Likewise, GusNIP produce prescriptions reach 37 states and the District of Columbia, covering all US regions, but there remains room to expand. Using momentum to mainstream produce prescriptions in health care may help engage desired groups broadly.

Future longitudinal studies using follow-up data could examine how identified characteristics and programmatic differences influence engagement, outcomes, and the extent to which these interact to influence who enrolls or reenrolls, who persists, and who benefits. Although measurement tools used in the National Training, Technical Assistance, Evaluation, and Information Center's shared measures are validated, self-reported measures may introduce biases.

PUBLIC HEALTH IMPLICATIONS

GusNIP produce prescription baseline surveys provide an opportunity to assess enrollment in this national Farm Bill–legislated food is medicine initiative. As produce prescription interventions evolve nationwide, particularly amid changes in the policy and funding landscape, it is important to understand who participates, who is not yet represented, and who could benefit most to support participants, programs, and communities. AJPH

ABOUT THE AUTHORS

Carmen Byker Shanks, Victoria A. Zigmont, Ruth Quattro, Christopher R. Long, Courtney A. Parks, Hollyanne Fricke, Elise Mitchell, Bailey Houghtaling, and Amy L. Yaroch are, or at the time of this study were, with the Center for Nutrition & Health Impact, Omaha, NE. Hilary Seligman is with the Departments of Medicine and of Epidemiology and Biostatistics, University of California, San Francisco. Sarah Stotz is with the Department of Food Science and Human Nutrition, Colorado State University, Fort Collins.

CORRESPONDENCE

Correspondence should be sent to Carmen Byker Shanks, 14301 FNB Pkwy, Suite 100, Omaha, NE 68154 (e-mail: cbshanks@centerfornutrition.org). Reprints can be ordered at https://www.ajph.org by clicking the "Reprints" link.

PUBLICATION INFORMATION

Full Citation: Byker Shanks C, Zigmont VA, Quattro R, et al. Characteristics of the people and communities served by GusNIP produce prescriptions: United States, 2020–2024. *Am J Public Health*. 2025;115(12):2015–2019.

Acceptance Date: September 5, 2025.

DOI: https://doi.org/10.2105/AJPH.2025.308293

ORCID iDs:

Carmen Byker Shanks https://orcid.org/0000-0002-9030-9938

Victoria A. Zigmont https://orcid.org/0000-0002-3747-4328

Christopher R. Long https://orcid.org/0000-0002-0574-7790

Courtney A. Parks https://orcid.org/0000-0002-8989-667X

Elise Mitchell https://orcid.org/0009-0002-5741-7176

Hilary Seligman https://orcid.org/0000-0003-2292-5189

Sarah Stotz https://orcid.org/0000-0003-4107-3313

CONTRIBUTORS

C. Byker Shanks, V. A. Zigmont, and R. Quattro conceptualized the study and led article development. C. Byker Shanks, V. A. Zigmont, C. R. Long, C. A. Parks, H. Fricke, E. Mitchell, B. Houghtaling, H. Seligman, S. Stotz, and A. L. Yaroch performed data quality assurance. V. A. Zigmont performed statistical analysis. R. Quattro led the geographic information systems work. C. R. Long, C. A. Parks, H. Fricke, E. Mitchell, B. Houghtaling, H. Seligman, S. Stotz, and A. L. Yaroch critically revised the article. All authors guided survey development, data protocols, and data acquisition; interpreted the data; and reviewed and approved the final version of the article.

ACKNOWLEDGMENTS

The National Incentive Program Training, Technical Assistance, Evaluation, and Information Center is supported by the US Department of Agriculture (USDA) National Institute of Food and Agriculture, Gus Schumacher Nutrition Incentive Program (GusNIP; grant 2019-70030-30415/project accession No. 1020863, grant 2023-70435-38766/project accession No. 1029638, and grant 2023-70414-40461/project accession No. 1031111).

We extend our sincere appreciation to GusNIP produce prescription grantees, their partners, and participants for their vital contributions.

Note. Any opinions, findings, conclusions, or recommendations expressed in this publication are those of the authors and should not be construed to represent any official USDA or US government determination or policy.

CONFLICTS OF INTEREST

The authors have no conflicts of interest to disclose.

HUMAN PARTICIPANT PROTECTION

The University of Nebraska Medical Center's institutional review board deemed this research exempt and not human participants research (2020-2022;#0665-20-EX).

REFERENCES

1. Harper Z, Alvarado AV, Katz SE, et al. Examining food security, fruit and vegetable intake, and cardiovascular disease risk outcomes of produce prescription (PPR) programs: a systematic review. *J Nutr Educ Behav*. 2024;56(11):794–821. https://doi.org/10.1016/j.jneb.2024.06.012
2. Hager K, Shi P, Li Z, et al. Evaluation of a produce prescription program for patients with diabetes: a longitudinal analysis of glycemic control. *Diabetes Care*. 2023;46(6):1169–1176. https://doi.org/10.2337/DC22-1645
3. The Gus Schumacher Nutrition Incentive Program Nutrition Incentive Hub, Nutrition Incentive Program Training, Technical Assistance, Evaluation, and Information Center. Impact findings Y4: September 1, 2022 to August 31, 2023. 2024. Available at: https://nutritionincentivehub.org/media/ev5aet4n/year-4-gusnip-impact-findings-report-2024.pdf. Accessed October 16, 2024.
4. US Department of Agriculture. The Gus Schumacher Nutrition Incentive Program—produce prescription (The Gus Schumacher Nutrition Incentive

Program-PPR). August 4, 2025. Available at: https://www.nifa.usda.gov/gusnip-request-applications-resources-ppr. Accessed August 13, 2025.

5. Budd Nugent N, Byker Shanks C, Seligman H, et al. Accelerating evaluation of financial incentives for fruits and vegetables: a case for shared measures. *Int J Environ Res Public Health*. 2021;18(22):12140. https://doi.org/10.3390/ijerph182212140
6. Thompson FE, Midthune D, Kahle L, Dodd KW. Development and evaluation of the National Cancer Institute's dietary screener questionnaire scoring algorithms. *J Nutr*. 2017;147(6):1226–1233. https://doi.org/10.3945/JN.116.246058
7. Blumberg J, Bialostosky K, Hamilton WL, Briefel RR. The effectiveness of a short form of the Household Food Security Scale. *Am J Public Health*. 1999;89(8):1231–1234. https://doi.org/10.2105/AJPH.89.8.1231
8. Moriarty DG, Zack MM, Kobau R. The Centers for Disease Control and Prevention's Healthy Days measures—population tracking of perceived physical and mental health over time. *Health Qual Life Outcomes*. 2003;1:37. https://doi.org/10.1186/1477-7525-1-37
9. US Department of Agriculture. EFNEP basics for coordinators: The Expanded Food and Nutrition Education Program (EFNEP). April 1, 2016. Available at: https://www.nifa.usda.gov/sites/default/files/resource/EFNEP%20Basics%20-%20New%20Coordinator%20Guide%20-%20rev%2004.01.2016.pdf. Accessed August 13, 2025.
10. US Department of Health and Human Services; US Department of Agriculture. Dietary guidelines for Americans, 2020–2025. December 2020. Available at: https://www.dietaryguidelines.gov/sites/default/files/2021-03/Dietary_Guidelines_for_Americans-2020-2025.pdf. Accessed October 3, 2025.
11. Wang DD, Li Y, Bhupathiraju SN, et al. Fruit and vegetable intake and mortality: results from 2 prospective cohort studies of US men and women and a meta-analysis of 26 cohort studies. *Circulation*. 2021;143(17):1642–1654. https://doi.org/10.1161/circulationaha.120.048996

Hardship and Hope: The Relationship Between Unconditional Prenatal and Infant Cash Transfers, Economic Stability, and Maternal Mental Health and Well-Being

Mona Hanna, MD, MPH, H. Luke Shaefer, PhD, Eric Finegood, PhD, Sumit Agarwal, MD, PhD, MPH, Yasamean Zamani-Hank, PhD, MPH, and Jenny LaChance, MS

See also Kerker, p. 1954.

AJPH December 2025, Vol. 115, No. 12

Objectives. To examine the impact of Rx Kids—a community-wide and unconditional prenatal and infant cash transfer program in Flint, Michigan—on economic stability, maternal mental health, and well-being.

Methods. Using a difference-in-differences framework, we compared outcomes for surveyed Flint mothers who gave birth before and after Rx Kids implementation to those outside the city.

Results. Relative to comparisons, mothers exposed to Rx Kids saw improvements in hardship, mental health, and well-being—notably, a 4.2-percentage-point reduction in the risk of eviction ($P < .05$) and a 14.0-percentage-point reduction in screening positive for postpartum depression ($P < .05$). Program exposure was associated with increased trust in institutions and feeling loved, hopeful, respected, and valued.

Conclusions. Rx Kids, the United States' first, to our knowledge, community-wide prenatal and infant cash transfer program, is associated with improved economic stability, mental health, and well-being. Rx Kids' place-based scale provides a replicable model for efficiently addressing perinatal poverty and improving health. (*Am J Public Health*. 2025;115(12):2020–2029. https://doi.org/10.2105/AJPH.2025.308244)

While the United States spends more on health care than any peer nation,[1] there is a paucity of investment in the health and well-being of mothers and infants. The United States is 1 of only 7 countries without a paid maternity leave policy,[2] the only high-income nation without some form of universal health insurance,[1] and an outlier in its high child poverty rate.[3]

This translates into a public health and global competitiveness crisis, with the health, well-being, and survival of mothers and infants in the United States generally much worse than in peer countries.[4–6] With highly disparate outcomes for historically marginalized groups,[7] extant efforts to improve perinatal health—including maternal mental health, maternal morbidity and mortality, and infant birth outcomes—have largely failed to address the underlying societal underinvestment in mothers and infants.

Poverty spikes to its highest level throughout the life course perinatally, as income drops and expenses rise.[8,9] At a time of profound neurodevelopmental consequences, perinatal economic insecurity exacerbates housing instability, nutrition insecurity, and other forms of material hardship, with major implications for maternal and infant health.[10] It contributes to poor maternal mental health, including psychological distress, depression, hopelessness, shame, and limited parenting capacity and bandwidth.[11–14]

Housing instability is common during the perinatal period; up to one third of low-income individuals move during pregnancy,[15,16] and between 4% and 9% experience homelessness.[17] Housing instability is linked with preterm birth, low birth weight, neonatal intensive care admission, delivery complications, and inadequate prenatal care.[17,18] Even the threat of eviction is associated with adverse birth outcomes.[19,20] Postnatally, families with babies and toddlers are the most at-risk age group for eviction,[19] implicating a broad range of health and development consequences.

In addition, mothers and infants in poor communities face particular challenges from long-standing, place-based inequities. These manifest in built environments that impede health, with unsafe housing, limited access to healthy foods, community violence, health care barriers, diminished social cohesion, low trust in institutions, and other adversities.[21–25]

Recognizing the economic and developmental vulnerability of the perinatal period—both at the individual and community level—and that the United States experiences worse maternal and infant health outcomes than its high-income peers, the perinatal period is an opportune moment for prevention and support. Built on global evidence on large-scale government prenatal and child cash transfers and inspired by the COVID-19 pandemic–era expanded Child Tax Credit's success,[26] the nation's first, to our knowledge, community-wide and unconditional prenatal and infant cash transfer program was developed and implemented in Flint, Michigan, as a place-based effort to proactively invest in the health and well-being of mothers and infants.

In a city with one of the country's highest child poverty rates and chronically disparate racial maternal and infant health outcomes, Rx Kids launched in January 2024 as a "prescription for health, hope, and opportunity."[27] All City of Flint expectant mothers are eligible to receive a 1-time transfer of $1500 after midpregnancy and $500 per month for 12 months postnatally. Rx Kids has achieved near-universal aggregate take-up (Y. Zamani-Hank, written communication, November 25, 2024) and expanded to other communities. Administered by the nonprofit GiveDirectly, the program is led by Michigan State University–Hurley Children's Hospital Pediatric Public Health Initiative in collaboration with Poverty Solutions at the University of Michigan.

The program's conceptual model (Figure 1) proposes two upstream mechanisms—improved economic stability and a reimagined social contract—by which prenatal and infant cash transfers can have an impact on health and well-being. Cash-transfer–related improvements to economic stability are expected to improve maternal mental health and well-being[11,28–31] and other proximal family-level determinants of maternal and child health, including food security[32,33] and housing stability.[34] The universal, unconditional design minimizes stigma and shame[35] and fosters a relationship built on dignity, deservingness, and trust, with the goal of building a reimagined social contract. We expect Rx Kids' design and messaging, centered on love, hope, and celebration, to improve trust and faith in health care and government, thus leading to improved well-being, health-promoting behaviors, and take-up of other supports.

To our knowledge, this program is the first of its kind and this is the first study to examine the effects of Rx Kids on several maternal self-reported outcomes, using a survey developed in collaboration with community partners and administered to mothers who delivered at the largest regional birthing hospital. The aim of this study was to determine whether exposure to Rx Kids is associated with improvements in mothers' self-report of economic stability, mental health, and well-being.

METHODS

Rx Kids was implemented in Flint, which has a population just under 80 000[36] and approximately 1000 births annually.[37] Because of historic and structural factors, including a recent drinking water crisis,[38] Genesee County's impoverished population is concentrated in Flint, where 40% of residents and 59% of children live in poverty.[39] Racially diverse, 57% of the population identify as Black or African American, and 34% identify as non-Hispanic White.[40]

Design

The sampling frame included all mothers who gave birth at Hurley Medical Center (HMC), a large public hospital in Genesee County, between July 1, 2023, and June 30, 2024 (n = 2073). HMC accounts for 69.4% of Flint births and 47.7% of all county births. A list including addresses, phone numbers, and e-mails for all births was generated from Epic electronic medical records (EMR). Mothers who were aged younger than 18 years on their child's date of birth, those who experienced stillbirths or neonatal death, and those residing outside Michigan were excluded. Parents of multiples received 1 invitation.

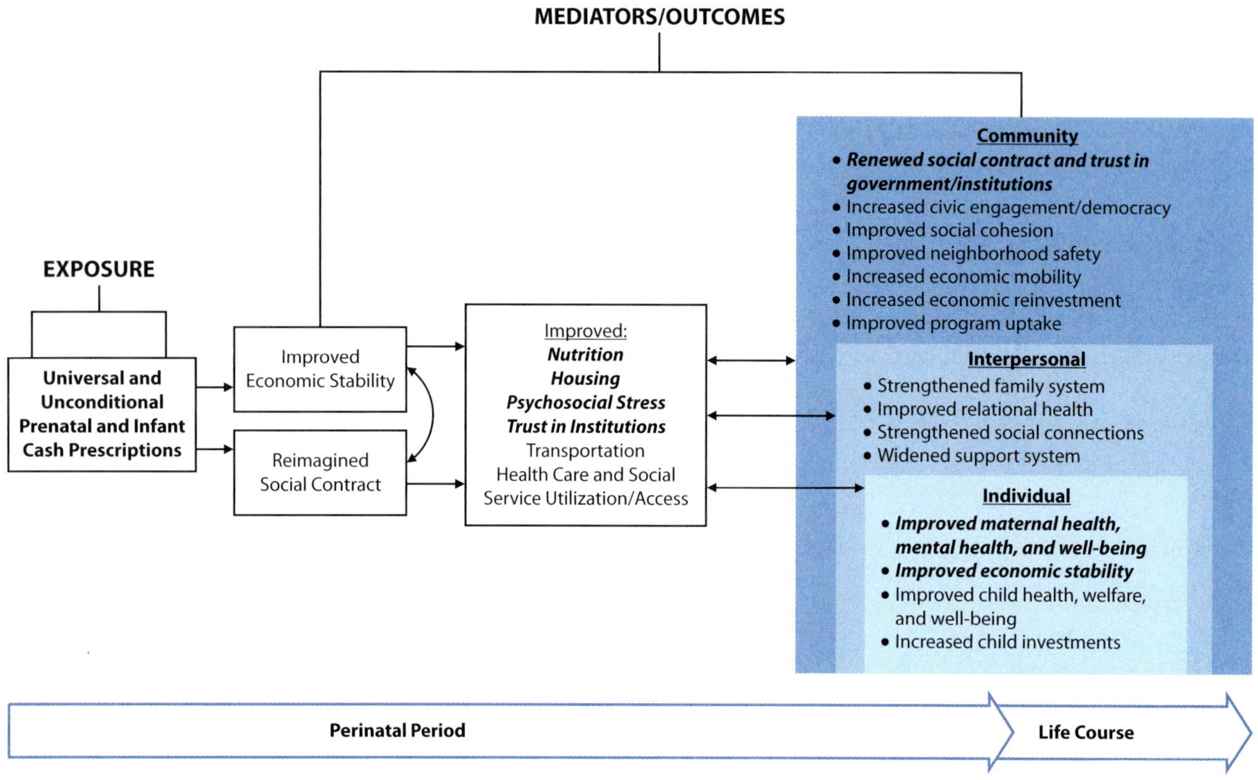

FIGURE 1— Rx Kids Conceptual Model

Note. Bold and italic variables are measured in this analysis.

Residential status (within vs outside the City of Flint) was geocoded. Based on the child's date of birth (year 2023 vs 2024) and family's residence (Flint vs outside Flint), we categorized potential participants into four cohorts: 2023 non-Flint, 2024 non-Flint, 2023 Flint, and 2024 Flint. The only cohort eligible for Rx Kids was 2024 Flint. Children of mothers from the 2023 cohorts were born, on average, 1 year earlier than those from the 2024 cohorts. Children's ages ranged within each of the four cohorts.

Procedure

All eligible participants were mailed an invitation—which did not mention Rx Kids—to complete the survey. The same day, e-mails were sent to participants with valid e-mail addresses. The communications contained informed consent information, a survey link, and a unique, 9-digit code to ensure participants only took the survey once. A text message was sent approximately 7 days later, followed by 3 reminder texts and 2 phone calls the following month. Administered through REDCap electronic data capture tools at Michigan State University,[41,42] the survey was designed for completion in less than 30 minutes. After completion, respondents received a $50 electronic gift card.

A total of 2073 mothers were invited to take the survey (Appendix Table A, available as a supplement to the online version of this article at https://ajph.org). Health system data were available for 2026 of those mothers, and n = 1037 (51%) completed the survey after consenting. The 2024 Flint cohort had the highest response rate (54%). Survey nonrespondents appeared more likely to have public health insurance than respondents, suggesting nonrespondents may be somewhat more disadvantaged. Appendix Table B reports demographic characteristics for all cohorts. Roughly two thirds of Flint respondents self-reported their race as Black, while nearly 25% self-reported their race as non-Hispanic White. These are approximately reversed for non-Flint respondents. Flint respondents were more likely to be unmarried or unpartnered than those outside Flint, while the non-Flint cohorts reported higher educational attainment and income, on average. Flint 2024 mothers were most likely to report very low income and reported lower incomes than the Flint 2023 cohort, which had a somewhat lower response rate.

This suggests any observed improvements in hardship or mental health outcomes may be modestly biased downward because the Flint 2024 subsample is lower-income and therefore potentially more likely to report material hardship and poor mental health outcomes.

Measures

All outcome measures are defined in Appendix Table C.

Hardship. Housing hardship questions were drawn from Pilkauskas et al., asking respondents if they owed back rent or mortgage and, if so, how much they owed.[43] We calculated the average amount owed among all respondents and the average amount owed if greater than $1. Reported values greater than $9000 were excluded as they appeared to report mortgage principal balances. For eviction, respondents were asked if they were "evicted or your landlord forced you to leave your home or apartment for not paying the rent or mortgage?" Responses were coded affirmatively if evicted after birth to account for the timing of Rx Kids transfers.

For food insecurity, an adapted 2-question measure[44] and 1 item asking respondents whether they had "enough of the kinds of food we want"[33] were included. Three additional hardship questions covered diaper use, availability of cash for emergencies, and perceived freedom to spend cash. We recoded outcomes into dichotomous variables (Table C).

Maternal mental health and well-being. The 10-item Center for Epidemiologic Studies Depression scale (CES-D-10) measured depression.[45] We assessed anxiety using 2 items from the Generalized Anxiety Disorder scale (GAD-7).[46,47] We used a Likert scale for self-reported mental health, scored as 1 for good, very good, or excellent, and 0 if fair or poor. We coded the 6-item Perceived Hope Score[48,49] as 1 if a "high score" of 30 or greater, and 0 otherwise. A high score represents an average answer of "agree" or "strongly agree" to each item.

We created 5 items to assess maternal feelings of being loved, valued, respected, empowered, and hopeful. We adapted 2 questions from the Organization for Economic Co-operation and Development Survey on Trust in Public Institutions, rating trust in health care and government on a scale of 1 to 10.[50] We considered respondents to have high trust if they responded with 9 or 10.

Analysis

Our difference-in-differences analysis accounted for variation across time, inside and outside Flint. We included all 2024 Flint respondents in the treatment group irrespective of program participation (an intent-to-treat approach). Multivariable difference-in-differences models used ordinary least squares regression (linear probability models with binary outcomes) because of problems with interaction terms in nonlinear models.[51] Logistic regression specifications showed directionally similar results (Appendix Table D). To generate the difference-in-differences estimate, each model included a dummy variable for Flint (Flint = 1; non-Flint = 0), time (2024 = 1; 2023 = 0) and an interaction term (Flint*Time). The primary coefficient was Flint*Time, which tested whether the differences in outcomes for mothers who gave birth at HMC in Flint before (2023) and after (2024) Rx Kids implementation were different from the trends in outcomes for ineligible non-Flint mothers in 2023 and 2024. Other control variables included maternal age, number of children, race and ethnicity, educational attainment, marital status, and income. Statistical tests were 2-tailed with a level of significance set at $P < .05$. We conducted supplemental significance testing using the Benjamini–Hochberg procedure to account for multiple hypothesis testing.

The key assumption in our difference-in-differences analysis was that—absent Rx Kids—outcomes would have evolved similarly for mothers within and just outside of Flint between 2023 and 2024. This assumption requires that no other interventions coincided with Rx Kids that affected Flint and nearby non-Flint mothers differentially. We queried multisector leaders, and no changes were identified in economic conditions, and particularly in prenatal and infant supports or services during this time.[52,53]

RESULTS

Table 1 presents unadjusted material hardship estimates. Flint 2024 mothers improved compared with Flint 2023 to a statistically significant degree on 5 of 11 hardship measures. In the other 6, Flint 2024 respondents improved compared with Flint 2023, but the change was not statistically significant.

Mothers exposed to Rx Kids were behind $177 less on rent or mortgage payments than Flint 2023 mothers; of those behind, Rx Kids–exposed moms owed significantly less than their counterparts. Only 1 Flint 2024 mother (0.5% of sample) reported being evicted since childbirth, a substantial drop from Flint 2023. Flint mothers exposed to Rx Kids saw a statistically significant 12.5-percentage-point

AJPH December 2025, Vol. 115, No. 12

TABLE 1— Maternal Reports on Economic Stability Among New Mothers in Flint, MI, and Surrounding Region: 2023–2024

	2023 Non-Flint	2024 Non-Flint	2023 Flint	2024 Flint
No.	361	340	145	190
Owes back rent or mortgage, %	9.2	13.0	22.5	14.8
Average back rent or mortgage owed, $	90	184	332	155*
Average back rent or mortgage owed if > $1, $	997	1438	1475	1011*
Evicted after birth, %	2.8	1.8	5.5	0.5**
Food did not last, %	21.4	18.9	31.8	26.5
Worry about food, %	27.8	24.8	36.6	35.3
Not enough foods we want, %	40.3	40.4	46.9	34.4*
Fewer diapers than would like, %	16.4	13.8	29.0	23.0
Not buy something to buy diapers instead, %	26.6	20.6	40.1	36.4
Free to choose how to spend cash, %	74.4	67.9	65.7	77.9*
Enough cash emergencies, %	61.0	61.5	37.8	41.0

Source. Analysis of survey responses from Hurley Medical Center Maternal Well-Being Survey.
*$P < .05$; **$P < .01$. Statistical significance for difference between 2023 Flint and 2024 Flint cohorts.

decline in the proportion reporting they did "not have enough of the kinds of foods we want," compared with Flint 2023.

Table 2 reports descriptive estimates on maternal mental health and well-being. Rx Kids–exposed mothers were 13.0 percentage points less likely to screen positive for postpartum depression than Flint 2023 (CES-D-10 score ≥ 10).[45] Rx Kids–exposed moms were 12.8 percentage points less likely to report feeling nervous, anxious, or on edge than 2023 Flint, and 8.4 percentage points less likely to report "not being able to stop or control worrying" (GAD-7).[46,47] Moms exposed to Rx Kids were more likely to rate their general mental health as "excellent" or "very good," compared with 2023 Flint, although non-Flint mothers saw a

TABLE 2— Maternal Well-Being and Trust in Institutions Among New Mothers in Flint, MI, and Surrounding Region: 2023–2024

	2023 Non-Flint, %	2024 Non-Flint, %	2023 Flint, %	2024 Flint, %
No.	361	340	145	190
CES-D-10 depression score ≥ 10	35.3	33.0	46.2	33.2*
GAD-7 question 1 (Feeling nervous, anxious, or on edge)	24.2	19.8	31.7	18.9**
GAD-7 question 2 (Not being able to stop or control worrying)	20.5	17.1	27.3	18.9*
Mental health good, very good, or excellent	64.0	72.3	61.5	72.3*
Perceived Hope Scale score ≥ 30	47.3	52.3	41.5	56.6**
Feel loved	84.1	85.4	68.8	80.4*
Have hope	72.8	74.6	62.9	76.2**
Feel respected	66.7	65.7	55.6	69.8**
Feel valued	64.0	65.5	53.1	68.8*
Feel empowered	51.0	56.0	46.0	57.4*
High trust in health care	13.3	13.6	22.9	31.7
High trust in government	4.2	4.6	9.2	14.8

Note. CES-D-10 = Center for Epidemiologic Studies Depression scale; GAD = Generalized Anxiety Disorder scale.
Source. Analysis of survey responses from Hurley Medical Center Maternal Well-being Survey.
*$P < .05$; **$P < .01$. Statistical significance for difference between 2023 Flint and 2024 Flint cohorts.

similar improvement. Rx Kids–exposed mothers were more likely to report feeling loved (11.6 percentage points), hopeful (13.3 percentage points), respected (14.2 percentage points), valued (15.7 percentage points), and empowered (11.4 percentage points), compared with 2023 Flint moms.

Table 3 reports on multivariable (adjusted) difference-in-differences analyses testing the association between Rx Kids exposure (Flint 2024) and outcomes presented in Tables 1 and 2. The Flint*Time (2024) term reports the relationship between differences in the outcome for Flint 2023 and Flint 2024, compared with differences between 2023 and 2024 non-Flint mothers. Appendix Table F reports full output.

Nine of 11 coefficients in Table 3 on material hardship and economic stability are in line with improvements associated with Rx Kids, while two show no change. Six show statistically significant improvements. Rx Kids exposure is associated with a statistically significant 14.0-percentage-point decrease in reporting not having enough of the kinds of food respondents want. It was associated with a 13.0-percentage-point decrease in owing past-due rent or mortgage. Among those carrying greater than $1 past due, there was a $1004 decrease in the amount due. Program exposure was associated with a 4.2-percentage-point decrease in the risk of eviction after childbirth. Finally, program exposure was linked to a 19.0-percentage-point increase in mothers feeling free to choose how to spend the cash they have.

Rx Kids exposure is associated with a 14.0-percentage-point decreased risk of screening positive for postpartum depression. It is associated with a 12-percentage-point increase in having a high perceived hope score, although the change was not statistically significant ($P < .1$). Rx Kids exposure was linked to an 11-percentage-point increase in the likelihood that a mother reported feeling loved, a 13-percentage-point increase in having hope, a 15-percentage-point increase in feeling respected, and a 12-percentage-point increase in feeling valued; all were statistically significant. Finally, program exposure was linked to a statistically significant 10-percentage-point increase in reporting high trust in health care, and point estimates were in line with a 6.4-percentage-point ($P < .1$) increase in high trust in government, but not statistically significant at the $P < .05$ level.

After accounting for testing of multiple hypotheses, estimates remained statistically significant at a false discovery rate of 10% (Appendix Table E). Appendix Figure A graphically demonstrates the relationship between two key outcomes

TABLE 3— Association Between Exposure to the Rx Kids Program and Outcomes Among New Mothers in Flint, MI, and Surrounding Region: 2023–2024

Outcome	b (95% CI)
Material hardship and economic well-being	
Food did not last	−0.05 (−0.11, 0.01)
Worry about food	0.00 (−0.06, 0.06)
Not enough foods we want	−0.14 (−0.20, −0.08)
Owes back rent or mortgage	−0.13 (−0.17, −0.09)
Back rent or mortgage owed, $	−301.76 (−371.16, −232.36)
Back rent or mortgage owed for if > $1, $	−1004.41 (−1254.34, −754.48)
Evicted after birth	−0.04 (−0.06, −0.02)
Fewer diapers than would like	−0.05 (−0.10, 0.00)
Not buy something needed to buy diapers instead	0.00 (−0.06, 0.06)
Free to choose how to spend cash	0.19 (0.13, 0.25)
Enough cash emergencies	0.05 (−0.01, 0.11)
Maternal mental health and well-being	
CES-D-10 depression score ≥ 10	−0.14 (−0.20, −0.08)
GAD-7 question 1 (Feeling nervous, anxious, or on edge)	−0.08 (−0.16, 0.00)
GAD-7 question 2 (Not being able to stop or control worrying)	−0.06 (−0.11, −0.01)
Mental health good, very good, or excellent	−0.20 (−0.51, 0.11)
Perceived Hope Scale score ≥ 30	0.12 (0.05, 0.19)
Feel loved	0.11 (0.06, 0.16)
Have hope	0.13 (0.07, 0.19)
Feel respected	0.15 (0.09, 0.21)
Feel valued	0.12 (0.06, 0.18)
Feel empowered	0.09 (0.02, 0.16)
Trust in institutions	
High trust in health care	0.10 (0.05, 0.15)
High trust in government	0.06 (0.03, 0.09)

Note. CES-D-10 = Center for Epidemiologic Studies Depression scale; CI = confidence interval; GAD = Generalized Anxiety Disorder scale. This multivariable difference-in-differences analysis used ordinary least squares regression.
Source. Analysis of survey responses from Hurley Medical Center Maternal Well-Being Survey.

and Rx Kids exposure, holding control variables at their means. In 2023, Flint mothers were roughly as likely to report eviction as non-Flint mothers. In 2024, Flint mothers were substantially less likely to report eviction than non-Flint mothers. Similarly, for postpartum depression, Flint mothers in 2023 were far more likely to screen positive than non-Flint mothers. In 2024, this disparity was completely erased.

DISCUSSION

The perinatal period is the poorest across the life course, and living in poor places exacerbates the pathogenicity of poverty. A prenatal and infant cash transfer program, Rx Kids launched in the city with one of the nation's highest child poverty rates[39] in a never-done-before, to our knowledge, effort to address the maternal and infant health crisis. Driven by the interconnected pathways of improved economic stability and a reimagined social contract, study results show substantive improvements in several often-intractable domains of material hardship (housing security, nutrition), maternal mental health (depression), maternal well-being (loved, hopeful, respected, valued), and trust in institutions.

Findings were consistent with global and domestic evidence on prenatal and child cash transfers and aligned with insights from Rx Kids participant surveys (n = 112; 56% response rate;[27] n = 534; 53% response rate[54]) that revealed improvements in family financial security, maternal and infant health, stress reduction, health care services access, and parenting confidence.[27,54] This study, however, further delineated Rx Kids' impact with temporal and geographic controls by comparing outcomes for Flint mothers before and after program implementation to differences in outcomes for noneligible mothers living outside Flint.

The hardship improvements seen in housing security, and particularly eviction, are important because these outcomes have profound impacts on the health and well-being of both mother and child. That families in Flint were less likely to be evicted than their much-higher-income non-Flint counterparts in 2024, who were not eligible for Rx Kids, is striking.

The maternal mental health and well-being findings are also notable. Not only did Rx Kids–exposed mothers report a major decrease in postpartum depression—with far-reaching implications for maternal and infant health—but they also felt more loved, respected, and hopeful, and expressed more trust in institutions. Buffered from economic hardship, the increase in hope—defined as optimism with belief that one has agency—reflects a powerful determinant of well-being; hopelessness has been linked to depression, and to a rising number of "deaths of despair," and even vulnerability to misinformation, mistrust, and polarization.[55] Increased trust in institutions is especially consequential, considering this intervention launched where governmental betrayal was central to a public health crisis[38] that resulted in a further corrosion of trust.[56] These findings capture the underpinning of a reimagined social contract—what it means to be part of a society and a community that cares and provides for each other.

Consequentially, across both sets of outcomes presented, Flint mothers went from markedly worse off in comparison with non-Flint mothers in 2023 to virtually identical outcomes compared with non-Flint mothers in 2024. Rx Kids may be helping a community with lower income and education levels "catch up" to its wealthier and more highly educated neighbors. As a panacea of sorts that proactively treats the pathogen of perinatal poverty, programs like Rx Kids may improve the economic stability, health, and well-being of entire disadvantaged places, while infusing hope to reimagine the social contract and bolster democracy.

Limitations

The analysis assumed that the EMR address accurately represents the mother's living situation. However, because of the nature of self-reported address information, some Rx Kids recipients may be coded incorrectly. In this analysis, we are only able to report "intent-to-treat" (those eligible for the intervention) estimates rather than "treatment-on-the-treated" (eligibles who received the benefit) estimates. Because of the very high take-up, though, these rates (i.e., the intent-to-treat and the treatment-on-the-treated) should be relatively similar. In an ideal difference-in-differences analysis, the treatment and control groups would be more homogenous, and more than 1 preintervention period would be observed to assess whether the assumption of parallel trends holds. The parallel trends assumption is fundamentally untestable because the counterfactual trend for the exposed group is unobserved; our results should thus be interpreted in the context of the assumptions of the difference-in-differences methodology. A test of parallel trends in the preperiod is neither necessary nor sufficient to establish the validity of difference-in-differences.[57]

Given that the control group had higher income and educational attainment on average, it is even more striking that Rx Kids may have substantially narrowed the gap between Flint and non-Flint mothers on many outcomes in 2024. While it is possible that some other change in the policy landscape was driving these results, no other relevant changes were identified. The 2024 Flint cohort had a somewhat higher survey response rate than other cohorts, and respondents were somewhat less disadvantaged than nonrespondents, which may have impacted the findings. However, available data indicate that the treatment group was the most disadvantaged of all cohorts, indicating that, if anything, there was a downward bias in the probability of seeing impacts. Finally, our data were self-reported survey responses; however, there was no other data source on mothers' perceptions of these outcomes; thus, it is the best-available representation of mothers' perceived financial stressors and well-being.

Future Directions

This is the first in a series of surveys in Flint that will report on a consistent set of outcomes with cohorts of mothers exposed to Rx Kids. Analysis of future surveys will allow for comparison with this analysis. Rx Kids' universal design, with its near-100% take-up, further permits robust research using geocoded administrative data sources using difference-in-differences analysis comparing temporal and geographic trends. Research on administrative data is in process for many of the potential outcomes in Figure 1, including maternal and infant health, health care utilization, child welfare, voter participation, societal savings, and economic reinvestment. To further delineate the proposed mechanisms of change for key outcomes, in-depth qualitative research is underway. Other research includes examining the dose–response of cash transfers on desired outcomes, longitudinal follow-up, and replication of the survey in other Rx Kids communities.

Public Health Implications

As the United States' first, to our knowledge, community-wide prenatal and infant cash transfer program, the scale and design of Rx Kids fills a maternal and infant health research and policy gap, with implications for multiple sectors, including health care, public health, housing, early childhood, racial equity, social services, civil society, national security, and global competitiveness. The results described herein demonstrate the potential for this model to have a positive impact on the economic security, mental health, and well-being of families and entire communities. The place-based and population-level scale mimics government-level interventions, providing a replicable model[58] for efficiently and effectively investing in maternal and infant health and well-being. AJPH

ABOUT THE AUTHORS

Mona Hanna and Eric Finegood are with Michigan State University–Hurley Children's Hospital Pediatric Public Health Initiative, Charles Stewart Mott Department of Public Health, Michigan State University College of Human Medicine, Flint. H. Luke Shaefer is with the Gerald R. Ford School of Public Policy and Poverty Solutions, University of Michigan, Ann Arbor. Sumit Agarwal is with the University of Michigan Medical School and School of Public Health, University of Michigan, Ann Arbor. Yasamean Zamani-Hank is with the Department of Family Medicine, Charles Stewart Mott Department of Public Health, and Department of Epidemiology and Biostatistics, College of Human Medicine, Michigan State University, East Lansing. Jenny LaChance is with Michigan State University–Hurley Children's Hospital Pediatric Public Health Initiative, Hurley Medical Center, Flint.

CORRESPONDENCE

Correspondence should be sent to Mona Hanna, MD, MPH, Michigan State University–Hurley Children's Hospital Pediatric Public Health Initiative, 200 E 1st St, Flint, MI 48502 (e-mail: hannamon@msu.edu). Reprints can be ordered at https://www.ajph.org by clicking the "Reprints" link.

PUBLICATION INFORMATION

Full Citation: Hanna M, Shaefer HL, Finegood E, Agarwal S, Zamani-Hank Y, LaChance J. Hardship and hope: the relationship between unconditional prenatal and infant cash transfers, economic stability, and maternal mental health and well-being. *Am J Public Health*. 2025;115(12):2020–2029.

Acceptance Date: July 4, 2025.

DOI: https://doi.org/10.2105/AJPH.2025.308244

ORCID iDs:

Mona Hanna https://orcid.org/0000-0003-1887-4710

Eric Finegood https://orcid.org/0009-0006-1203-7750

Sumit Agarwal https://orcid.org/0000-0002-7938-139X

CONTRIBUTORS

M. Hanna, H. L. Shaefer, and J. LaChance conceptualized and designed the study, analyzed data, and drafted the article. E. Finegood and Y. Zamani-Hank designed the study and analyzed data. S. Agarwal analyzed data and drafted the article. All authors helped interpret data and critically reviewed and revised the article.

ACKNOWLEDGMENTS

This research was supported by W. K. Kellogg Foundation (grant P-6019931-2023).

The authors thank Mallory Goldsworthy, Katlin Harwood-Schelb, Maya Wolock, Katherine Negele, and Michigan State University–Pediatric Public Health Initiative summer interns (class of 2024): Spotless Amponsah, Alexis Jaggi, Gloria Mshana, Ella Ryan, and Nour Tellow for their help implementing the survey, and thank Arianna Foster for data analysis support. We thank Sarah Miller, Natasha Pilkauskas, and Greg Duncan for helpful comments on an earlier version of this study.

Note. The contents are those of the authors and do not necessarily represent the official views of, nor an endorsement by, W. K. Kellogg Foundation.

CONFLICTS OF INTEREST

The authors have no conflicts of interest to report.

HUMAN PARTICIPANT PROTECTION

This research was approved by the Hurley Medical Center institutional review board (2187211). All survey participants provided informed consent.

REFERENCES

1. Gunja MZ, Gumas ED, Williams II RD. *US Health Care from a Global Perspective, 2022: Accelerating Spending, Worsening Outcomes*. The

Commonwealth Fund. 2023. Available at: https://doi.org/10.26099/8ejy-yc74. Accessed January 20, 2025.

2. Miller CC. The world 'has found a way to do this': the US lags on paid leave. *New York Times.* June 22, 2023. Available at: https://www.nytimes.com/2021/10/25/upshot/paid-leave-democrats.html. Accessed January 21, 2025.

3. Collyer S, Curran M, Garfinkel I, Harris D, Richardson D, Wimer C. A step in the right direction: the expanded Child Tax Credit would move the United States' high child poverty rate closer to peer nations. Columbia University, Center on Poverty and Social Policy and UNICEF Innocenti, Global Office of Research and Foresight. 2022. Available at: https://poverty-and-social-policy.site.drupaldisttest.cc.columbia.edu/sites/default/files/content/Publications/Child-Tax-Credit-and-Relative-Poverty-CPSP-UNICEF-2022.pdf. Accessed January 21, 2025.

4. Gunja MZ, Gumas ED, Masitha R, Zephyrin LC. Insights into the US maternal mortality crisis: an international comparison. The Commonwealth Fund. 2024. Available at: https://www.commonwealthfund.org/publications/issue-briefs/2024/jun/insights-us-maternal-mortality-crisis-international-comparison. Accessed January 21, 2025.

5. Woolf SH, Chapman DA. Excess US deaths attributable to high all-cause mortality rates among youths aged 0 to 19 years. *JAMA Pediatr.* 2024;178(9):942–944. https://doi.org/10.1001/jamapediatrics.2024.1869

6. Bronstein JM, Wingate MS, Brisendine AE. Why is the US preterm birth rate so much higher than the rates in Canada, Great Britain, and Western Europe? *Int J Health Serv.* 2018;48(4):622–640. https://doi.org/10.1177/0020731418786360

7. Hill L, Rao A, Artiga S, Ranji U. Racial disparities in maternal and infant health: current status and efforts to address them. Kaiser Family Foundation. 2024. Available at: https://www.kff.org/racial-equity-and-health-policy/issue-brief/racial-disparities-in-maternal-and-infant-health-current-status-and-efforts-to-address-them. Accessed January 21, 2025.

8. Stanczyk AB. The dynamics of US household economic circumstances around a birth. *Demography.* 2020;57(4):1271–1296. https://doi.org/10.1007/s13524-020-00897-1

9. Hamilton C, Harris D, Wimer C, Kimberlin S, Collyer S, Garfinkel I. The case for a federal birth grant: a plan to reduce poverty for newborns and their families. Columbia University Center on Poverty and Social Policy. 2023:9. Available at: https://povertycenter.columbia.edu/sites/povertycenter.columbia.edu/files/content/Publications/Case-for-federal-birth-grant-CPSP-2023.pdf. Accessed October 24, 2024.

10. World Health Organization, United Nations Children's Fund, World Bank Group. *Nurturing Care for Early Childhood Development: A Framework for Helping Children Survive and Thrive to Transform Health and Human Potential.* World Health Organization. 2018. Available at: https://www.who.int/publications/i/item/9789241514064. Accessed January 27, 2025.

11. Masarik AS, Conger RD. Stress and child development: a review of the Family Stress Model. *Curr Opin Psychol.* 2017;13:85–90. https://doi.org/10.1016/j.copsyc.2016.05.008

12. Lange BCL, Dáu ALBT, Goldblum J, Alfano J, Smith MV. A mixed methods investigation of the experience of poverty among a population of low-income parenting women. *Community Ment Health J.* 2017;53(7):832–841. https://doi.org/10.1007/s10597-017-0093-z

13. Ridley M, Rao G, Schilbach F, Patel V. Poverty, depression, and anxiety: causal evidence and mechanisms. *Science.* 2020;370(6522):eaay0214. https://doi.org/10.1126/science.aay0214

14. Jefferson EEY. Will it ever change? Lack of parental leave and its detrimental effects on maternal wellbeing. *Lancet Reg Health Am.* 2023;25:100572. https://doi.org/10.1016/j.lana.2023.100572

15. Zender R, Bachand AM, Reif JS. Exposure to tap water during pregnancy. *J Expo Anal Environ Epidemiol.* 2001;11(3):224–230. https://doi.org/10.1038/sj.jea.7500163

16. Bell ML, Belanger K. Review of research on residential mobility during pregnancy: consequences for assessment of prenatal environmental exposures. *J Expo Sci Environ Epidemiol.* 2012;22(5):429–438. https://doi.org/10.1038/jes.2012.42

17. DiTosto JD, Holder K, Soyemi E, Beestrum M, Yee LM. Housing instability and adverse perinatal outcomes: a systematic review. *Am J Obstet Gynecol MFM.* 2021;3(6):100477. https://doi.org/10.1016/j.ajogmf.2021.100477

18. Leifheit KM, Schwartz GL, Pollack CE, et al. Severe housing insecurity during pregnancy: association with adverse birth and infant outcomes. *Int J Environ Res Public Health.* 2020;17(22):8659. https://doi.org/10.3390/ijerph17228659

19. Graetz N, Gershenson C, Hepburn P, Porter SR, Sandler DH, Desmond M. A comprehensive demographic profile of the US evicted population. *Proc Natl Acad Sci U S A.* 2023;120(41):e2305860120. https://doi.org/10.1073/pnas.2305860120

20. Khadka A, Fink G, Gromis A, McConnell M. In utero exposure to threat of evictions and preterm birth: evidence from the United States. *Health Serv Res.* 2020;55(suppl 2):823–832. https://doi.org/10.1111/1475-6773.13551

21. Shannon MM, Clougherty JE, McCarthy C, et al. Neighborhood violent crime and perceived stress in pregnancy. *Int J Environ Res Public Health.* 2020;17(15):5585. https://doi.org/10.3390/ijerph17155585

22. Nowak AL, Giurgescu C. The built environment and birth outcomes: a systematic review. *MCN Am J Matern Child Nurs.* 2017;42(1):14–20. https://doi.org/10.1097/NMC.0000000000000299

23. Messer LC, Maxson P, Miranda ML. The urban built environment and associations with women's psychosocial health. *J Urban Health.* 2013;90(5):857–871. https://doi.org/10.1007/s11524-012-9743-1

24. Bole A, Bernstein A, White MJ, Council on Environmental Health and Climate Change, Section on Minority Health, Equity, and Inclusion. The built environment and pediatric health. *Pediatrics.* 2024;153(1):e2023064773. https://doi.org/10.1542/peds.2023-064773

25. Edin KJ, Shaefer HL, Nelson TJ. *The Injustice of Place: Uncovering the Legacy of Poverty in America.* 1st ed. New York, NY: HarperCollins Publishers, Mariner Imprint; 2023.

26. Shaefer HL, Hanna M, Harris D, Richardson D, Laker M. Protecting the health of children with universal child cash benefits. *Lancet.* 2024;404(10469):2380–2391. https://doi.org/10.1016/S0140-6736(24)02366-3

27. Rx Kids. Key insights from the first citywide maternal and infant cash prescription program. Rx Kids: a prescription for health, hope, and opportunity. August 14, 2024. Available at: https://rxkids.org/key-insights-from-the-first-citywide-maternal-and-infant-cash-prescription-program. Accessed November 8, 2024.

28. Ryu S, Fan L. The relationship between financial worries and psychological distress among US adults. *J Fam Econ Issues.* 2023;44(1):16–33. https://doi.org/10.1007/s10834-022-09820-9

29. Batra A, Jackson K, Hamad R. Effects of the 2021 expanded Child Tax Credit on adults' mental health: a quasi-experimental study. *Health Aff (Millwood).* 2023;42(1):74–82. https://doi.org/10.1377/hlthaff.2022.00733

30. Kovski N, Pilkauskas NV, Michelmore K, Shaefer HL. Unconditional cash transfers and mental health symptoms among parents with low incomes: evidence from the 2021 Child Tax Credit. *SSM Popul Health.* 2023;22:101420. https://doi.org/10.1016/j.ssmph.2023.101420

31. Evans WN, Garthwaite CL. Giving mom a break: the impact of higher EITC payments on maternal health. *Am Econ J Econ Policy.* 2014;6(2):258–290. https://doi.org/10.1257/pol.6.2.258

32. Pilkauskas NV, Michelmore K, Kovski N, Shaefer HL. The expanded Child Tax Credit and economic wellbeing of low-income families. *J Popul Econ.* 2024;37(4):68. https://doi.org/10.1007/s00148-024-01047-2

33. Liebman J, Carlson K, Novick E, Portocarrero P. The Chelsea Eats Program: experimental impacts. Rappaport Institute for Greater Boston, Harvard Kennedy School. 2022:64. Available at: https://www.hks.harvard.edu/sites/default/files/Taubman/RIGB/Chelsea%20Eats%20Experimental%20Impacts%20120622.pdf. Accessed October 8, 2024.

34. Pilkauskas NV, Michelmore K, Kovski N. The effects of the 2021 Child Tax Credit on housing affordability and the living arrangements of families with low incomes. *Demography.* 2024;61(4):1069–1096. https://doi.org/10.1215/00703370-11458327

35. UNICEF and the Overseas Development Institute. Universal child benefits: policy issues and options. 2020. Available at: https://www.unicef.org/reports/universal-child-benefits-2020. Accessed January 27, 2025.

36. US Census Bureau, US Department of Commerce. Age and sex. 2024. Available at: https://data.census.gov/table/ACSST1Y2023.S0101?g=050XX00US26049_160XX00US2629000. Accessed October 16, 2024.

37. State of Michigan. Five-year average live births by race or ancestry of mother and age of mother Flint City, Genesee County, Michigan 2018–2022. 2023. Available at: https://vitalstats.michigan.gov/osr/chi/Births14/BxTablesADA/IndicatorObject.asp?Char=208&Row=RACE&Col=STANDARD&Stat=NxFxD&Average=A&TableType=G&RowGroup=RACE_FIXED&COLGROUP=AGE&JS=NO&AreaCode=0473&AreaType=M. Accessed October 15, 2024.

38. Hanna-Attisha M, LaChance J, Sadler RC, Champney Schnepp A. Elevated blood lead levels in children associated with the Flint drinking water crisis: a spatial analysis of risk and public health response. *Am J Public Health.* 2016;106(2):283–290. https://doi.org/10.2105/AJPH.2015.303003

39. US Census Bureau, US Department of Commerce. Poverty status in the past 12 months. 2024. Available at: https://data.census.gov/table/ACSST1Y2023.S1701?g=050XX00US26049_160XX00US2629000. Accessed October 16, 2024.

40. US Census Bureau, US Department of Commerce. Selected characteristics of the total and native populations in the United States. 2024. Available at: https://data.census.gov/table/ACSST1Y2023.S0601?q=race&g=050XX00US26049_160XX00US2629000. Accessed October 16, 2024.

41. Harris PA, Taylor R, Minor BL, REDCap Consortium, et al. The REDCap Consortium: building an international community of software platform partners. *J Biomed Inform.* 2019;95:103208. https://doi.org/10.1016/j.jbi.2019.103208

42. Harris PA, Taylor R, Thielke R, Payne J, Gonzalez N, Conde JG. Research electronic data capture (REDCap)—a metadata-driven methodology and workflow process for providing translational research informatics support. *J Biomed Inform.* 2009;42(2):377–381. https://doi.org/10.1016/j.jbi.2008.08.010

43. Pilkauskas NV, Michelmore K, Kovski N, Shaefer HL. The expanded Child Tax Credit and economic wellbeing of low-income families. *J Popul Econ.* 2024;37(4). https://doi.org/10.1007/s00148-024-01047-2

44. Hager ER, Quigg AM, Black MM, et al. Development and validity of a 2-item screen to identify families at risk for food insecurity. *Pediatrics.* 2010;126(1):e26–e32. https://doi.org/10.1542/peds.2009-3146

45. Andresen EM, Malmgren JA, Carter WB, Patrick DL. Screening for depression in well older adults: evaluation of a short form of the CES-D (Center for Epidemiologic Studies Depression Scale). *Am J Prev Med.* 1994;10(2):77–84.

46. Kroenke K, Spitzer RL, Williams JBW, Monahan PO, Löwe B. Anxiety disorders in primary care: prevalence, impairment, comorbidity, and detection. *Ann Intern Med.* 2007;146(5):317–325. https://doi.org/10.7326/0003-4819-146-5-200703060-00004

47. Spitzer RL, Kroenke K, Williams JBW, Löwe B. A brief measure for assessing generalized anxiety disorder: the GAD-7. *Arch Intern Med.* 2006;166(10):1092–1097. https://doi.org/10.1001/archinte.166.10.1092

48. Krafft AM, Martin-Krumm C, Fenouillet F. Adaptation, further elaboration, and validation of a scale to measure hope as perceived by people: discriminant value and predictive utility vis-à-vis dispositional hope. *Assessment.* 2019;26(8):1594–1609. https://doi.org/10.1177/1073191117700724

49. Krafft AM, Martin-Krumm C, Fenouillet F. Perceived Hope Scale. APA PsycTests. November 2019. https://doi.org/10.1037/t74017-000

50. Organization for Economic Co-operation and Development. *OECD Trust Survey Design and Technical Documentation*. 2024:57. Available at: https://www.oecd.org/content/dam/oecd/en/publications/support-materials/2024/07/oecd-survey-on-drivers-of-trust-in-public-institutions-2024-results_eeb36452/2023%20Trust%20Survey%20-%20Technical%20annex.pdf. Accessed January 13, 2025.

51. Ai C, Norton EC. Interaction terms in logit and probit models. *Econ Lett.* 2003;80(1):123–129. https://doi.org/10.1016/S0165-1765(03)00032-6

52. Wooldridge JM. *Econometric Analysis of Cross Section and Panel Data.* 2nd ed. Cambridge, Massachusetts: MIT Press; 2010.

53. Jeffries N, Zaslavsky AM, Diez Roux AV, et al. Methodological approaches to understanding causes of health disparities. *Am J Public Health.* 2019;109(suppl 1):S28–S33. https://doi.org/10.2105/AJPH.2018.304843

54. Rx Kids. Rx Kids Participant Survey Results. January 28, 2025. Available at: https://rxkids.org/rx-kids-survey-results-november-2024. Accessed January 30, 2025.

55. Graham C. Hope & despair: implications for life outcomes & policy. *Behav Sci Policy.* 2023;9(2):47–52. https://doi.org/10.1177/23794607231222529

56. Morckel V, Terzano K. Legacy city residents' lack of trust in their governments: an examination of Flint, Michigan residents' trust at the height of the water crisis. *J Urban Aff.* 2019;41(5):585–601. https://doi.org/10.1080/07352166.2018.1499415

57. Kahn-Lang A, Lang K. The promise and pitfalls of differences-in-differences: reflections on 16 and Pregnant and other applications. *J Bus Econ Stat.* 2020;38(3):613–620. https://doi.org/10.1080/07350015.2018.1546591

58. Hanna M, Shaefer HL, Fogle H, et al. Scaling up prenatal and infant cash prescriptions to eradicate deep infant poverty in the United States. Brookings Institution. 2024. Available at: https://www.brookings.edu/articles/prenatal-and-infant-cash-prescriptions-to-eradicate-deep-infant-poverty-united-states. Accessed January 10, 2025.

Air Pollutants and Breast Cancer Risk: A Parallel Analysis of Five Large US Prospective Cohorts

Alexandra J. White, PhD, Jaime E. Hart, ScD, Sabah M. Quraishi, PhD, Deborah B. Bookwalter, ScD, Marina R. Sweeney, PhD, Elizabeth W. Spalt, MS, Michael S. Hendryx, PhD, Veronica L. Irvin, PhD, Dorothy S. Lane, MD, Aladdin H. Shadyab, PhD, Shawnita Sealy-Jefferson, PhD, Marian L. Neuhouser, PhD, Eric A. Whitsel, MD, Joel D. Kaufman, MD, Francine Laden, ScD, and Dale P. Sandler, PhD

See also Terry, p. 1957.

Objectives. To determine whether outdoor air pollution exposure is associated with breast cancer incidence.

Methods. Residential-level concentrations of nitrogen dioxide (NO_2, parts per billion [ppb]), fine particulate matter ($PM_{2.5}$; ≤ 2.5 μ/m^3) and ozone (ppb) in the United States were estimated for participants of the Nurses' Health Studies, Women's Health Initiative Clinical Trials and Observational Study Cohort, and Sister Study using high-resolution spatiotemporal models. Cox proportional hazards regression estimated cohort-specific hazard ratios (HRs) and 95% confidence intervals (CIs), and a random effects model determined summary HRs, overall and by estrogen receptor (ER)/progesterone receptor (PR) subtype and census region.

Results. NO_2 was positively associated with overall breast cancer incidence (n = 28 811 cases; HR = 1.03; 95% CI = 1.00, 1.05), with little variation by subgroups. $PM_{2.5}$ was associated with higher incidence of ER-/PR- tumors (n = 2367 cases; HR = 1.14; 95% CI = 1.04, 1.24; *P*-heterogeneity < .001) and with higher overall incidence in the Midwest (HR = 1.15; 95% CI = 1.01, 1.32; *P*-heterogeneity = .01). Ozone was not associated with overall incidence, but was associated with ER-/PR- tumors (n = 3406 cases; HR = 1.10; 95% CI = 1.00, 1.21; *P*-heterogeneity = .03).

Conclusions. In this largest US study to date, we confirmed an association between NO_2 and breast cancer, and we present novel associations of $PM_{2.5}$ and ozone with ER-/PR- tumors. (*Am J Public Health*. 2025;115(12):2030–2043. https://doi.org/10.2105/AJPH.2025.308247)

The incidence of breast cancer in the United States has been generally increasing since the mid-1980s.[1] Most established risk factors for breast cancer are related to reproductive and lifestyle factors and largely reflect associations with estrogen receptor (ER)-positive disease.[2,3] Research on environmental risk factors suggests that chemical and pollutant exposures contribute to breast cancer incidence, particularly for women who may experience higher susceptibility.[4,5]

Outdoor air pollution exposure (e.g., particulate matter [PM], nitrogen oxides [NO_x, NO_2], ozone [O_3]) has been classified by the International Agency for Research on Cancer as a Group 1 carcinogen, based on evidence for fine particulate matter ($PM_{2.5}$; ≤ 2.5 μ/m^3) and lung cancer.[6] Air pollution is hypothesized to affect carcinogenesis through altered gene expression, inflammation, and immune and oxidative stress responses.[6] Air pollution also includes compounds with endocrine-disrupting properties[7] and thus may be particularly relevant to breast cancer given its relationship to hormonal factors.

Previous studies of NO_2 and breast cancer, including 3 meta-analyses, provide evidence of a modest association

AJPH December 2025, Vol. 115, No. 12

(hazard ratios [HR], rate ratios, and odds ratios of 1.02–1.06 per 10-μg/m^3 increase in exposure).[8–13] Although earlier meta-analyses have observed null associations for $PM_{2.5}$ and breast cancer,[9,13] more recent studies, including a meta-analysis of 11 cohort studies, have observed positive associations (HR = 1.03–1.14 per 5-μg/m^3 increase in exposure).[10,11,14–17] The few studies of ozone have been null.[10,18,19]

Despite a growing literature, well-powered studies considering tumor heterogeneity are limited.[16,17,19–23] Although the geographic heterogeneity of air pollution is well documented,[23,24] regional differences in observed associations are not well established.[16,19,23] The aim of this study was to conduct parallel analyses using data from 5 large, prospective US cohorts to evaluate the associations between NO_2, $PM_{2.5}$, ozone, and incident breast cancer, overall and by tumor subtype and geographic region, and to summarize findings across cohorts.

METHODS

Study cohorts included the Nurses' Health Study (NHS), the Nurses' Health Study II (NHSII), the Sister Study (SIS), the Women's Health Initiative Clinical Trials (WHI-CT), and the Women's Health Initiative Observational Study (WHI-OS). The NHS recruited 121 700 female nurses from 11 US states in 1976 who were 30 to 55 years of age.[25] The NHSII recruited 116 430 female nurses from 14 US states in 1989 who were 25 to 42 years of age.[25] By the mid-1990s, participants in the NHS and NHSII lived in all 50 states. A total of 161 808 postmenopausal women (aged 50–79 years) enrolled in 1 or more of the overlapping, randomized WHI-CT of menopausal hormone therapy, calcium and vitamin D supplementation, and diet modification, or in the WHI-OS from 1993 to 1998.[26–28] Participants in the WHI-CT and WHI-OS were recruited from 40 clinical centers nationwide, located in 23 states and Washington, DC. WHI-CT participants who participated in the hormone therapy arm were initially assigned to 1 of 4 treatments: estrogen, estrogen control, estrogen plus progestin, or estrogen plus progestin control. From 2003 to 2009, the SIS recruited 50 884 women (aged 35–74 years) from all 50 states and Puerto Rico with at least 1 full or half-sister with a previous diagnosis of breast cancer.[29]

Outcome Assessment

In all studies, incident breast cancer was reported by participants during routine follow-up and verified by medical records (as well as physician adjudication for all studies except the SIS) and by pathology reports when available. This analysis was limited to diagnoses confirmed by medical record or death certificate–National Death Index records; for the SIS, unconfirmed diagnoses were censored.

Exposure Assessment

We generated biweekly air pollutant concentrations at all participant residential addresses using a synthesized suite of regional, spatiotemporal models derived from a combination of data from 1500 regulatory monitors, more than 900 research monitors at residential and community locations, and more than 200 geographic covariates developed for large-scale epidemiological research and calculated at each monitoring and residential location.[30,31] For NO_2, gradient monitoring was additionally conducted near roadways. Air pollutant models accounted for complex spatiotemporal dependencies in a land use and spatial smoothing framework.[32,33] We used the cross-validation method to evaluate air pollutant model predictive performance ($R^2 = 0.87$ for NO_2, $R^2 = 0.89$ for $PM_{2.5}$, and $R^2 = 0.73$ for ozone).[30] NO_2 and ozone concentrations were available at the earliest starting in January 1990, and $PM_{2.5}$ concentrations were available beginning in January 1999.

We calculated person-months of follow-up from cohort- and pollutant-specific analytic baselines (e.g., starting in 1992 for NO_2 and ozone in the NHS and NHSII) through breast cancer diagnosis, death, loss to follow-up, or end of follow-up in 2016 to 2017 (May 2016 for NHS and NHSII, June 2017 for SIS, and 2017 for WHI-CT and WHI-OS; Figure A, available as a supplement to the online version of this article at http://www.ajph.org). Women with a diagnosis of breast cancer prior to the analytic baseline were excluded, as well as those with uncertain timing (n = 3920 for NHS, n = 21 for NHSII, n = 79 for SIS, n = 101 for WHI-CT, n = 5444 for WHI-OS). Women diagnosed with other types of cancer were retained in the analysis. We analyzed air pollutant concentrations using a long-term exposure estimate calculated as time-varying 24-month rolling averages weighted by address history. Person-months were included when at least 23 prior months of estimates were available. Follow-up began at the earliest in 1992 for NO_2 and ozone, and in 2001 for $PM_{2.5}$. For the SIS, enrollment started later than in the other cohorts (2003–2009); pollutant estimates were available starting at the time of enrollment, with the 24-month average at baseline based on self-reported and

LexisNexis-derived residential histories.[34] For the WHI-CT and WHI-OS, pollutant estimates prior to enrollment were extended back to 1990.

Covariate Assessment

For each cohort, we ascertained information on demographic and socioeconomic characteristics, medical and reproductive history, and behavioral risk factors (e.g., smoking status, alcohol intake, and physical activity) at the time of analytic baseline.[25–29] Routine follow-up questionnaires updated reproductive factors, behavioral risk factors, and medical diagnoses. We updated menopausal status throughout follow-up for those who were premenopausal at the analytic baseline. Census region was updated throughout follow-up for all participants.

The neighborhood socioeconomic status (nSES) index was developed based on data from the 2000 US Census[35] and the 2005–2009 and 2007–2011 cycles of the American Community Survey,[36,37] with a higher value indicating greater neighborhood deprivation.[38] This index was estimated for the analytic baseline address and updated for 1999–2000 addresses for the WHI, NHSI, and NHSII.

Statistical Analysis

Cohorts contributed individual-level data and were analyzed in parallel using the same statistical models to produce cohort-specific results that were then summarized across cohorts. The analysis was restricted to women with available data on air pollutant exposure (unavailable for women living outside the contiguous United States), race and ethnicity, educational attainment, census region of residence, and nSES (Figure B, available as a supplement to the online version of this article at http://www.ajph.org). We calculated Spearman correlation coefficients for the associations between each of the pollutants and nSES.

We used Cox proportional hazards models to examine the association between each air pollutant and breast cancer incidence, overall and by tumor invasiveness (invasive; ductal carcinoma in situ), ER status (overall and invasive only), joint ER and PR (progesterone receptor) status (overall and invasive only), and ER and PR status among premenopausal and postmenopausal women separately. We calculated HRs and 95% confidence intervals (CIs) for a 10 parts per billion (ppb) increase in NO_2 and ozone and a 5-µg/m^3 increase in $PM_{2.5}$. We assessed linearity using likelihood ratio tests comparing the model with only the linear term to the model with linear and restricted cubic spline terms, and no violations were identified. For each cohort, the data set was structured with 1 record for each person-month of follow-up, and all models were stratified by age. In the NHS and NHSII, we used age and calendar month as stratifying variables and used an indicator variable as the time scale. In the SIS, the time scale was calendar month. In the WHI-CT and WHI-OS, the time scale was time on study because sharing of calendar time was restricted, and models were further stratified by masked (nonordered) enrollment year to adjust for temporal effects.

We selected the covariate adjustment set using a directed acyclic graph (Figure C, available as a supplement to the online version of this article at http://www.ajph.org), which included self-reported race and ethnicity (Black including Hispanic/Latina; non-Black Hispanic/Latina; non-Hispanic White; "Other," including Asian/Pacific Islander and American Indian), educational attainment (high school or less; some college or associate's degree; bachelor's degree or higher), nSES score (continuous), and time-varying census region (Northeast, Midwest, South, West). In the WHI-CT, all models were also adjusted for hormone therapy treatment arm (estrogen, estrogen control, estrogen plus progestin, estrogen plus progestin control).

For each air pollutant, we calculated summary effect estimates using a random effects model that pooled study-specific effect estimates that were adjusted for the primary covariate adjustment set. We examined heterogeneity in the HRs estimated across studies using the Cochran Q test.

We evaluated effect measure modification by several covariates (race and ethnicity, analytic baseline nSES quartile, time-varying primary census region, body mass index [BMI], and menopausal status, time-varying for those premenopausal at enrollment). We evaluated modification by race and ethnicity and nSES, as air pollution exposure in the United States is inequitably distributed, with racial and ethnic minorities and those living in areas of lower SES experiencing higher exposure.[39,40] We considered geographic region to evaluate potential heterogeneity by pollution composition[23] and menopausal status given that previous studies observed variability.[15,41,42] We evaluated modification by BMI because particulate matter constituents can act as endocrine-disrupting chemicals,[7] which are lipophilic and accumulate in adipose tissue.[43] To assess modification within studies, we used likelihood ratio tests to compare models with and without pollutant by covariate

AJPH December 2025, Vol. 115, No. 12

cross-product terms. For the summary estimate, we used the contrast test method[44] (P-heterogeneity) to evaluate heterogeneity across subtypes and subgroups.

Sensitivity analyses included (1) a 10-year lag analysis; (2) a model coadjusting for the other air pollutants (e.g., NO_2 model adjusted for $PM_{2.5}$ and ozone); (3) an expanded adjustment set, which included the following breast cancer risk factors: smoking status, alcohol intake, physical activity, BMI, age at first birth, parity, breastfeeding, oral contraceptive use, age at menopause, postmenopausal hormone use (in addition to the hormone therapy arm in the WHI-CT), and family history of breast cancer (mother or sister); and (4) use of cumulative average air pollutant exposure (overall and restricted to time-varying age younger than 60 years). At the start of follow-up, cumulative averages were calculated using all available air pollutant estimates prior to baseline and were updated to reflect the average value throughout follow-up in a time-dependent manner.

RESULTS

Mean follow-up time overall was 17.51 years (range = 9.76 [SIS] to 23.34 [NHSII]). The NO_2 and ozone analyses included 28 811 cases and the $PM_{2.5}$ analysis included 20 197 cases; study characteristics are shown in Table 1. Most correlations between NO_2 and $PM_{2.5}$ were moderate, whereas ozone was inversely correlated with NO_2 and $PM_{2.5}$ (Figure D, available as a supplement to the online version of this article at http://www.ajph.org).

A small positive association with overall breast cancer was observed for a 10-ppb increase in NO_2 exposure ($HR_{summary}$ = 1.03; 95% CI = 1.00, 1.05; Table 2). Although the HR was most consistently elevated for ER and PR positive tumors, there was no significant heterogeneity by ER and PR status or by invasiveness (Table A, available as a supplement to the online version of this article at http://www.ajph.org). Furthermore, little variability was observed by menopausal status, race and ethnicity, geographic region, nSES, or BMI (Figure 1; Table B, available as a supplement to the online version of this article at http://www.ajph.org), although elevated associations were observed for those living in the Midwest ($HR_{summary}$ = 1.07; 95% CI = 1.00, 1.14) and in the lowest category of nSES ($HR_{summary}$ = 1.06; 95% CI = 1.01, 1.11; Table B).

Overall, a 5-μg/m^3 increase in $PM_{2.5}$ exposure was not associated with breast cancer overall ($HR_{summary}$ = 0.99; 95% CI = 0.96, 1.02; Table 2) or with ER+/PR+ breast cancer. However, we observed a positive association with ER-/PR- tumors ($HR_{summary}$ = 1.14; 95% CI = 1.04, 1.24; P-heterogeneity < .001). When stratifying by region, we observed an overall breast cancer association in the Midwest ($HR_{summary}$ = 1.15; 95% CI = 1.01, 1.32), but not other regions (P-heterogeneity = 0.01; Figure 1, Table B). No differences were observed by invasiveness (Table A) or other factors (Figure 1, Table B).

No association was observed for ozone (10-ppb increase) and breast cancer overall (Table 2). However, an elevated association was observed for ER-/PR- tumors ($HR_{summary}$ = 1.10; 95% CI = 1.00, 1.21; P-heterogeneity = .04). No significant differences were observed by tumor invasiveness (Table A) or other factors (Figure 1), although an inverse association was observed among women in the Midwest ($HR_{summary}$ = 0.88; 95% CI = 0.79, 0.98; P-heterogeneity = .13; Table B).

Results for all 3 pollutants remained similar when we used a 10-year lag, adjusting for the other pollutants or for the model adjusting for breast cancer risk factors (Table C, available as a supplement to the online version of this article at http://www.ajph.org) and when cumulative average exposures were used instead of the rolling average (Table D, available as a supplement to the online version of this article at http://www.ajph.org). Including the SIS self-reported breast cancer cases did not change the findings.

DISCUSSION

In this parallel analysis of 5 large US cohorts, with over 28 000 breast cancer cases combined, we observed a 3% increase in overall breast cancer incidence for a 10-ppb increase in NO_2 outdoor concentrations. We also found that a 5-μg/m^3 increase in $PM_{2.5}$ outdoor concentrations was associated with a higher incidence of HR negative breast cancer as well as overall breast cancer among participants living in the Midwest.

Our finding of a modest increase in the incidence of breast cancer in relation to NO_2 is consistent with the literature. Three recent meta-analyses all concluded that a 10-μg/m^3 increase in NO_2 was associated with a 2% increase in breast cancer risk (95% CI = 1.01, 1.04[9,13] and 1.00, 1.03[12]). Gabet et al. estimated that a decrease in average NO_2 from 17.4 μg/m^3 to 6.3 μg/m^3 (fifth percentile) based on an HR of 1.02 would result in a 3% decrease in the number of breast cancer cases, or 1677 fewer cases in France annually.[9] Based on an estimated 316 950 cases of female breast cancer expected to be

AJPH December 2025, Vol. 115, No. 12

TABLE 1— Selected Analytic Baseline Characteristics of Participants in 5 US-Based Cohorts: United States, 1992–2017

Characteristics[a]	NHS	NHSII	SIS	WHI-CT	WHI-OS
NO_2					
Analytic no.	108 642	113 743	49 126	64 117	80 833
Analytic baseline year(s)	1992	1992	2003–2008	1993–1998	1993–1998
24-mo avg (ppb), median (IQR)	11.4 (7.5–17.2)	11.9 (7.9–17.4)	8.5 (5.8–11.9)	14.1 (9.7–19.2)	14.0 (9.8–19.0)
$PM_{2.5}$					
Analytic no.	97 759	111 597	49 126	59 844	75 315
Analytic baseline year(s)	2001	2001	2003–2008	2001	2001
24-mo avg ($\mu g/m^3$), median (IQR)	12.0 (10.3–14.0)	12.9 (11.0–14.5)	10.8 (8.8–12.4)	12.9 (10.5–14.9)	13.0 (10.6–15.0)
Ozone					
Analytic no.	108 642	113 743	49 126	64 117	80 833
Analytic baseline year(s)	1992	1992	2003–2008	1993–1998	1993–1998
24-mo avg (ppb), median (IQR)	24.8 (22.8–27.0)	24.7 (22.7–26.9)	26.6 (24.5–28.7)	24.0 (21.4–26.1)	24.1 (21.7–26.2)
Total follow-up time, mean	19.72	23.34	9.76	14.61	13.61
Age, y, %					
< 40	0.0	64.4	4.1	0.0	0.0
40–49	14.0	35.6	23.9	0.0	0.0
50–59	41.5	0.0	39.1	34.7	32.3
60–69	39.2	0.0	26.8	46.2	44.0
70–79	5.3	0.0	6.0	19.1	23.7
Age, y, mean ±SD	58.7 ±0.2	37.4 ±0.7	55.7 ±0.0	62.8 ±0.0	63.5 ±0.4
nSES score, mean ±SD[b]	−0.32 ±0.0	−0.22 ±0.9	−0.38 ±0.0	−0.45 ±0.1	−0.60 ±0.1
Census region, %					
Northeast	53.8	34.8	17.1	23.6	23.6
Midwest	17.8	33.4	27.4	22.6	22.4
South	14.7	17.3	33.7	25.9	26.1
West	13.7	14.6	21.8	27.9	27.9
Race and ethnicity, %					
Black	2.0	1.8	8.5	10.3	8.1
Hispanic/Latina	0.9	0.9	3.0	4.5	4.2
White (not of Hispanic origin)	95.2	93.4	85.3	82.9	85.2
Other	2.0	3.8	3.3	2.3	2.5
Educational attainment, %					
High school or less	0.0	0.0	15.1	24.0	21.2
Some college/associate's	77.5[c]	0.0	33.8	39.8	36.5
Bachelor's or higher	22.5	100[d]	51.1	36.2	42.3
Mother and sisters with breast cancer, %					
0	85.2	89.1	0.0	87.7	86.4
1	13.5	10.5	73.7	11.2	12.3
≥ 2	1.2	0.5	26.3	1.1	1.3
Smoking status, %					
Never	43.0	64.7	55.8	50.3	49.9
Former	39.4	22.3	36.0	40.7	42.5
Current	17.4	12.9	8.2	7.8	6.2
Missing	0.2	0.1	< 0.1	1.1	1.4

Continued

TABLE 1— Continued

Characteristics[a]	NHS	NHSII	SIS	WHI-CT	WHI-OS
Alcohol intake, drinks/week, %					
Nondrinker	33.5	37.8	18.4	28.4	28.8
< 1	18.1	17.2	35.4	34.5	31.7
1 to < 7	21.5	39.5	32.4	25.8	26.1
≥ 7	12.4	5.2	13.7	10.5	12.7
Missing	14.5	0.3	0.1	0.8	0.7
Total physical activity, %					
< 5 MET-hours/week	25.7	24.9	36.7	38.7	32.2
5 to < 10	14.2	17.5	16.7	16.2	16.8
10 to < 20	18.4	22.2	21.9	19.8	25.3
≥ 20	27.3	35.3	24.7	15.5	24.6
Missing	14.4	0.1	< 0.1	9.8	1.2
Body mass index, kg/m^2, %					
< 25	49.6	65.3	40.6	27.1	40.4
25–29	31.5	20.5	31.5	35.6	33.7
≥ 30	18.7	13.9	27.6	36.8	24.8
Missing	0.2	0.3	0.3	0.5	1.1
Age at menarche, y, %					
< 12	22.4	24.5	20.3	21.7	21.9
12–13	56.8	57.3	56.3	54.7	55.0
≥ 14	20.0	17.9	23.4	23.2	22.6
Missing	0.8	0.3	< 0.1	0.4	0.4
Parity, %					
Nulliparous	5.9	25.6	18.2	10.7	12.5
1–2 births	34.9	53.6	51.3	31.5	35.1
≥ 3 births	57.1	20.9	30.4	57.3	51.7
Missing	2.1	0.0	< 0.1	0.5	0.7
Age at first birth, y, %					
Nulliparous	5.9	25.6	18.2	10.7	12.5
< 20	0.8	5.0	13.1	14.6	11.2
20–24	46.9	23.7	31.2	38.7	36.7
≥ 25	44.3	45.2	37.4	26.7	29.5
Missing	2.1	0.5	0.1	9.4	10.1
Breastfeeding, %					
Nulliparous	5.9	25.6	18.2	10.7	12.5
Parous, breastfed < 1 mo	29.1	12.9	29.3	37.1	36.2
1–6 mo	27.6	11.9	18.1	25.5	25.2
≥ 7 mo	22.5	39.6	34.3	25.2	24.3
Missing	15.0	10.0	0.1	1.5	1.8
Oral contraceptive use, %					
Never	51.2	15.5	15.6	56.7	59.6
Ever	48.8	84.4	84.4	43.3	40.4
Missing	0.0	0.2	< 0.1	< 0.1	0.0

Continued

TABLE 1— Continued

Characteristics[a]	NHS	NHSII	SIS	WHI-CT	WHI-OS
Age at menopause, y, %					
Premenopausal	19.6	96.9	33.5	0.0	0.0
< 40	3.9	1.6	5.2	9.2	8.9
40–49	26.5	1.4	21.1	36.1	37.3
≥ 50	46.2	< 0.1	40.2	46.5	49.7
Missing	3.8	0	<0.1	8.3	4.1
PMH use, %[e]					
Never	52.1	97.2	54.4	48.4	39.3
Former	15.8	0.2	34.7	17.6	13.9
Current	28.7	2.6	10.5	34.0	46.7
Missing	3.4	< 0.1	0.4	0.1	0.1

Note. IQR = interquartile range; MET = metabolic equivalent; NHS = Nurses' Health Study; NHSII = Nurses' Health Study II; NO_2 = nitrogen dioxide; nSES = neighborhood socioeconomic status; $PM_{2.5}$ = fine particulate matter ≤ 2.5 μ/m³g; PMH = postmenopausal hormone; ppb = parts per billion; SIS = Sister Study; WHI-CT = Women's Health Initiative Clinical Trials; WHI-OS = Women's Health Initiative Observational Study. Participant numbers were as follows: n = 416 537 for NO_2 and ozone analyses, n = 393 547 for $PM_{2.5}$ analysis.
[a]Analytic population excludes those with missing air pollution, census region, nSES score, race and ethnicity, or educational attainment.
[b]Higher scores represent greater neighborhood deprivation.
[c]Registered nurses are required to have, at minimum, an associate's degree. Therefore, NHS participants who did not report their educational attainment were categorized as having received at least some college.
[d]Educational attainment was not collected by NHSII; participants were assumed to have at least a bachelor's degree.
[e]PMH use excluded hormone use related to the treatment arm in WHI-CT.

diagnosed in the United States in 2025,[1] a 3% reduction would result in 9500 fewer cases. NO_2, which results from combustion processes, is a component of traffic-related air pollution. Although not considered a mutagen, NO_2 may serve as a cancer promoter or as a proxy for other traffic-related chemicals, such as polycyclic aromatic hydrocarbon (PAH) exposure, which are not routinely monitored.[12,45] PAHs can induce inflammation and oxidative stress, and some have demonstrated estrogen agonist or antagonist (i.e., endocrine-disrupting) properties.[7,46]

With more than 2300 ER-/PR- cases, we observed an approximately 14% higher incidence of ER-/PR- tumors per 5-μg/m³ increase in $PM_{2.5}$. Of the few studies that have evaluated $PM_{2.5}$ and breast cancer subtype heterogeneity, results have been largely underpowered,[19–23] including previous analyses in both the NHSII[21] and SIS.[23] In the Multiethnic Cohort, a 26% increase in ER-/PR- breast cancer (case n = 543; 95% CI = 0.83, 1.91) was observed for $PM_{2.5}$, although the estimate was also elevated for ER+ or PR+ cancer (case n = 2413; HR = 1.17, 95% CI = 0.96, 1.42) .[17] Other studies found no associations for either hormone receptor positive or negative tumors,[21–23] and 1 study observed an association only for ER+ tumors.[16]

We also observed a 15% increase in overall breast cancer risk for $PM_{2.5}$ exposure among Midwestern women, which is similar to results from the Black Women's Health Study (18% increase per interquartile range [2.87 μg/m³]).[19] In an earlier analysis in the SIS, an association between $PM_{2.5}$ and invasive breast cancer was observed only for participants living in the West.[23] Although not shown, with the additional cases and new exposure model used in this analysis, results from the SIS were consistent with those from the combined cohorts.

$PM_{2.5}$ is a heterogeneous mixture with demonstrated genotoxic potential,[6] and it has been associated with early markers of breast cancer susceptibility.[47,48] Components include metals (e.g., arsenic, cadmium); PAHs; secondary inorganic aerosols such as nitrate (NO_3^-), ammonium (NH_4^+), and sulfate (SO_4^{2-}); and other compounds and elements.[24] There is some limited evidence suggesting an association between airborne cadmium[49,50] and arsenic[50] and ER-/PR- breast cancers. Further well-powered studies to consider both $PM_{2.5}$ components, including from specific sources such as wildfires,[51] and hormone receptor negative tumors are needed.

Regional variation in the $PM_{2.5}$ component mixture could explain in part the geographic variability observed here. There is evidence that both

TABLE 2— Associations of Spatiotemporally Modeled NO_2, $PM_{2.5}$, and Ozone With Incident Breast Cancer, Overall and by Hormone Receptor Status With Follow-Up Through 2016–2017: United States, 1992–2017

	Overall				ER+ or PR+		ER-/PR-		
	Person-Years	Cases	Crude HR (95% CI)[a]	Adjusted HR (95% CI)[b]	Cases	Adjusted HR (95% CI)[b]	Cases	Adjusted HR (95% CI)[b]	P^c
10-ppb increase in NO_2									
NHS	2 142 217	9 267	1.04 (1.01, 1.08)	1.03 (0.99, 1.07)	5 898	1.00 (0.96, 1.05)	1 053	0.92 (0.83, 1.02)	.14
NHSII	2 654 911	5 772	1.05 (1.01, 1.10)	1.05 (0.99, 1.10)	3 610	1.04 (0.97, 1.10)	737	0.95 (0.83, 1.09)	.24
SIS	479 594	3 044	1.04 (0.95, 1.13)	1.04 (0.95, 1.14)	2 528	1.09 (0.99, 1.20)	387	0.87 (0.67, 1.12)	.09
WHI-CT	937 031	4 879	0.99 (0.94, 1.04)	0.98 (0.93, 1.04)	3 639	0.97 (0.91, 1.03)	541	1.12 (0.97, 1.29)	.06
WHI-OS	1 100 157	5 907	1.02 (0.98, 1.07)	1.03 (0.98, 1.08)	4 410	1.03 (0.98, 1.09)	700	0.93 (0.82, 1.07)	.15
Summary				1.03 (1.00, 1.05)		1.02 (0.99, 1.05)		0.96 (0.89, 1.04)	.15
Q test				0.54		0.29		0.19	
5-$\mu g/m^3$ increase in $PM_{2.5}$									
NHS	1 277 322	5 242	0.98 (0.93, 1.04)	1.00 (0.94, 1.06)	3 523	0.97 (0.90, 1.05)	557	1.06 (0.89, 1.26)	.39
NHSII	1 669 694	4 326	0.96 (0.89, 1.02)	0.97 (0.90, 1.04)	2 869	0.89 (0.82, 0.98)	522	1.25 (1.03, 1.52)	.002
SIS	479 594	3 044	0.97 (0.88, 1.06)	0.96 (0.86, 1.06)	2 528	0.95 (0.84, 1.06)	387	1.06 (0.81, 1.38)	.43
WHI-CT	648 537	3 518	0.98 (0.91, 1.04)	0.99 (0.92, 1.06)	2 780	0.98 (0.91, 1.07)	391	1.16 (0.96, 1.41)	.12
WHI-OS	762 475	4 077	1.00 (0.94, 1.07)	1.02 (0.95, 1.09)	3 183	0.99 (0.91, 1.07)	513	1.16 (0.97, 1.38)	.1
Summary				0.99 (0.96, 1.02)		0.96 (0.93, 1.00)		1.14 (1.04, 1.24)	< .001
Q test				0.85		0.46		0.75	
10-ppb increase in ozone									
NHS	2 142 217	9 267	0.97 (0.91, 1.04)	0.98 (0.92, 1.05)	5 898	1.05 (0.97, 1.14)	1 053	1.10 (0.92, 1.32)	.64
NHSII	2 654 911	5 772	0.96 (0.89, 1.04)	1.00 (0.92, 1.08)	3 610	0.99 (0.89, 1.10)	737	1.27 (1.02, 1.58)	.04
SIS	479 594	3 044	0.93 (0.84, 1.03)	0.93 (0.84, 1.03)	2 528	0.91 (0.81, 1.02)	387	1.05 (0.79, 1.39)	.35
WHI-CT	937 031	4 879	0.99 (0.91, 1.06)	0.99 (0.91, 1.07)	3 639	0.99 (0.90, 1.09)	541	1.02 (0.82, 1.29)	.79
WHI-OS	1 100 157	5 907	0.97 (0.90, 1.04)	0.97 (0.90, 1.04)	4 410	0.94 (0.86, 1.02)	700	1.04 (0.85, 1.28)	.34
Summary				0.98 (0.94, 1.01)		0.98 (0.93, 1.03)		1.10 (1.00, 1.21)	.04
Q test				0.82		0.22		0.67	

Note. CI = confidence interval; ER = estrogen receptor; HR = hazard ratio; HT = hormone therapy; NHS = Nurses' Health Study; NHSII = Nurses' Health Study II; NO_2 = nitrogen dioxide; nSES = neighborhood socioeconomic status; $PM_{2.5}$ = fine particulate matter ≤ 2.5 μ/m^3; ppb = parts per billion; PR = progesterone receptor; SIS = Sister Study; WHI-CT = Women's Health Initiative Clinical Trials; WHI-OS = Women's Health Initiative Observational Study.

[a]Crude model adjusted for age (as a stratifying variable) and calendar month (or calendar year for WHI-CT and WHI-OS).

[b]Adjusted model additionally adjusted for census region (time-varying; Northeast, Midwest, South, West), nSES (continuous), race and ethnicity (Black, Hispanic, non-Hispanic White, Other), educational attainment (high school or less, some college/associate's, bachelor's or higher), HT arm (WHI-CT only: estrogen, estrogen control, estrogen plus progestin, estrogen plus progestin control).

[c]For individual cohort estimates, the *P* value is for the likelihood ratio test comparing models with and without a pollutant × covariate cross-product term; for the summary estimate, the *P* value is the contrast test method *P*-heterogeneity.

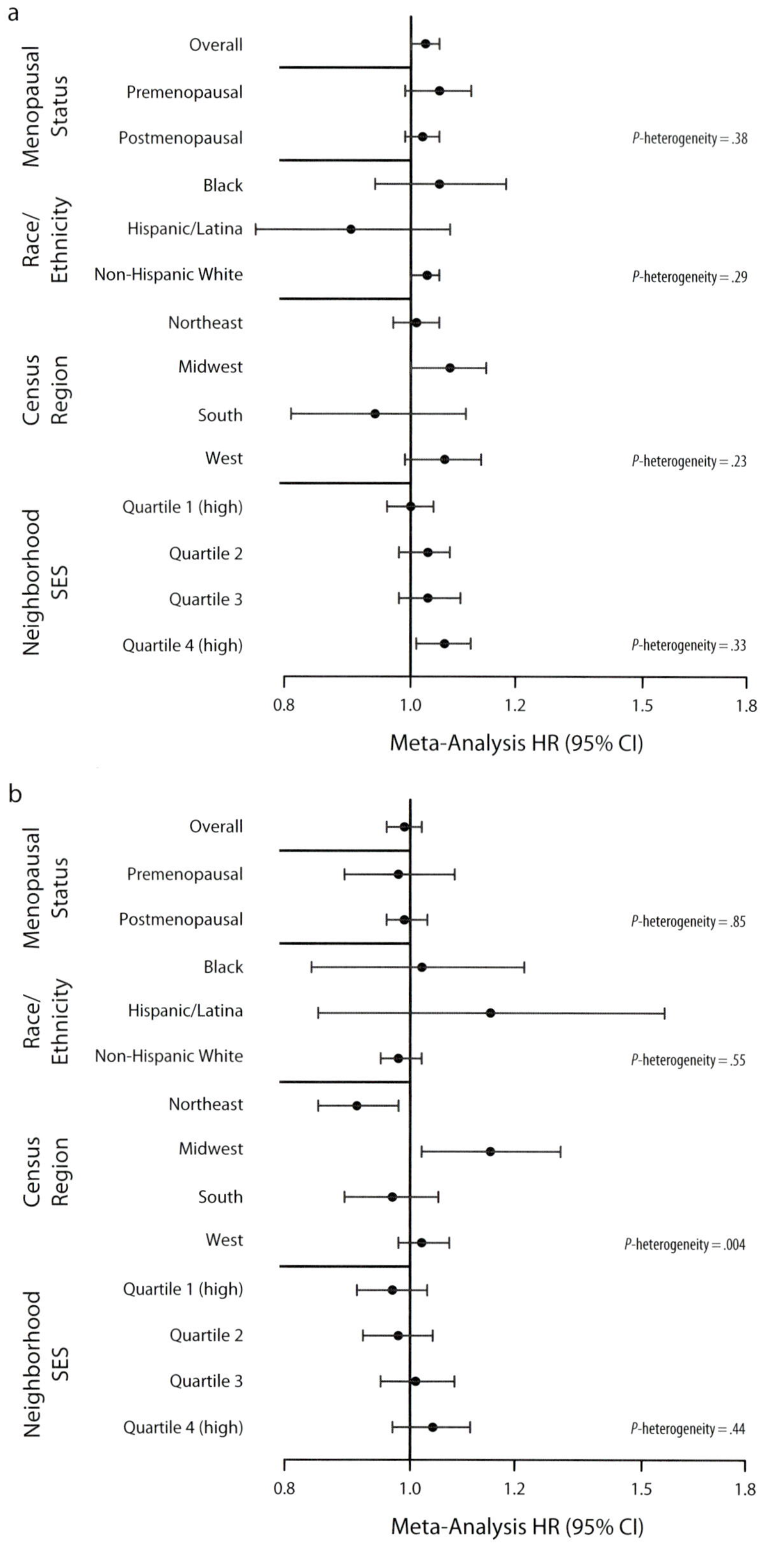

FIGURE 1— Associations Between Incident Breast Cancer and (a) NO_2, (b) $PM_{2.5}$, and (c) Ozone, Overall and Stratified by Potential Modifiers: United States, 1992–2017

Note. CI = confidence interval; HR = hazard ratio; NO_2 = nitrogen dioxide; $PM_{2.5}$ = fine particulate matter ≤ 2.5 μ/m^3; SES = socioeconomic status.

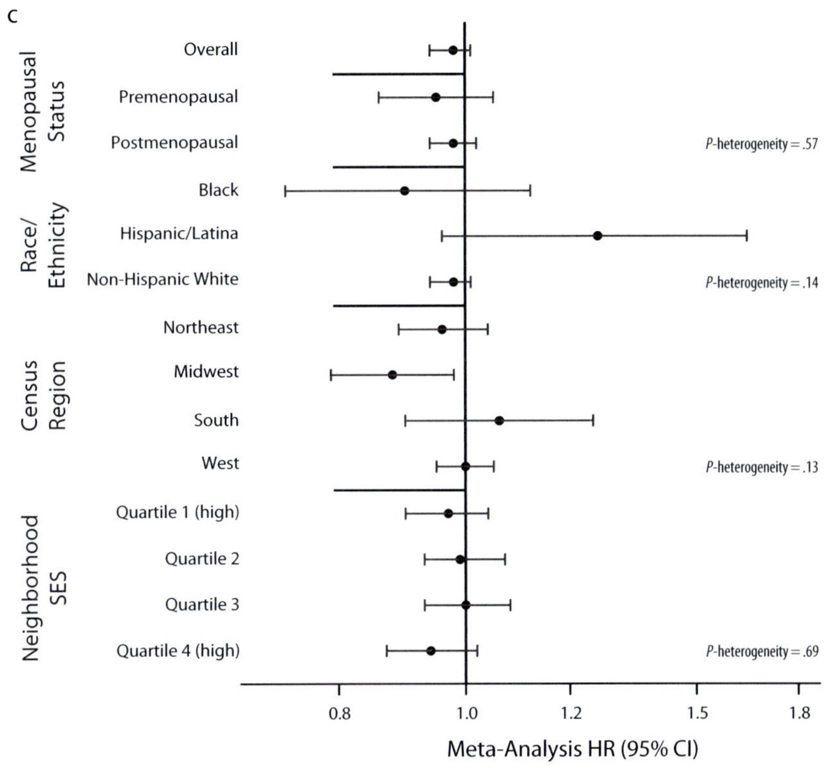

FIGURE 1— Continued

nitrate and ammonium concentrations were higher in the Midwest than in the other census regions in 2000.[52] Both nitrate and ammonium have been associated with higher levels of inflammatory markers[53,54] and with a higher proportion of breast epithelial-to-stroma tissue,[47] both of which are risk factors for breast cancer.[55–57]

Although our observed lack of association for ozone and breast cancer overall is consistent with previously published studies,[10,18,19] our finding of an association between ozone and ER-/PR- breast cancer is novel. Ozone exposure may induce oxidative stress, although the carcinogenicity of ozone remains uncertain.[58]

Our sensitivity analyses, evaluating a 10-year lag and a cumulative average exposure, produced very similar results to those for our overall models, with a small association for NO_2 with overall breast cancer. Given that carcinogenesis is a multistage process, including tumor initiation and tumor promotion,[59] and that associations were not stronger when we explored a 10-year lag, our findings suggest that NO_2 likely acts as a promoter but not an initiator. These findings could also be reflective of a high correlation in exposure across time, which may make it difficult to disentangle the impact of timing of exposure.

This study is the largest analysis of air pollution and breast cancer in the United States, with more than 28 000 cases across 5 cohorts, including the largest number of ER-/PR- cases. However, US air pollution levels are lower than in other populous countries[60]; indeed, the average concentrations observed here are lower than current regulatory guidelines (53 ppb annually).[61] In Asia, where pollution levels are higher, studies of air pollution and breast cancer are limited.[14,62] More research in these areas is needed to determine whether observed associations with breast cancer, assessed at largely low concentrations of air pollutants, extend to higher exposures.[51]

Strengths and Limitations

An important strength of this study is the use of the same high-resolution exposure model across all cohorts[30] for estimating pollutant concentrations. We used the same statistical models with the same covariates in each of the 5 cohorts to improve comparability across studies. Many prior studies, including some of the largest ones,[10,15,16,23] have relied solely on participants' baseline addresses to evaluate air pollution exposure, which likely results in nondifferential misclassification of exposure and potentially biased effect estimates, whereas here we have considered exposure at all addresses throughout follow-up.[63,64] We considered different ways to model time-varying exposure (rolling vs cumulative average), and the results were similar for both, lending support to the robustness of our findings. We also included multiple US-wide cohort studies that provided a wide range of geographic coverage and permitted the evaluation of regional heterogeneity of exposure-effect relationships, which addresses the potential impact of differences in $PM_{2.5}$ composition across US census regions.[16,19,23]

The $PM_{2.5}$ data were not available at the time of recruitment for all of the cohorts because extensive monitoring by the US Environmental Protection Agency (EPA) was not established until 1999.[30] Thus, the follow-up period for the $PM_{2.5}$ analysis, which began in 2001 at the earliest, postdated recruitment by 3 to 8 years for the WHI-CT and WHI-OS, by 12 years for the NHSII, and by 25 years for the NHS. It is therefore possible that more rapidly growing tumors were diagnosed prior to the start of analytic follow-up and were not included here. This could result in a bias toward the null for our findings because of a depletion of susceptibles.[65] However, our positive findings for $PM_{2.5}$ were limited to an association for ER-/PR- tumors, which tend to be more aggressive than ER+ or PR+ tumors.[66] Additionally, exposure data were available for the entire SIS follow-up period because of the later study enrollment dates, and we observed similar results across studies.

We were unable to account for exposures at locations other than the residence, nor did we have information on the time spent outdoors. We anticipate that any misclassification of exposure would be nondifferential with respect to the outcome. We were also not able to capture exposures during several critical windows of susceptibility (e.g., puberty, pregnancy) related to breast development.[67] For example, cigarette smoke, which contains similar constituents to air pollution such as PAHs and heavy metals,[24,68,69] has been associated with breast cancer risk more robustly in women who started smoking as teenagers[70] or before their first pregnancy.[71] This suggests that exposure to $PM_{2.5}$ before first birth may be of particular importance, although this has been challenging to address in current cohorts because of the timing of availability of air pollution exposure models, which largely draw on routine EPA monitoring data. Younger cohorts will be better poised to address the impacts of early life exposure.

Public Health Implications

This is the largest analysis of outdoor air pollution concentrations and breast cancer incidence in the United States and the largest study globally to consider tumor subtypes. Consistent with prior studies, NO_2 was associated with a small increase in breast cancer incidence overall. Higher concentrations of $PM_{2.5}$ and ozone were both associated with ER-/PR- tumors, which have few established risk factors and higher case fatality rates compared with hormone receptor positive tumors. Although our risk estimates were modest, air pollution may contribute to large numbers of breast cancer cases given high incidence rates and ubiquitous exposures. Furthermore, the potential impact of exposure could be greater in countries or regions with higher concentrations of air pollutants. AJPH

ABOUT THE AUTHORS

Alexandra J. White and Dale P. Sandler are with the Epidemiology Branch, National Institute of Environmental Health Sciences, Research Triangle Park, NC. Jaime E. Hart and Francine Laden are with the Department of Environmental Health, Harvard T. H. Chan School of Public Health, Boston, MA. At the time of this work, Sabah M. Quraishi was with the Department of Environmental and Occupational Health Sciences, University of Washington School of Public Health, Seattle, WA. Deborah B. Bookwalter is with Public Health and Epidemiology Practice, Westat, Rockville, MD. Marina R. Sweeney is with Social & Scientific Systems, a DLH Holdings Company, Durham, NC. Elizabeth W. Spalt and Joel D. Kaufman are with the Department of Environmental and Occupational Health Sciences, University of Washington School of Public Health, Seattle. Michael S. Hendryx is with the Department of Environmental and Occupational Health, Indiana University School of Public Health, Bloomington. Veronica L. Irvin is with the College of Health, Oregon State University, Corvallis. Dorothy S. Lane is with the Department of Family, Population, and Preventive Medicine, Stony Brook University, Stony Brook, NY. Aladdin H. Shadyab is with the Herbert Wertheim School of Public Health and Human Longevity Science, University of California San Diego, La Jolla. Shawnita Sealy-Jefferson is with the Division of Epidemiology, College of Public Health, The Ohio State University, Columbus. Marian L. Neuhouser is with the Division of Public Health Sciences, Fred Hutchinson Cancer Center and School of Public Health, University of Washington, Seattle. Eric A. Whitsel is with the Department of Epidemiology, Gillings School of Global Public Health, University of North Carolina, Chapel Hill.

CORRESPONDENCE

Correspondence should be sent to Alexandra J. White, PhD, Epidemiology Branch, National Institute of Environmental Health Sciences, National Institutes of Health, 111 T.W. Alexander Dr, Durham, NC 27709 (e-mail: alexandra.white@nih.gov). Reprints can be ordered at http://www.ajph.org by clicking the "Reprints" link.

PUBLICATION INFORMATION

Full Citation: White AJ, Hart JE, Quraishi SM, et al. Air pollutants and breast cancer risk: a parallel analysis of five large US prospective cohorts. *Am J Public Health*. 2025;115(12):2030–2043.

Acceptance Date: July 11, 2025.

DOI: https://doi.org/10.2105/AJPH.2025.308247

ORCID iDs:

Alexandra J. White https://orcid.org/0000-0003-2455-2945

Sabah M. Quraishi https://orcid.org/0000-0002-3052-3385

Marina R. Sweeney https://orcid.org/0000-0003-3546-2937

Elizabeth W. Spalt https://orcid.org/0009-0008-3470-9954

Veronica L. Irvin https://orcid.org/0000-0001-6337-9108

Shawnita Sealy-Jefferson https://orcid.org/0000-0002-8449-4903

Joel D. Kaufman https://orcid.org/0000-0003-4174-9037

Francine Laden https://orcid.org/0000-0002-2813-2174

Dale P. Sandler https://orcid.org/0000-0002-6776-0018

CONTRIBUTORS

A. J. White conceptualized the study, contributed to resources, supervised the study, wrote the original draft, and contributed to reviewing and editing. J. E. Hart, M. L. Neuhouser, E. A. Whitsel, J. D. Kaufman, and F. Laden contributed to resources and to reviewing and editing. S. M. Quraishi, E. W. Spalt, M. S. Hendryx, V. L. Irvin, D. S. Lane, A. H. Shadyab, and S. Sealy-Jefferson contributed to reviewing and editing. D. B. Bookwalter contributed to formal analysis and methodology and contributed to reviewing and editing. M. R. Sweeney contributed to reviewing and editing. D. P. Sandler conceptualized the study and contributed to resources and to reviewing and editing.

ACKNOWLEDGMENTS

This work was supported by the National Institute of Environmental Health Sciences (NIEHS; R01ES027696, R56ES026528, R01ES023500, P30ES007033, R01ES02588, and P30ES000002); the National Institutes of Health (NIH; 1UG3OD023271-01 and 4UH3OD023271-03); the Intramural Research Program of the NIH at NIEHS (Z01-ES044005 and Z1AES103332); the National Institute of Aging (P01AG055367); the National Heart, Lung, and Blood Institute (R01 HL071759, 75N92021D00001, 75N92021D00002, 75N92021D00003, 75N92021D00004, and 75N92021D00005); the Kresge Foundation (grant no. 243365); the Celia Strickland Austin and G. Kenneth Austin III Endowed Professor in Public Health at Oregon State University (V. L. I.); and the US Environmental Protection Agency (EPA; RD831697, RD-83830001, RD83479601, and R83374101).

We thank Kari Moore for her contributions to creating and compiling the census measures.

Preliminary findings from this work were presented at the American Society of Preventive Oncology annual conference in 2024.

Note. The views expressed in this document are solely those of the authors and do not necessarily represent those of the NIH, NCI, NHLBI, NIA, NIEHS, EPA, or the Kresge Foundation. The funders had no involvement in the study design, data analysis, interpretation, and writing of the manuscript or in the decision to submit the manuscript for publication. This article has not been formally reviewed by the EPA.

CONFLICTS OF INTEREST

The authors declare that they have no conflicts of interest related to this work to disclose.

HUMAN PARTICIPANT PROTECTION

Women's Health Initiative Clinical Trials and Observational Study: all women provided written informed consent at baseline, and the protocol and consent forms were approved by the institutional review board (IRB) for each participating institution. Nurses' Health Study and Nurses' Health Study II: the IRB of Brigham and Women's Hospital approved both studies, and all participants provided informed consent through the return of the initial questionnaire. Sister Study: the IRB of the National Institute of Environmental Health Sciences and the Copernicus Group IRB approved the study; all participants provided written consent.

REFERENCES

1. Siegel RL, Kratzer TB, Giaquinto AN, Sung H, Jemal A. Cancer statistics, 2025. *CA Cancer J Clin.* 2025;75(1):10–45. https://doi.org/10.3322/caac.21871
2. American Cancer Society. Breast cancer risk factors you cannot change. Available at: https://www.cancer.org/cancer/types/breast-cancer/risk-and-prevention/breast-cancer-risk-factors-you-cannot-change.html. Accessed November 29, 2023.
3. American Cancer Society. Lifestyle-related breast cancer risk factors. Available at: https://www.cancer.org/cancer/types/breast-cancer/risk-and-prevention/lifestyle-related-breast-cancer-risk-factors.html. Accessed November 29, 2023.
4. Rodgers KM, Udesky JO, Rudel RA, Brody JG. Environmental chemicals and breast cancer: an updated review of epidemiological literature informed by biological mechanisms. *Environ Res.* 2018;160:152–182. https://doi.org/10.1016/j.envres.2017.08.045
5. Zeinomar N, Oskar S, Kehm RD, Sahebzeda S, Terry MB. Environmental exposures and breast cancer risk in the context of underlying susceptibility: a systematic review of the epidemiological literature. *Environ Res.* 2020;187:109346. https://doi.org/10.1016/j.envres.2020.109346
6. Loomis D, Grosse Y, Lauby-Secretan B, et al. The carcinogenicity of outdoor air pollution. *Lancet Oncol.* 2013;14(13):1262–1263. https://doi.org/10.1016/s1470-2045(13)70487-x
7. Darbre PD. Overview of air pollution and endocrine disorders. *Int J Gen Med.* 2018;11:191–207. https://doi.org/10.2147/IJGM.S102230
8. Amadou A, Praud D, Coudon T, et al. Long-term exposure to nitrogen dioxide air pollution and breast cancer risk: a nested case-control within the French E3N cohort study. *Environ Pollut.* 2023;317:120719. https://doi.org/10.1016/j.envpol.2022.120719
9. Gabet S, Lemarchand C, Guenel P, Slama R. Breast cancer risk in association with atmospheric pollution exposure: a meta-analysis of effect estimates followed by a health impact assessment. *Environ Health Perspect.* 2021;129(5):57012. https://doi.org/10.1289/EHP8419
10. Hvidtfeldt UA, Chen J, Rodopoulou S, et al. Breast cancer incidence in relation to long-term low-level exposure to air pollution in the ELAPSE Pooled Cohort. *Cancer Epidemiol Biomarkers Prev.* 2023;32(1):105–113. https://doi.org/10.1158/1055-9965.EPI-22-0720
11. Poulsen AH, Hvidtfeldt UA, Sorensen M, et al. Air pollution with NO(2), PM(2.5), and elemental carbon in relation to risk of breast cancer- a nationwide case-control study from Denmark. *Environ Res.* 2023;216(pt 3):114740. https://doi.org/10.1016/j.envres.2022.114740
12. Praud D, Deygas F, Amadou A, et al. Traffic-related air pollution and breast cancer risk: a systematic review and meta-analysis of observational studies. *Cancers (Basel).* 2023;15(3):927. https://doi.org/10.3390/cancers15030927
13. Wei W, Wu BJ, Wu Y, Tong ZT, Zhong F, Hu CY. Association between long-term ambient air pollution exposure and the risk of breast cancer: a systematic review and meta-analysis. *Environ Sci Pollut Res Int.* 2021;28(44):63278–63296. https://doi.org/10.1007/s11356-021-14903-5
14. Huang YJ, Lee PH, Chen LC, Lin BC, Lin C, Chan TC. Relationships among green space, ambient fine particulate matter, and cancer incidence in Taiwan: a 16-year retrospective cohort study. *Environ Res.* 2022;212(pt C):113416. https://doi.org/10.1016/j.envres.2022.113416
15. Terre-Torras I, Recalde M, Diaz Y, et al. Air pollution and green spaces in relation to breast cancer risk among pre and postmenopausal women: a mega cohort from Catalonia. *Environ Res.* 2022;214(pt 1):113838. https://doi.org/10.1016/j.envres.2022.113838
16. White AJ, Fisher JA, Sweeney MR, et al. Ambient fine particulate matter and breast cancer incidence in a large prospective US cohort. *J Natl Cancer Inst.* 2024;116(1):53–60. https://doi.org/10.1093/jnci/djad170
17. Wu AH, Wu J, Tseng C, et al. Air pollution and breast cancer incidence in the multiethnic cohort study. *J Clin Oncol.* 2025;43(3):273–284. https://doi.org/10.1200/JCO.24.00418
18. Bai L, Shin S, Burnett RT, et al. Exposure to ambient air pollution and the incidence of lung cancer and breast cancer in the Ontario Population Health and Environment Cohort. *Int J Cancer.* 2020;146(9):2450–2459. https://doi.org/10.1002/ijc.32575
19. White AJ, Gregoire AM, Niehoff NM, et al. Air pollution and breast cancer risk in the Black Women's Health Study. *Environ Res.* 2021;194:110651. https://doi.org/10.1016/j.envres.2020.110651
20. Cheng I, Tseng C, Wu J, et al. Association between ambient air pollution and breast cancer risk: The Multiethnic Cohort Study. *Int J Cancer.* 2020;146(3):699–711. https://doi.org/10.1002/ijc.32308
21. Hart JE, Bertrand KA, DuPre N, et al. Long-term particulate matter exposures during adulthood and risk of breast cancer incidence in the Nurses' Health Study II Prospective Cohort. *Cancer Epidemiol Biomarkers Prev.* 2016;25(8):1274–1276. https://doi.org/10.1158/1055-9965.EPI-16-0246
22. Lemarchand C, Gabet S, Cenee S, Tvardik N, Slama R, Guenel P. Breast cancer risk in relation to ambient concentrations of nitrogen dioxide and particulate matter: results of a population-based case-control study corrected for potential selection bias (the CECILE study). *Environ Int.*

2021;155:106604. https://doi.org/10.1016/j.envint.2021.106604

23. White AJ, Keller JP, Zhao S, Carroll R, Kaufman JD, Sandler DP. Air pollution, clustering of particulate matter components, and breast cancer in the Sister Study: a US-wide cohort. *Environ Health Perspect.* 2019;127(10):107002. https://doi.org/10.1289/EHP5131
24. Bell ML, Dominici F, Ebisu K, Zeger SL, Samet JM. Spatial and temporal variation in PM(2.5) chemical composition in the United States for health effects studies. *Environ Health Perspect.* 2007;115(7):989–995. https://doi.org/10.1289/ehp.9621
25. Bao Y, Bertoia ML, Lenart EB, et al. Origin, methods, and evolution of the three Nurses' Health Studies. *Am J Public Health.* 2016;106(9):1573–1581. https://doi.org/10.2105/AJPH.2016.303338
26. Design of the Women's Health Initiative clinical trial and observational study. The Women's Health Initiative Study Group. *Control Clin Trials.* 1998;19(1):61–109.
27. Anderson GL, Manson J, Wallace R, et al. Implementation of the Women's Health Initiative study design. *Ann Epidemiol.* 2003;13(9 suppl):S5–S17. https://doi.org/10.1016/s1047-2797(03)00043-7
28. Hays J, Hunt JR, Hubbell FA, et al. The Women's Health Initiative recruitment methods and results. *Ann Epidemiol.* 2003;13(9 suppl):S18–S77. https://doi.org/10.1016/s1047-2797(03)00042-5
29. Sandler DP, Hodgson ME, Deming-Halverson SL, et al. The Sister Study Cohort: baseline methods and participant characteristics. *Environ Health Perspect.* 2017;125(12):127003. https://doi.org/10.1289/EHP1923
30. Kirwa K, Szpiro AA, Sheppard L, et al. Fine-scale air pollution models for epidemiologic research: insights from approaches developed in the Multi-Ethnic Study of Atherosclerosis and Air Pollution (MESA Air). *Curr Environ Health Rep.* 2021;8(2):113–126. https://doi.org/10.1007/s40572-021-00310-y
31. Brown JA, Ish JL, Chang C-J, et al. Outdoor air pollution exposure and uterine cancer incidence in the Sister Study. *J Natl Cancer Inst.* 2024;116(6):948–956. https://doi.org/10.1093/jnci/djae031
32. Keller JP, Olives C, Kim SY, et al. A unified spatiotemporal modeling approach for predicting concentrations of multiple air pollutants in the Multi-Ethnic Study of Atherosclerosis and Air Pollution. *Environ Health Perspect.* 2015;123(4):301–309. https://doi.org/10.1289/ehp.1408145
33. Sampson PD, Richards M, Szpiro AA, et al. A regionalized national universal kriging model using partial least squares regression for estimating annual PM(2.5) concentrations in epidemiology. *Atmos Environ (1994).* 2013;75:383–392. https://doi.org/10.1016/j.atmosenv.2013.04.015
34. Medgyesi DN, Fisher JA, Flory AR, et al. Evaluation of a commercial database to estimate residence histories in the Los Angeles Ultrafines Study. *Environ Res.* 2021;197:110986. https://doi.org/10.1016/j.envres.2021.110986
35. US Census Bureau. Decennial Census of Population and Housing Datasets. 2000. Available at: https://www.census.gov/programs-surveys/decennial-census/data/datasets.2000.html. Accessed November 28, 2023.
36. US Census Bureau. American Community Survey 5-Year Data 2009. Available at: https://www.census.gov/data/developers/data-sets/acs-5year/2009.html. Accessed November 28, 2023.
37. US Census Bureau. 2007-2011 American Community Survey 5-Year Estimate. Available at: https://www.census.gov/newsroom/releases/archives/news_conferences/20121203_acs5yr.html. Accessed November 28, 2023.
38. Moore K, Diez Roux AV, Auchincloss A, et al. Home and work neighbourhood environments in relation to body mass index: the Multi-Ethnic Study of Atherosclerosis (MESA). *J Epidemiol Community Health.* 2013;67(10):846–853. https://doi.org/10.1136/jech-2013-202682
39. Liu J, Clark LP, Bechle MJ, et al. Disparities in air pollution exposure in the United States by race/ethnicity and income, 1990-2010. *Environ Health Perspect.* 2021;129(12):127005. https://doi.org/10.1289/EHP8584
40. Hajat A, Hsia C, O'Neill MS. Socioeconomic disparities and air pollution exposure: a global review. *Curr Environ Health Rep.* 2015;2(4):440–450. https://doi.org/10.1007/s40572-015-0069-5
41. Villeneuve PJ, Goldberg MS, Crouse DL, et al. Residential exposure to fine particulate matter air pollution and incident breast cancer in a cohort of Canadian women. *Environ Epidemiol.* 2018;2(3):e021. https://doi.org/10.1097/EE9.0000000000000021
42. Andersen ZJ, Ravnskjær L, Andersen KK, et al. Long-term exposure to fine particulate matter and breast cancer incidence in the Danish Nurse Cohort Study. *Cancer Epidemiol Biomarkers Prev.* 2017;26(3):428–430. https://doi.org/10.1158/1055-9965.EPI-16-0578
43. Brown RH, Ng DK, Steele K, Schweitzer M, Groopman JD. Mobilization of environmental toxicants following bariatric surgery. *Obesity (Silver Spring).* 2019;27(11):1865–1873. https://doi.org/10.1002/oby.22618
44. Wang M, Spiegelman D, Kuchiba A, et al. Statistical methods for studying disease subtype heterogeneity. *Stat Med.* 2016;35(5):782–800. https://doi.org/10.1002/sim.6793
45. White AJ, Bradshaw PT, Hamra GB. Air pollution and breast cancer: a review. *Curr Epidemiol Rep.* 2018;5(2):92–100. https://doi.org/10.1007/s40471-018-0143-2
46. Moorthy B, Chu C, Carlin DJ. Polycyclic aromatic hydrocarbons: from metabolism to lung cancer. *Toxicol Sci.* 2015;145(1):5–15. https://doi.org/10.1093/toxsci/kfv040
47. Ish JL, Abubakar M, Fan S, et al. Outdoor air pollution and histologic composition of normal breast tissue. *Environ Int.* 2023;176:107984. https://doi.org/10.1016/j.envint.2023.107984
48. Niehoff NM, Keil AP, Jones RR, Fan S, Gierach GL, White AJ. Outdoor air pollution and terminal duct lobular involution of the normal breast. *Breast Cancer Res.* 2020;22(1):100. https://doi.org/10.1186/s13058-020-01339-x
49. Kresovich JK, Erdal S, Chen HY, Gann PH, Argos M, Rauscher GH. Metallic air pollutants and breast cancer heterogeneity. *Environ Res.* 2019;177:108639. https://doi.org/10.1016/j.envres.2019.108639
50. Liu R, Nelson DO, Hurley S, Hertz A, Reynolds P. Residential exposure to estrogen disrupting hazardous air pollutants and breast cancer risk: the California Teachers Study. *Epidemiology.* 2015;26(3):365–373. https://doi.org/10.1097/EDE.0000000000000277
51. White AJ. Growing evidence for the role of air pollution in breast cancer development. *J Clin Oncol.* 2025;43(3):244–247. https://doi.org/10.1200/JCO-24-01987
52. Amini H, Danesh-Yazdi M, Di Q, et al. Hyperlocal super-learned $PM_{2.5}$ components across the contiguous US. Preprint posted online December 28, 2022. https://doi.org/10.21203/rs.3.rs-1745433/v2
53. Kjerulff B, Thisted Horsdal H, Kaspersen K, et al. Medium term moderate to low-level air pollution exposure is associated with higher C-reactive protein among healthy Danish blood donors. *Environ Res.* 2023;233:116426. https://doi.org/10.1016/j.envres.2023.116426
54. Liu C, Cai J, Qiao L, et al. The acute effects of fine particulate matter constituents on blood inflammation and coagulation. *Environ Sci Technol.* 2017;51(14):8128–8137. https://doi.org/10.1021/acs.est.7b00312
55. Abubakar M, Fan S, Bowles EA, et al. Relation of quantitative histologic and radiologic breast tissue composition metrics with invasive breast cancer risk. *JNCI Cancer Spectr.* 2021;5(3):pkab015. https://doi.org/10.1093/jncics/pkab015
56. Vellal AD, Sirinukunwattan K, Kensler KH, et al. Deep learning image analysis of benign breast disease to identify subsequent risk of breast cancer. *JNCI Cancer Spectr.* 2021;5(1):pkaa119. https://doi.org/10.1093/jncics/pkaa119
57. Lou MWC, Drummond AE, Swain CTV, et al. Linking physical activity to breast cancer via inflammation, part 2: the effect of inflammation on breast cancer risk. *Cancer Epidemiol Biomarkers Prev.* 2023;32(5):597–605. https://doi.org/10.1158/1055-9965.EPI-22-0929
58. Poma A, Colafarina S, Aruffo E, et al. Effects of ozone exposure on human epithelial adenocarcinoma and normal fibroblasts cells. *PLoS One.* 2017;12(9):e0184519. https://doi.org/10.1371/journal.pone.0184519
59. Hill W, Weeden CE, Swanton C. Tumor promoters and opportunities for molecular cancer prevention. *Cancer Discov.* 2024;14(7):1154–1160. https://doi.org/10.1158/2159-8290.CD-24-0128
60. Cohen AJ, Brauer M, Burnett R, et al. Estimates and 25-year trends of the global burden of disease attributable to ambient air pollution: an analysis of data from the Global Burden of Diseases Study 2015. *Lancet.* 2017;389(10082):1907–1918. https://doi.org/10.1016/S0140-6736(17)30505-6
61. US Environmental Protection Agency. NAAQS Table. Available at: https://www.epa.gov/criteria-air-pollutants/naaqs-table#2. Accessed June 4, 2024.
62. Li YC, Chiou JY, Lin CL, Wei JC, Yeh MH. The association between air pollution level and breast cancer risk in Taiwan. *Medicine (Baltimore).* 2021;100(19):e25637. https://doi.org/10.1097/MD.0000000000025637
63. Hamra GB. Invited commentary: is bias towards the null from nondifferential misclassification wishful thinking? *Am J Epidemiol.* 2022;191(8):1496–1497. https://doi.org/10.1093/aje/kwac091
64. Yland JJ, Wesselink AK, Lash TL, Fox MP. Misconceptions about the direction of bias from nondifferential misclassification. *Am J Epidemiol.* 2022;191(8):1485–1495. https://doi.org/10.1093/aje/kwac035
65. Kehm RD, Lloyd SE, Burke KR, Terry MB. Advancing environmental epidemiologic methods to

confront the cancer burden. *Am J Epidemiol.* 2025;194(1):195–207. https://doi.org/10.1093/aje/kwae175

66. Putti TC, El-Rehim DM, Rakha EA, et al. Estrogen receptor-negative breast carcinomas: a review of morphology and immunophenotypical analysis. *Mod Pathol.* 2005;18(1):26–35. https://doi.org/10.1038/modpathol.3800255
67. Terry MB, Michels KB, Brody JG, et al. Environmental exposures during windows of susceptibility for breast cancer: a framework for prevention research. *Breast Cancer Res.* 2019;21(1):96. https://doi.org/10.1186/s13058-019-1168-2
68. Li Y, Hecht SS. Carcinogenic components of tobacco and tobacco smoke: a 2022 update. *Food Chem Toxicol.* 2022;165:113179. https://doi.org/10.1016/j.fct.2022.113179
69. Schnelle-Kreis J, Sklorz M, Orasche J, Stölzel M, Peters A, Zimmermann R. Semi volatile organic compounds in ambient PM2.5: seasonal trends and daily resolved source contributions. *Environ Sci Technol.* 2007;41(11):3821–3828. https://doi.org/10.1021/es060666e
70. Egan KM, Stampfer MJ, Hunter D, et al. Active and passive smoking in breast cancer: prospective results from the Nurses' Health Study. *Epidemiology.* 2002;13(2):138–145. https://doi.org/10.1097/00001648-200203000-00007
71. Andersen ZJ, Jorgensen JT, Gron R, Brauner EV, Lynge E. Active smoking and risk of breast cancer in a Danish nurse cohort study. *BMC Cancer.* 2017;17(1):556. https://doi.org/10.1186/s12885-017-3546-4

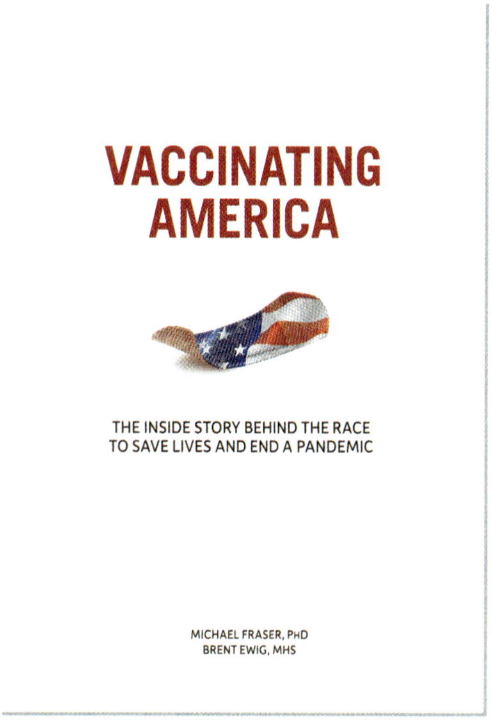

Examining Trends in Substance Use Behaviors Among Women With Primary and Secondary Syphilis: United States, 2018–2023

Julie Rushmore, DVM, PhD, David A. Jackson, MD, MPH, Jeremy A. Grey, PhD, Elizabeth A. Torrone, PhD, MSPH, and Emily R. Learner, PhD, MPH

See also Rowan et al., p. 1960.

Objectives. To examine recent trends in substance use among women with primary and secondary (P&S) syphilis in the United States.

Methods. We reviewed case notifications sent to the Centers for Disease Control and Prevention via the National Notifiable Diseases Surveillance System for women and girls aged 15 years and older with P&S syphilis from 2018 to 2023. We calculated percentages of behaviors associated with substance use during the past year (having sex while intoxicated or high, having sex with a person who injects drugs, or methamphetamine use) by year, race/ethnicity, and region.

Results. Our analysis included 51 209 P&S syphilis cases. Most women and girls (86%) were of reproductive age. Behaviors were stable temporally and regionally, but methamphetamine use was highest in the West (30%). All behaviors were reported more frequently among non-Hispanic White women than non-Hispanic Black or Hispanic women.

Conclusions. Although substance use behaviors were frequently reported, trends were stable, indicating that the proportion of women reporting these behaviors did not scale with recent national increases in P&S syphilis among women. Universal syphilis screening of reproductive age women and girls could be evaluated as an option to reduce syphilis among them along with adverse outcomes, including congenital syphilis. (*Am J Public Health.* 2025;115(12):2044–2052. https://doi.org/10.2105/AJPH.2025.308254)

AJPH December 2025, Vol. 115, No. 12

Reported primary and secondary (P&S) syphilis cases among women and girls in the United States increased nearly 200% in recent years, from 4995 cases in 2018 to 13 763 cases in 2023, with case rates more than doubling during that time frame: from 3.7 cases per 100 000 persons in 2018 to 8.1 cases per 100 000 persons in 2023.[1] In women, P&S syphilis can cause significant morbidity, including sores, rashes, fatigue, and fever. If untreated, syphilis can lead to severe neurologic, ocular, and otic manifestations—including changes in mentation, vision, or hearing—and, in rare cases, death.[2] Additionally, syphilis among pregnant women may lead to congenital syphilis, which can cause adverse pregnancy outcomes, including low birth weight, brain and nerve disorders, miscarriage, stillbirth, or early infant death.[3] In the United States, increases in congenital syphilis mirror increases in syphilis among women,[4] with reported congenital syphilis cases increasing by more than 10 times during 2013 to 2023, from 362 cases in 2013 to 3882 cases in 2023, and case rates rising rapidly from 9.2 cases per 100 000 live births in 2013 to 105.8 cases per 100 000 live births in 2023.[1] Congenital syphilis is preventable through timely testing and appropriate treatment of maternal syphilis during pregnancy.[5]

Although many studies explore factors associated with syphilis transmission among men, particularly among men who have sex with men,[6] less is understood about factors associated with syphilis in the growing epidemic among women in the United States. Understanding factors associated with syphilis among women is critical given the severity of sequelae among women and the potential negative outcomes of congenital syphilis. Furthermore, preventing syphilis among women is an effective way to prevent congenital syphilis.[4] Recent trends suggest that methamphetamine use, having sex while intoxicated or high, and having sex with people who inject drugs are factors that may be associated with recent syphilitic infections among women,[1,7,8] potentially because of links between substance use and sexual behaviors that increase risk of syphilis transmission (e.g., condomless sex, anonymous sex, anal sex, transactional sex).[8,9] Surveillance data also show regional and racial/ethnic differences in P&S syphilis case rates, indicating that factors affecting infection may also vary regionally and by race/ethnicity.[1]

We examined national trends in demographic (i.e., race/ethnicity), behavioral (i.e., substance use, sexual activity), and geographic (i.e., region) factors among US women with P&S syphilis from 2018 to 2023. Understanding the temporal relationships among these factors and P&S syphilis in women can help guide interventions aimed at reducing P&S syphilis among women and, by extension, congenital syphilis.

METHODS

We reviewed P&S syphilis case notifications provided to the Centers for Disease Control and Prevention from 51 jurisdictions (50 states and the District of Columbia) via the National Notifiable Diseases Surveillance System from 2018 to 2023. P&S syphilis case notifications include information about case demography and reported behaviors, including substance use within the past 12 months—which is obtained during local health department case investigations. Our analysis included women and girls aged 15 years or older who were reported as non-Hispanic White, Hispanic/Latina, or non-Hispanic Black/African American; these 3 racial/ethnic groups made up approximately 86% of all cases of P&S syphilis among women from 2018 to 2023. Although our analysis was not limited to women of reproductive age (i.e., 15–44 years), more than 85% of included cases fell within these age parameters.

We calculated the annual percentage of syphilis cases reported with select behaviors associated with substance use during the past 12 months: having sex while intoxicated or high (yes/no), having sex with a person who injects drugs (PWID; yes/no), and using methamphetamine (yes/no). We stratified results by race/ethnicity (Hispanic/Latina, non-Hispanic Black/African American, non-Hispanic White), and US Census region (Midwest, Northeast, South, West). We focused on methamphetamine use because a higher percentage (17%) of women with P&S syphilis used methamphetamine in 2022 than other substances (e.g., cocaine use: 5%, heroin use: 5%, crack use: 3%).[10]

We calculated the percentage of women reporting each behavior separately. We counted a "yes" response for a behavior in the numerator of the percentage. For having sex while intoxicated or high and having sex with a PWID, the denominator included all cases reported with a "yes" or "no" response for the given behavior. We excluded cases with missing or unknown responses from the denominator for that behavior. For methamphetamine use, some jurisdictions may have collected data in a "check all that apply" format for a list of substance use options (e.g., heroin, crack) and may not have routinely reported "no" responses to each individual substance use variable. Therefore, for methamphetamine use, missing data could indicate either (1) the woman reported she did not use that substance, or (2) it is unknown whether the woman used that substance.

Thus, we considered missing responses for this variable to be "no" responses and included them in the denominator if there was an indication that the jurisdiction may have collected the variable in a "check all that apply" manner (e.g., the case had a "yes" response for another substance use variable and did not have a response to any of the other substance use variables). When we imputed "no" responses from missing data in cases for which substance use was presumed to have been collected via a "check all that apply" approach, the number of women who reported methamphetamine use remained unchanged (n = 5854), and the number of women who did not report methamphetamine use increased from n = 15 725 to n = 27 565. This approach of imputing "no" from missing data in these cases resulted in a larger denominator and a lower proportion of methamphetamine use than would excluding all missing data.

Because our objective was to describe trends in reported behaviors among all P&S syphilis cases in women, we visually examined trends in the proportion of behaviors for the 3 racial/ethnic groups by region over time. We did not perform statistical testing or calculate 95% confidence intervals because our surveillance data comprise all available counts of reported syphilis cases among women nationally (i.e., it was not a sample). We provided numerators and denominators for each percentage.

To examine the influence of potential bias introduced by missing behavioral data, we conducted a sensitivity analysis in which we included only P&S syphilis cases among women and girls aged 15 years or older from jurisdictions with high completion (defined as at least 60% completion) of the 3 behaviors of interest: having sex while intoxicated or high, having sex with a PWID, and using methamphetamine. We then calculated the annual percentage of cases engaging in each of these 3 behaviors in the high-completion data set, stratified by race/ethnicity and region, and visually examined whether trends changed meaningfully to assess the robustness of our findings.

We performed all analyses in R, version 4.2.2 (RStudio, Boston, MA).

RESULTS

Our analysis included 51 209 reported cases of P&S syphilis among Hispanic/Latina, non-Hispanic Black/African American, and non-Hispanic White women and girls aged 15 years or older from 2018 to 2023; these cases were reported by 51 unique jurisdictions (Table 1). Most cases (86%) were of reproductive age (i.e., 15–44 years); more specifically, most were aged between 20 and 39 years (69%). Approximately 45% of cases were reported as non-Hispanic White, followed by non-Hispanic Black/African American (37%) and then Hispanic/Latina (18%). The geographic distribution of cases was uneven, with most cases occurring in the South (48%), followed by the West (28%), Midwest (17%), and Northeast (8%). The number of cases increased over time, with 4450 (9%) cases in 2018, and 11 658 (23%) cases in 2023.

Across all study years, we identified 36% of cases among US women as having had sex while intoxicated or high (Table 1; Figure 1). This percentage was relatively stable over time and ranged from 34% to 39%. We observed no meaningful differences when stratifying by region. By contrast, stratification by race/ethnicity demonstrated that women who were non-Hispanic White were more frequently reported as having sex while intoxicated or high (47%) over the study duration than were Hispanic/Latina women (29%) and non-Hispanic Black/African American women (29%).

We identified approximately 12% of cases among US women as having sex with a PWID across all study years (Table 1; Figure 2). The percentage was stable from 2018 to 2023 (range = 10%–15% nationally) and generally consistent across regions. Non-Hispanic White individuals (23%) had the highest indication of having sex with a PWID, followed by Hispanic/Latina individuals (8%) and then non-Hispanic Black/African American individuals (2%).

Among US women with reported cases of syphilis across all study years, we identified 18% as using methamphetamine within the past 12 months (Table 1; Figure 3). These findings were stable from 2018 to 2023, ranging from 16% to 20% nationally. Regionally, the percentage of methamphetamine use was highest in the West at 30% (n = 2546), which was double the percentage in the South (15%; n = 2642) and Midwest (15%; n = 615); the percentage in the Northeast was markedly lower than any other region (2%; n = 51). Additionally, non-Hispanic White individuals had the highest overall indication of methamphetamine use (30%), followed by Hispanic/Latina individuals (16%) and non-Hispanic Black or African American individuals (4%).

Our sensitivity analysis, which limited the analysis to cases from jurisdictions with high completion (i.e., at least 60% completion of the 3 behavioral variables of interest), included 24 761 cases from 24 jurisdictions. Most cases were from Southern jurisdictions (67%; n = 16 540), followed by the Northeastern (15%; n = 3651), Western (13%; n = 3172), and Midwestern (6%; n = 1398) jurisdictions. We did not observe any meaningful differences between trends generated from the full data set versus data generated from high-completion jurisdictions (Figures A–C, available as a supplement to the online version of this article at http://www.ajph.org).

DISCUSSION

We examined US trends of having sex while intoxicated or high, having sex with a PWID, and methamphetamine use among women with P&S syphilis to assess whether regional or demographic factors were associated with key behaviors linked to syphilis transmission. From 2018 to 2023, more than one third of cases (36%) reported having sex while intoxicated or high, and approximately 12% and 18% reported having sex with a PWID or methamphetamine use, respectively. Percentages of all 3 behaviors were stable over time. Additionally, methamphetamine use varied considerably by region, with the highest percentage of methamphetamine use among cases in

TABLE 1— Reported Substance Use and Related Sexual Behaviors Among Women With Primary and Secondary Syphilis, by Demographic Characteristics: United States, 2018–2023

Variable	Total, No. (Column %)[a]	Reported Having Sex While Intoxicated/High, No. (Row %)[b]	Reported Having Sex With a PWID, No. (Row %)[b]	Reported Methamphetamine Use, No. (Row %)[b]
Age, y				
15–19	3509 (7)	663 (26)	86 (4)	153 (6)
20–24	8999 (18)	2198 (34)	457 (7)	659 (11)
25–29	10013 (20)	2447 (37)	739 (12)	1146 (17)
30–34	9167 (18)	2386 (41)	858 (16)	1297 (22)
35–39	7263 (14)	1868 (42)	706 (17)	1110 (24)
40–44	5170 (10)	1169 (38)	432 (15)	752 (24)
45–54	5154 (10)	1092 (35)	346 (12)	607 (19)
55–64	1664 (3)	301 (28)	72 (7)	122 (12)
≥65	270 (1)	21 (12)	2 (1)	8 (5)
Region				
Midwest	8522 (17)	2336 (44)	782 (15)	615 (16)
Northeast	4014 (8)	817 (28)	207 (7)	51 (2)
South	24523 (48)	6516 (36)	1876 (10)	2642 (15)
West	14150 (28)	2476 (36)	833 (16)	2546 (30)
Race/ethnicity				
Hispanic or Latina	9303 (18)	1691 (29)	421 (8)	1098 (16)
Non-Hispanic Black/African American	18759 (37)	3829 (29)	267 (2)	444 (4)
Non-Hispanic White	23147 (45)	6625 (47)	3010 (23)	4312 (30)
Year				
2018	4450 (9)	1077 (34)	373 (13)	578 (18)
2019	5601 (11)	1469 (39)	524 (15)	758 (20)
2020	6810 (13)	1540 (35)	416 (10)	696 (16)
2021	10369 (20)	2305 (35)	610 (10)	1151 (18)
2022	12321 (24)	2932 (38)	902 (12)	1332 (17)
2023	11658 (23)	2822 (37)	873 (12)	1339 (18)

Note. PWID = people who inject drugs. The study size was n = 51 209.
[a]Totals in this column include cases with missing or unknown data.
[b]Percentages were calculated after removing missing or unknown responses from denominators.

the West (30%). We also observed differences in reported substance use behaviors by race/ethnicity. Although the rate of P&S syphilis among non-Hispanic Black women is 3 times the rate among non-Hispanic White women,[1] we found that non-Hispanic White women with P&S syphilis had the highest percentage of all 3 substance use behaviors.

These findings could indicate that other factors, such as systemic racial/ethnic disparities (e.g., barriers to health insurance and access to quality health care) continue to be important determinants of sexually transmitted infection (STI) transmission among non-Hispanic Black women.[9,11] Although data collection and reporting may vary by jurisdiction, our sensitivity analyses showed that excluding jurisdictions with less than 60% completeness for the behavioral data did not affect our overall findings. Taken together, the stable trends over time and across regions suggest that although women and girls with syphilis frequently report substance use behaviors, the proportion of those reporting these behaviors does not appear to scale with recent national increases in P&S syphilis among women.

Testing for and treating syphilis among women is essential for reducing the level of syphilis in this population and for lowering rates of congenital

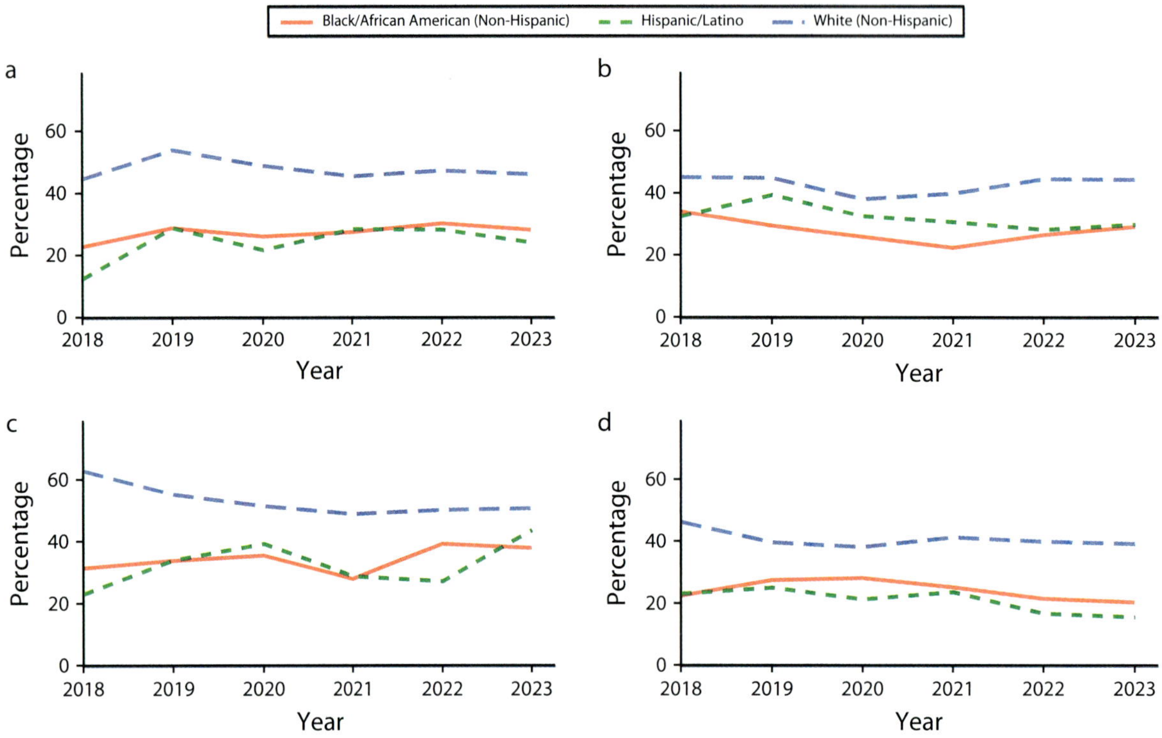

FIGURE 1— Trends of Having Sex While Intoxicated or High Among Women With Primary and Secondary Syphilis, Stratified by Race/Ethnicity and Region (a) South, (b) West, (c) Midwest, and (d) Northeast: United States, 2018–2023

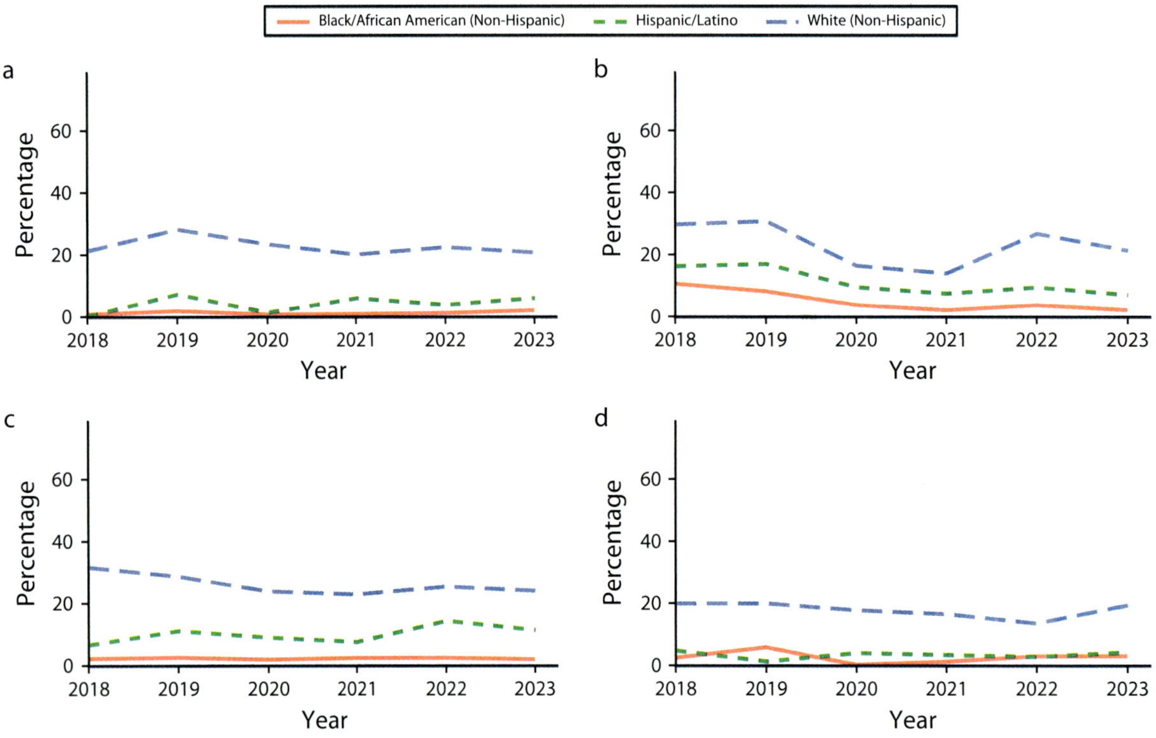

FIGURE 2— Trends of Having Sex With a Person Who Injects Drugs Among Women With Primary and Secondary Syphilis, Stratified by Race/Ethnicity and Region (a) South, (b) West, (c) Midwest, and (d) Northeast: United States, 2018–2023

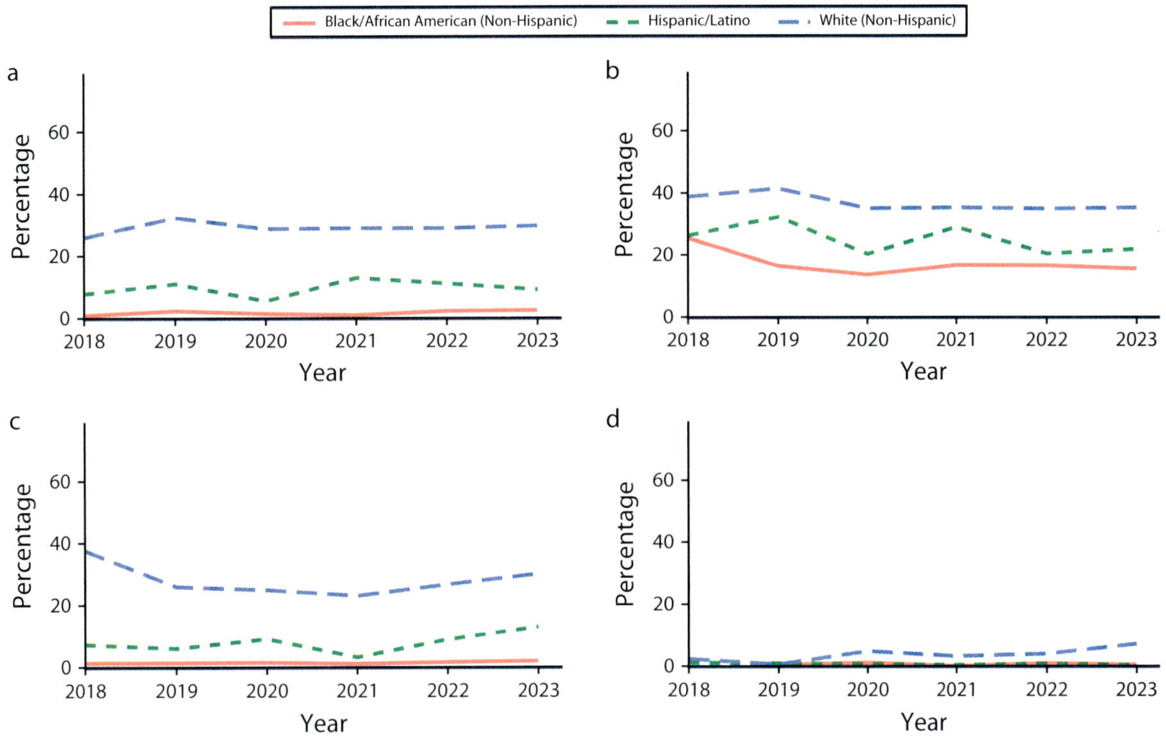

FIGURE 3— Trends of Methamphetamine Use Among Women With Primary and Secondary Syphilis Stratified by Race/Ethnicity and Region (a) South, (b) West, (c) Midwest, and (d) Northeast: United States, 2018–2023

syphilis. Current Centers for Disease Control and Prevention guidelines recommend screening women for syphilis if they have HIV, are pregnant, live in communities with high syphilis prevalence, or have individual risk factors (e.g., substance abuse, STIs during pregnancy, concurrent sexual partners, new sexual partner or partners, sexual partner or partners with an STI).[12,13] There are limitations to basing syphilis screening on individual risk factors.[14] For example, behaviors and exposures may change over time,[7] and for various reasons, women may choose not to disclose substance use or sexual behaviors that put them at risk for STIs.[15,16] Furthermore, many providers do not ask patients for comprehensive substance use and sexual health histories.[17,18] Given the relatively stable temporal and regional trends of P&S syphilis among women and the challenges associated with basing testing on individual risk factors, universal screening of reproductive age women could be evaluated as an option to help reduce syphilis among girls and women and lower rates of congenital syphilis.

Potential barriers to universal syphilis screening mirror those for HIV screening programs: time limitations, insufficient training, low patient acceptance, and follow-up care concerns.[19] Pilot programs of universal (opt-out) syphilis screening have identified, and successfully engaged in care, patients with active syphilis that would not have been screened based on individual risk factors alone.[20,21] Unlike HIV, which has extensive cost analyses of different screening approaches, the cost-effectiveness of universal screening for syphilis remains an open question.[20] Where feasible, syphilis screening programs could be linked to established universal HIV screening programs, tapping into existing infrastructure to reduce costs while maximizing feasibility and patient and provider acceptance.[21]

Women, and particularly women who use substances, may experience unique vulnerabilities to syphilitic infection and challenges to prevention. From 2018 to 2023, more than one third of women with P&S syphilis reported engaging in having sex while intoxicated or high, and 8% reported exchanging sex for money or drugs during the past year.[1] Substance use among female sex workers has been linked to increased workplace violence, condomless sex, and HIV infection.[22,23] Additionally, fear of criminal prosecution for exchanging sex or drug use has led many female sex workers to engage in riskier exchanges, increasing their vulnerabilities to violence, HIV, and STIs.[24–27]

AJPH December 2025, Vol. 115, No. 12

Pregnant women may face additional vulnerabilities and challenges. Recent evidence suggests that certain state-level policy changes may limit access to reproductive health services, potentially leading to missed STI diagnoses and opportunities to prevent congenital syphilis, particularly among women who are economically disadvantaged or who lack health insurance.[28] Additionally, states with policies that define substance use during pregnancy as child abuse and require health care professionals to report this behavior to child protective services often experience reductions and delays in prenatal care.[29] These policies may hinder syphilis testing and treatment among pregnant women who use substances, potentially contributing to higher rates of congenital syphilis.[16] Accordingly, pregnant women who use substances often report that they avoid health care because they are afraid of punitive actions, such as child protective services involvement and loss of child custody.[30] Finally, primary syphilis diagnoses may be missed among women, given that a pelvic examination could be needed to visualize a primary syphilitic lesion.[31]

Our results are consistent with previous work examining syphilis and substance use syndemics among women.[9] Specifically, we found high proportions of methamphetamine use from 2018 to 2023 among non-Hispanic White women with P&S syphilis in the West (37%), South (30%), and Midwest (28%), as well as Hispanic/Latina women with P&S syphilis in the West (25%) and non-Hispanic Black/African American women with P&S syphilis in the West (17%). Collaborations between STI prevention programs and partners that provide substance use disorder services could be important tools in combating this syndemic of STIs and substance use.[7–9] Collaborative interventions could promote STI testing and harm reduction services for overdose prevention at venues such as substance use treatment programs, syringe services programs, carceral settings, and emergency departments.[9] Where feasible, information on sexual contacts could be collected during partner services activities via disease intervention specialists. Additionally, residential substance use disorder treatment programs that offer services such as childcare, reproductive and sexual health care, legal services, and trauma-informed approaches to addiction treatment[32] may help address some of the unique needs of women who are pregnant or have children while they are seeking treatment for substance use.[9]

Limitations

There are several limitations to this study. First, stigma and criminalization fears may lead to underreporting of substance use and sexual behaviors. In particular, the prevalence of substance use may be underreported among pregnant women because of variations in disclosure, especially in areas with punitive policies for pregnant women who use substances.[30] Second, because of imputed "no" responses for relevant missing data (see Methods), our findings may be subject to misclassification error and thus may present overly conservative percentages for methamphetamine use among women with P&S syphilis.

Third, to allow adequate sample sizes after multiple levels of stratification, our analyses excluded 14% of cases not included in the 3 racial/ethnic groups with the largest number of cases. More work is under way to analyze trends for additional populations not presented here. Finally, given the observational nature of surveillance data, we could not determine causality between observed variables and syphilis.

Public Health Implications

Syphilis is a bacterial STI with potentially severe sequelae. Cases of P&S syphilis among women and cases of congenital syphilis have both increased substantially from 2018 to 2023 in the United States. Syphilis among women is both preventable and treatable, and congenital syphilis is preventable through timely screening and treatment of syphilitic infections among pregnant women. Although substance use behaviors were frequently reported, proportions of cases reporting these behaviors remained stable. This may suggest that other factors, such as sexual networks or community transmission levels, play a greater role in determining syphilis levels at the national scale.

Considering these findings and given inherent challenges in individual risk factor–based screening for syphilis, universal screening of reproductive age women could be evaluated as an option to help reduce levels of syphilis among women and congenital syphilis in the United States. Integrating expanded syphilis screening into the existing infrastructure of established universal HIV screening programs could help reduce costs while maximizing feasibility and patient and provider acceptance.[21] Standardizing provider-based sexual health history taking could further inform the impact of expanded screening strategies. AJPH

ABOUT THE AUTHORS

All authors are with the Division of STD Prevention, Centers for Disease Control and Prevention, Atlanta, GA.

CORRESPONDENCE

Correspondence should be sent to Julie Rushmore, 1600 Clifton Rd NE, Mailstop H24-4, Atlanta, GA 30329 (e-mail: jrushmore@cdc.gov). Reprints can be ordered at https://www.ajph.org by clicking the "Reprints" link.

PUBLICATION INFORMATION

Full Citation: Rushmore J, Jackson DA, Grey JA, Torrone EA, Learner ER. Examining trends in substance use behaviors among women with primary and secondary syphilis: United States, 2018–2023. *Am J Public Health*. 2025;115(12):2044–2052.

Acceptance Date: July 15, 2025.

https://doi.org/10.2105/AJPH.2025.308254

ORCID iDs:

Julie Rushmore https://orcid.org/0000-0002-2682-6893

David A. Jackson https://orcid.org/0000-0002-7528-121X

Jeremy A. Grey https://orcid.org/0000-0003-4889-1896

Emily R. Learner https://orcid.org/0000-0003-3778-8631

CONTRIBUTORS

J. Rushmore drafted the article. J. Rushmore, D. A. Jackson, and J. A. Grey analyzed data. All authors contributed substantially to the project design and conceptualization, edited the article, and approved the final version.

ACKNOWLEDGMENTS

We would like to thank surveillance staff in state, local, and territorial sexually transmitted infection programs and public health laboratories.

CONFLICTS OF INTEREST

The authors have no conflicts of interest to disclose.

HUMAN PARTICIPANT PROTECTION

This study used data routinely collected as part of public health surveillance and was therefore not subject to institutional review board approval for human participants' protection.

REFERENCES

1. Centers for Disease Control and Prevention. Sexually transmitted infections (STI) surveillance, 2023. November 12, 2024. Available at: https://www.cdc.gov/sti-statistics/annual/index.html. Accessed August 14, 2025.
2. Centers for Disease Control and Prevention. About syphilis. January 30, 2025. Available at: https://www.cdc.gov/syphilis/about/index.html. Accessed August 14, 2025.
3. Centers for Disease Control and Prevention. About congenital syphilis. January 31, 2025. Available at: https://www.cdc.gov/syphilis/about/about-congenital-syphilis.html. Accessed October 31, 2024.
4. Peterman TA, Su J, Bernstein KT, Weinstock H. Syphilis in the United States: on the rise? Expert *Rev Anti Infect Ther.* 2015;13(2):161–168. https://doi.org/10.1586/14787210.2015.990383
5. Cooper JM, Sánchez PJ. Congenital syphilis. *Semin Perinatol.* 2018;42(3):176–184. https://doi.org/10.1053/j.semperi.2018.02.005
6. Tsuboi M, Evans J, Davies EP, et al. Prevalence of syphilis among men who have sex with men: a global systematic review and meta-analysis from 2000–20. *Lancet Glob Health.* 2021;9(8):e1110–e1118. https://doi.org/10.1016/S2214-109X(21)00221-7
7. Centers for Disease Control and Prevention. Increased methamphetamine, injection drug, and heroin use among women and heterosexual men with primary and secondary syphilis—United States, 2013–2017. *MMWR Morb Mortal Wkly Rep.* 2019;68(6):144–148. https://doi.org/10.15585/mmwr.mm6806a4
8. Copen CE, Brookmeyer KA, Haderxhanaj LT, Hogben M, Torrone EA. Sexual risk behaviors among persons diagnosed with primary and secondary syphilis who reported high-risk substance use: data from the National Notifiable Diseases Surveillance System, 2018. *Sex Transm Dis.* 2022;49(2):99–104. https://doi.org/10.1097/OLQ.0000000000001546
9. Strathdee SA, Bristow CC, Gaines T, Shoptaw S. Collateral damage: a narrative review on epidemics of substance use disorders and their relationships to sexually transmitted infections in the United States. *Sex Transm Dis.* 2021;48(7):466–473. https://doi.org/10.1097/OLQ.0000000000001341
10. Centers for Disease Control and Prevention. Syphilis surveillance supplemental slides. April 28, 2025. Available at: https://www.cdc.gov/sti-statistics/syphilis-supplement/index.html. Accessed August 14, 2025.
11. Cohn T, Harrison CV. A systematic review exploring racial disparities, social determinants of health, and sexually transmitted infections in Black women. *Nurs Womens Health.* 2022;26(2):128–142. https://doi.org/10.1016/j.nwh.2022.01.006
12. Workowski KA, Bachmann LH, Chan PA, et al. Sexually transmitted infections treatment guidelines, 2021. *MMWR Recomm Rep.* 2021;70(4):1–187. https://doi.org/10.15585/mmwr.rr7004a1
13. US Preventive Services Task Force. Syphilis infection in nonpregnant adolescents and adults: screening. September 27, 2022. Available at: https://www.uspreventiveservicestaskforce.org/uspstf/recommendation/syphilis-infection-nonpregnant-adults-adolescents-screening. Accessed June 25, 2025.
14. Kimball AA, Torrone EA, Bernstein KT, et al. Predicting emergence of primary and secondary syphilis among women of reproductive age in US counties. *Sex Transm Dis.* 2022;49(3):177–183. https://doi.org/10.1097/OLQ.0000000000001573
15. Trivedi S, Williams C, Torrone E, Kidd S. National trends and reported risk factors among pregnant women with syphilis in the United States, 2012–2016. *Obstet Gynecol.* 2019;133(1):27–32. https://doi.org/10.1097/AOG.0000000000003000
16. Austin AE, O'Callaghan K, Rushmore J, Cramer R, McDonald R, Learner ER. States with a child abuse policy and mandated reporting policy for substance use during pregnancy have higher rates of congenital syphilis cases—United States, 2018–2022. *Am J Public Health.* In press.
17. Brookmeyer KA, Coor A, Kachur RE, Beltran O, Reno HE, Dittus PJ. Sexual history taking in clinical settings: a narrative review. *Sex Transm Dis.* 2021;48(6):393–402. https://doi.org/10.1097/OLQ.0000000000001319
18. Blevins CE, Anderson BJ, Caviness CM, Herman DS, Stein MD. Emerging adults' discussion of substance use and sexual behavior with providers. *J Health Commun.* 2019;24(2):121–128. https://doi.org/10.1080/10810730.2019.1583700
19. Arbelaez C, Wright EA, Losina E, et al. Emergency provider attitudes and barriers to universal HIV testing in the emergency department. *J Emerg Med.* 2012;42(1):7–14. https://doi.org/10.1016/j.jemermed.2009.07.038
20. Chadwick D, Williams H, Lane C, et al. Universal opt-out syphilis screening in a UK emergency department. *J Infect.* 2025;90(3):106444. https://doi.org/10.1016/j.jinf.2025.106444
21. Stanford KA, Hazra A, Friedman E, et al. Opt-out, routine emergency department syphilis screening as a novel intervention in at-risk populations. *Sex Transm Dis.* 2021;48(5):347–352. https://doi.org/10.1097/OLQ.0000000000001311
22. Wirtz AL, Peryshkina A, Mogilniy V, Beyrer C, Decker MR. Current and recent drug use intensifies sexual and structural HIV risk outcomes among female sex workers in the Russian Federation. *Int J Drug Policy.* 2015;26(8):755–763. https://doi.org/10.1016/j.drugpo.2015.04.017
23. Dunne EM, Dyer TP, Khan MR, Cavanaugh CE, Melnikov A, Latimer WW. HIV prevalence and risk behaviors among African American women who trade sex for drugs versus economic resources. *AIDS Behav.* 2014;18(7):1288–1292. https://doi.org/10.1007/s10461-014-0710-6
24. Wurth MH, Schleifer R, McLemore M, Todrys KW, Amon JJ. Condoms as evidence of prostitution in the United States and the criminalization of sex work. *J Int AIDS Soc.* 2013;16(1):18626. https://doi.org/10.7448/IAS.16.1.18626
25. Blunt D, Wolf A. Erased: the impact of FOSTA-SESTA and the removal of Backpage on sex workers. *Anti-Trafficking Rev.* 2020;(14):117–121. https://doi.org/10.14197/atr.201220148
26. Sherman SG, Nestadt DF, Silberzahn BE, Decker M, Park JN, Footer KH. The role of STIs in police as clients among street-based female sex workers in Baltimore City. *Sex Transm Dis.* 2021;48(1):12–18. https://doi.org/10.1097/OLQ.0000000000001292

27. Decker MR, Crago AL, Chu SK, et al. Human rights violations against sex workers: burden and effect on HIV. *Lancet.* 2015;385(9963):186–199. https://doi.org/10.1016/S0140-6736(14)60800-X
28. Davis KC, Fortino BR, O'Shea NG. Potential consequences of the *Dobbs v Jackson Women's Health Organization* decision. *Psychol Addict Behav.* 2024;38(2):161–166. https://doi.org/10.1037/adb0000986
29. Austin AE, Naumann RB, Simmons E. Association of state child abuse policies and mandated reporting policies with prenatal and postpartum care among women who engaged in substance use during pregnancy. *JAMA Pediatr.* 2022;176(11):1123–1130. https://doi.org/10.1001/jamapediatrics.2022.3396
30. Stone R. Pregnant women and substance use: fear, stigma, and barriers to care. *Health Justice.* 2015;3(1):1–15. https://doi.org/10.1186/s40352-015-0015-5
31. Holmes KK, Sparling PF, Stamm WE, et al., eds. *Sexually Transmitted Diseases.* 4th ed. New York, NY: McGraw-Hill Professional; 2008.
32. Bartholow LAM, Huffman RT. The necessity of a trauma-informed paradigm in substance use disorder services. *J Am Psychiatr Nurses Assoc.* 2023;29(6):470–476. https://doi.org/10.1177/10783903211036496

The Prevalence of Chronic Diseases Among Older Chinese Adults in the Past 2 Decades: A Study Based on the Chinese Longitudinal Healthy Longevity Survey, 2002–2022

Kai Cao, PhD, Qiushi Feng, PhD, Wenxin Tian, PhD, Minhui Liu, PhD, Daisheng Tang, PhD, Taojin Feng, MD, Xinyu Sun, MD, Yi Zeng, PhD, and Zhenglian Wang, PhD

Objectives. To comprehensively analyze the prevalence of chronic diseases (hypertension, lung disease, diabetes, stroke, cancer, and heart disease) among older Chinese people.

Methods. This study utilized data from 5 waves (2002, 2005, 2008, 2018, and 2022) of the Chinese Longitudinal Healthy Longevity Survey. We estimated prevalence rates using Poisson regression and Bayesian models from the DemoRates R-package and weighted according to the China population censuses.

Results. The prevalence of most chronic diseases decreased in the first period and then increased substantially in the second period. Interestingly, the COVID-19 pandemic saw a decrease in the prevalence of most chronic diseases. Notably, hypertension was the most prevalent chronic condition among older adults, with a prevalence rate as high as 45.27% in 2018, and cancer exhibited the most significant increase in prevalence during the second period, with an average annual increase of 11.03%.

Conclusions. Chronic disease prevalence among older Chinese adults exhibited dynamic and complex trends, influenced by socioeconomic factors, health care access, and public health emergencies. These findings highlight the importance of targeted interventions tailored to specific diseases, demographics, and regions. (*Am J Public Health*. 2025;115(12):2053–2061. https://doi.org/10.2105/AJPH.2025.308245)

AJPH December 2025, Vol. 115, No. 12

China's population is aging rapidly. As one of the most populous countries in the world, China faces a significant challenge in managing the escalating demands of health and well-being from its growing older population.[1] Chronic diseases, including lung disease, hypertension, diabetes, stroke, cancer, and heart disease, are the leading causes of death and disease burden among older Chinese adults.[2–4] These diseases not only affect individual quality of life but also place a heavy burden on health care systems and economies.[5,6] Chronic diseases have become a dominant factor affecting the health of the older population.[7] Prevention and management of the onset and progression of chronic diseases nowadays are critical strategies of public health to promote healthy aging and sustainable social development, especially in China.

The surveillance of chronic diseases among older adults has become an important research topic, and it has been shown that the burden of disease in older persons arises mainly from chronic diseases.[6] In China, chronic diseases among older people have become the top health concern among residents.[8] For example, according to the latest Global Burden of Disease estimates for 2021, the number of people aged 65 years and older with diabetes, cancer, chronic respiratory diseases, and cardiovascular diseases accounted for 29.08%, 39.48%, 47.69%, and 56.32% of the overall number of people with these diseases in China, respectively.[9] More worryingly, the available evidence suggests that the burden of chronic diseases in older people is likely to continue to grow.[10]

In China, monitoring the trends of chronic diseases is primarily done through the national system of disease control and prevention, which often relies on administrative data from registration and vital statistics, whereas large-scale chronic disease survey data at the community level are relatively rare.[11] The administrative data may have limitations such that they may not cover community-dwelling patients who have no access to or are not screened by the health system; thus, the survey data are acknowledged in the literature as a good complementary source.[12] Nationwide self-reported social surveys of older adults, in this sense, could contribute to the surveillance of chronic diseases in this regard, especially those covering oldest-old ages, which are often ignored in the current research.

China is undergoing an epidemiological transition.[13] In China, infectious disease mortality has decreased considerably over the last few decades as a result of improved health care, widespread vaccinations, and stronger public health measures.[14] However, the prevalence of chronic diseases is increasing, particularly among the elderly.[15] China has experienced an epidemiological change from infectious to chronic diseases in less time than many other countries, and this transition has escalated at unprecedented speed and scale.[16] At present, chronic diseases have become major threats to the health of Chinese inhabitants, bringing major challenges to the public health system.[5]

With this study, we aimed to examine the prevalence of chronic diseases among older adults aged 65 years and older in China, utilizing data from the 5 waves of the Chinese Longitudinal Healthy Longevity Survey (CLHLS) as well as the census data from 2000, 2010, and 2020. We analyzed the trend of the prevalence of chronic diseases over the past 2 decades, as well as the disparity across the young-old (aged 65–79 years) and oldest-old (aged ≥ 80 years) persons, gender, rural and urban areas, and different regions.

METHODS

We used data from 5 waves of the CLHLS, a nationally representative longitudinal survey of older adults in China. The 2002, 2005, 2008, 2018, and 2022 waves of the survey had 16 064, 15 638, 16 566, 15 874, and 17 078 respondents aged 65 years and older, respectively. The CLHLS employed a multistage, stratified cluster sampling design to achieve national representativeness. It randomly selected half of the counties and cities within 22 of the 31 provinces in mainland China, covering about 85% of the total Chinese population.[17] Since 2008, the study area has covered 23 provinces, with the addition of Hainan Province.[18] In the CLHLS, respondents were asked if they had been diagnosed with the following chronic diseases that are common among older Chinese adults: lung disease, hypertension, diabetes, stroke, cancer, and heart disease (Appendix A, available as a supplement to the online version of this article at https://ajph.org).[5] Although these were self-reported, more than 90% of these chronic diseases had been diagnosed by doctors.[18] To explore the temporal changes in the prevalence of chronic disease, we identified 3 different periods, namely the first period (2002–2008), the second period (2008–2018), and the COVID-19 pandemic period (2018–2022).

We used the DemoRates R-package (version 3.0, Zengyi Population Think Tank, Hangzhou, China) to estimate the single-age rates of chronic diseases separately by gender, rural and urban residence, and geographic regions from the data of the 5 CLHLS waves in 2002, 2005, 2008, 2018, and 2022. These single-age rates were then weighted by the census data of China from 2000, 2010, and 2020 to obtain the national prevalence by age groups, gender, rural and urban residence, and regions (Appendix B, available as a supplement to the online version of this article at https://ajph.org). We then compared the prevalence of chronic diseases in the 3 periods and tested for statistical significance.

RESULTS

We estimated the prevalence of chronic diseases among older adults in China by gender, age group, rural or urban residence, and three regions from 2002 to 2022 (Table A, available as a supplement to the online version of this article at https://ajph.org). We found that the ranking of chronic disease prevalence changed significantly over the past 2 decades. For older Chinese people aged 65 years and older, in 2002, the ranking was lung disease (22.19%), heart disease (18.62%), hypertension (17.70%), stroke (15.69%), diabetes (13.40%), and cancer (11.62%). However, in 2018, the highest prevalence was hypertension (45.27%), followed by heart disease (16.12%). We also observed a gradual decrease in the prevalence of lung disease and a gradual increase in hypertension. Although the prevalence of all chronic diseases decreased during the COVID-19 pandemic, the prevalence of hypertension remained high at 41.16%.

Figure 1 further shows the average annual increases in the prevalence of 6 chronic diseases among older Chinese people over 3 different periods. We found that in the first period (2008 vs 2002), the prevalence of 5 chronic diseases (except hypertension) trended downward. However, in the second period (2018 vs 2008), the prevalence of chronic diseases (except lung disease) trended upward, with cancer having the highest increase. Moreover, in the COVID-19 period (2022 vs 2018), the prevalence of hypertension, heart disease, lung disease, and diabetes showed a downward trend.

Excluding the special period of the COVID-19 pandemic, Figure 2 further shows the single-age average annual increases in the prevalence of chronic diseases among older Chinese adults in the first period (2008 vs 2002) and the second period (2018 vs 2008). In the first period, only the prevalence of hypertension increased by a mean of 5.39% in the total old age group (with a mean increase of 5.55% in the young-old group and 4.80% in the oldest-old group), while all other chronic diseases showed a decreasing trend. The decreases in cancer and diabetes were particularly impressive. In the second period, the prevalence of most chronic diseases increased at each single age, with the highest increase being 15.98%. The prevalence of cancer increased by an average of 11.03% in the total old age group, followed by diabetes at 10.42% and hypertension at 6.44%. Throughout the 2 periods, the gender disparity was not substantial.

Figure 3a illustrates the differences in the prevalence of chronic disease at 3 time points for oldest-old persons relative to young-old persons. In 2002, oldest-old persons had a lower prevalence than young-old persons for all chronic diseases except lung disease. In 2008, the oldest-old persons had a higher prevalence of lung disease and stroke than the young-old persons. In 2018, the prevalence of lung disease, stroke, heart disease, and hypertension was higher in oldest-old persons than in young-old persons. It is noteworthy that hypertension and heart disease ranked highest, both in the young-old and oldest-old persons. Figure 3b presents the gender differences in the prevalence of chronic diseases across the 3 time points. In 2002, women had a higher prevalence than men for all chronic diseases except lung disease. In 2008, relative to 2002, the gender differences increased significantly in the prevalence of lung disease, stroke, cancer, and heart disease, while the difference reversed in the prevalence of stroke and cancer. The gender differences in 2018 were similar to 2008; the prevalence of diabetes, heart disease, and hypertension was higher in women, while the prevalence of lung disease, cancer, and stroke was higher in men.

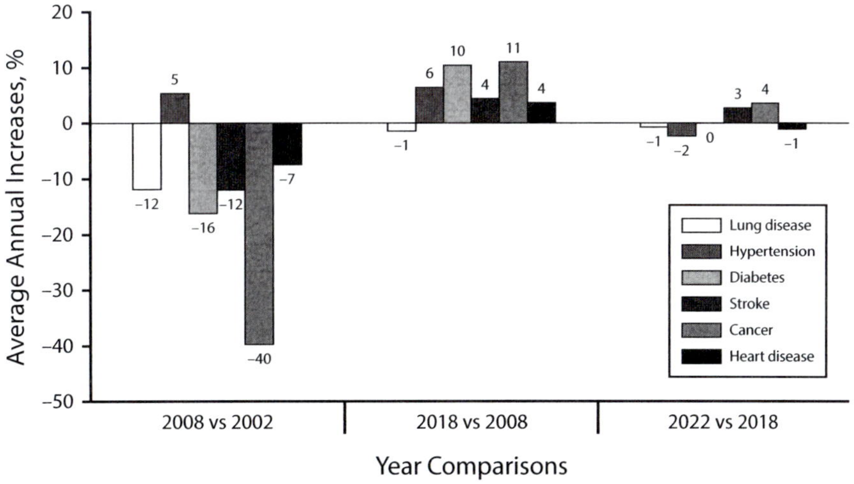

FIGURE 1— Comparisons of the Mean Annual Increases of the Age Structure Standardized Weighted Mean Prevalence Rates of Lung Disease, Hypertension, Diabetes, Stroke, Cancer, and Heart Disease in the Periods of 2002–2008, 2008–2018, and 2018–2022: China

Note. *P* values for period differences were all less than .001.

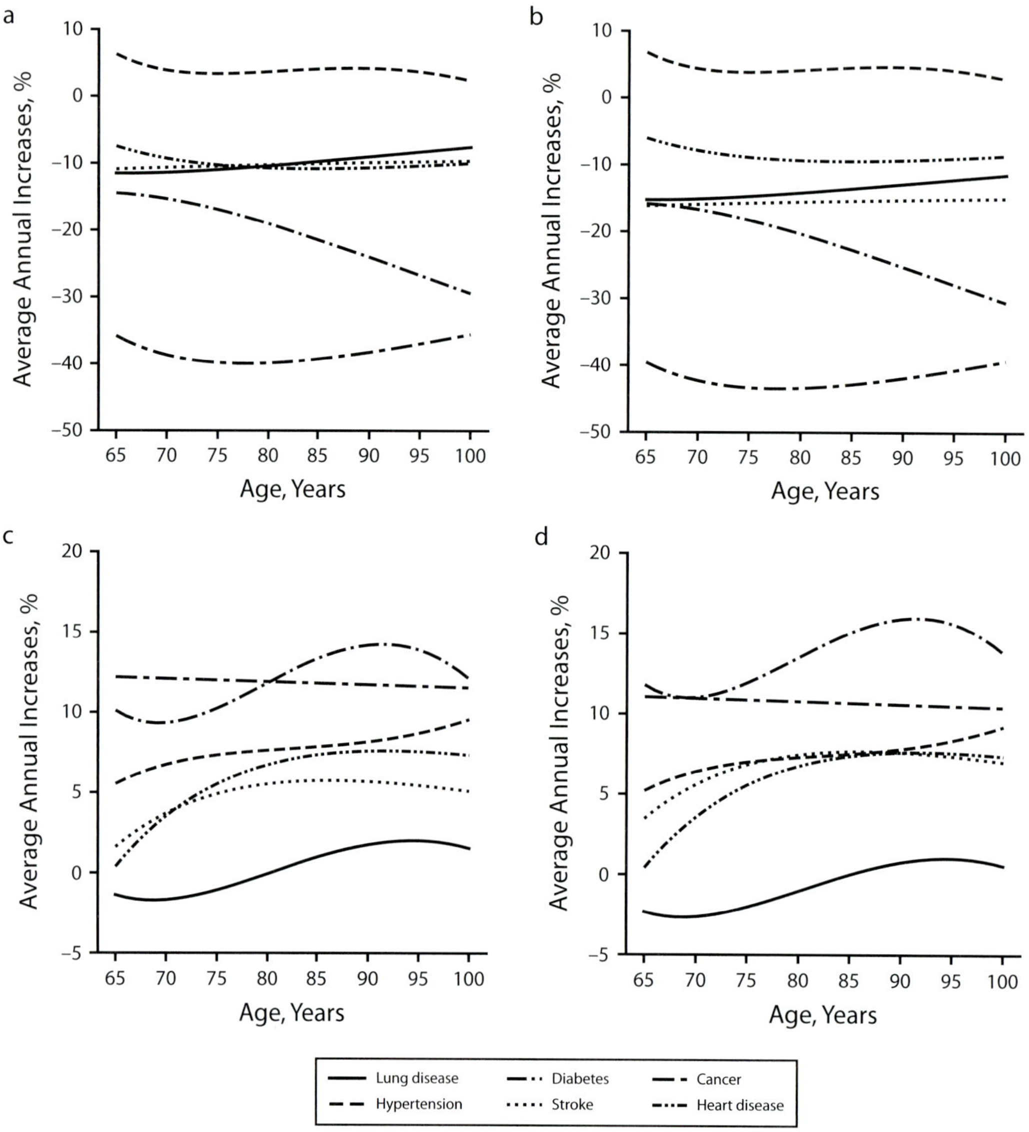

FIGURE 2— Comparisons of the Mean Annual Increases of the Single-Age-Specific Prevalence of Lung Disease, Hypertension, Diabetes, Stroke, Cancer, and Heart Disease for (a) Men in 2008 vs 2002, (b) Women in 2008 vs 2002, (c) Men in 2018 vs 2008, and (d) Women in 2018 vs 2008: China

Figure 3c reflects the rural–urban disparities in the prevalence of 6 chronic diseases across 3 time points. Notably, the prevalence of all chronic diseases was consistently higher in urban areas than in rural areas. For the different chronic diseases, the rural–urban disparity in the prevalence of lung disease showed a gradual increase over time. Conversely, this disparity showed a narrowing trend for hypertension.

Furthermore, the rural–urban disparities for diabetes, stroke, cancer, and heart disease increased dramatically in 2008 compared with 2002. Although these disparities narrowed in 2018, the disparities for diabetes, stroke, and cancer remained higher than those observed in 2002.

Figure 4 displays the regional differences of lung disease, and the regional differences of all chronic diseases are shown in Figures A to C (available as supplements to the online version of this article at https://ajph.org). The eastern regions generally exhibited the lowest prevalence of lung disease, whereas the prevalence of hypertension and cancer was relatively higher. However, it is worth noting that the prevalence of lung disease among oldest-old persons was highest in the eastern regions in 2002. Moreover, the northeastern

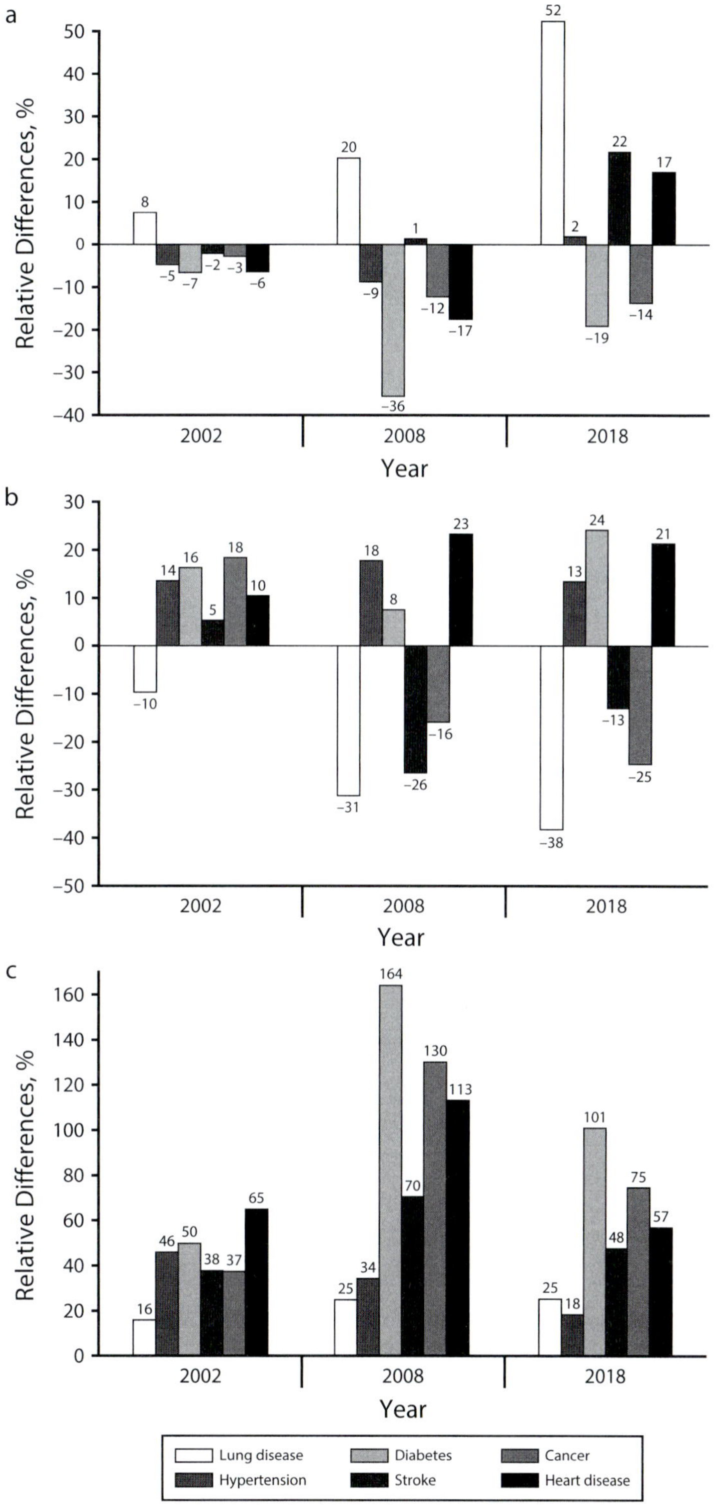

FIGURE 3— **Relative Differences of the Prevalence of Lung Disease, Hypertension, Diabetes, Stroke, Cancer, and Heart Disease in 3 Periods for (a) Oldest Old (Aged ≥ 80 Years) vs Young-Old (65–79 Years), (b) Women vs Men, and (c) Urban vs Rural Residence: China, 2002, 2008, and 2018**

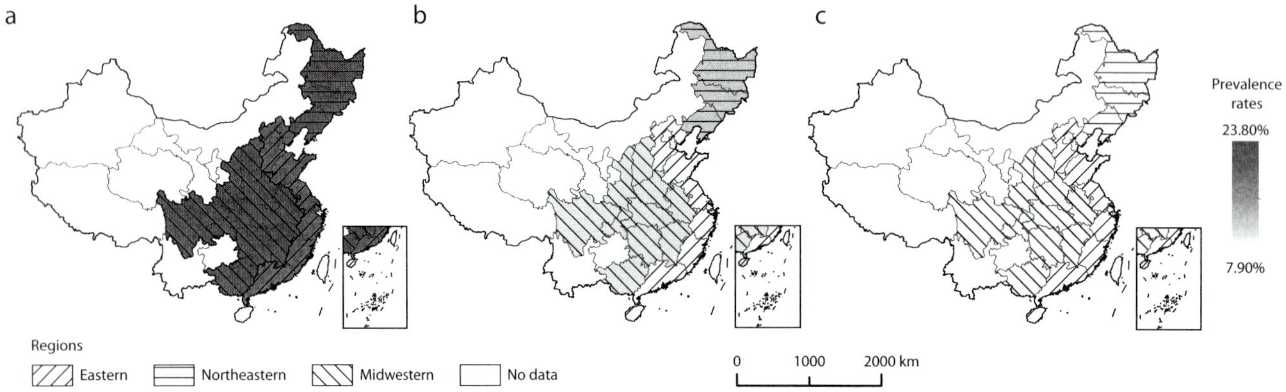

FIGURE 4— Regional Differences of the Prevalence of Lung Disease in (a) 2002, (b) 2008, and (c) 2018: China

Note. Regional differences in the prevalence of all 6 chronic diseases in 3 periods are shown in Figure A (available as a supplement to the online version of this article at https://ajph.org). The situations for the oldest-old (aged ≥ 80 years) groups and the young-old (aged 65–79 years) groups are presented in Figures B and C, respectively (available as supplements to the online version of this article at https://ajph.org). The Chinese Longitudinal Healthy Longevity Survey covered 22 of the 31 provinces in mainland China in 2002. Since 2008, the study area has covered 23 provinces, with the addition of Hainan Province.

regions showed the most pronounced decrease in the prevalence of lung disease but had the highest prevalence of stroke, diabetes, and heart disease. In addition, the midwestern regions had an overall lower prevalence of chronic diseases compared with other regions, with the exception of the highest prevalence of lung disease in 2018.

DISCUSSION

Recently, China has experienced an epidemiological transition. Furthermore, chronic diseases have become a main risk to the health of Chinese inhabitants, especially among the elderly. Meanwhile, China is also experiencing profound economic and social development. Over the past 2 decades, for example, the gross national income in China increased 1.67 times from 2002 to 2008, and 1.85 times from 2008 to 2018,[19] and the urbanization rate of the permanent resident population increased from 39.10% in 2002 to 64.72% in 2022.[20] These macro-level transformations certainly have complicated the ongoing epidemiological transition of China, including the dynamics in the prevalence of chronic disease among older people. These make it more imperative to conduct timely investigations on this topic.

One of our major findings is the significant impact of the COVID-19 pandemic on chronic disease prevalence in China. In 2022, during the pandemic, the prevalence or increase of all chronic diseases was lower than in the prepandemic period of 2018. Specifically, the prevalence of hypertension, heart disease, lung disease, and diabetes decreased, while the growth in prevalence for cancer and stroke decelerated. One possible reason for this stark difference could be that the pandemic-related reallocation of health care resources toward controlling COVID-19, coupled with lockdown measures, may have led to disruptions in chronic disease screening, ultimately contributing to a substantial decrease in diagnosed prevalence.[21]

More importantly, a twisted trend of chronic disease among older adults in China from 2002 to 2018 was revealed. Only the hypertension prevalence showed an upward trend during the first period (2002–2008), while the other 5 chronic diseases decreased in prevalence. Conversely, during the second period (2008–2018), the prevalence of chronic diseases (except lung disease) all increased substantially, among which cancer exhibited the most significant increase (with an average annual increase of 11.03%), followed by diabetes (10.42%). The decrease in the prevalence of most chronic diseases from 2002 to 2008 in China might be ascribed to improvements in health care quality and increased access to health care insurance in this period.[22] The universal health care insurance scheme in China, initiated in 1998, had a major impact on chronic disease prevention and management.[23] In 2008, after a decade of development, it is reasonable to see that chronic diseases were better controlled in older adults with increased access to and quality of health care.

On the other hand, the observed subsequent rise in chronic disease prevalence during the second period (2008–2018) revealed a more complicated scenario. One of the potential contributors is the improvement in educational attainment among older adults during this period, with a 63.9% increase from 2008 to 2018 compared with a mere 1.5% increase from 2002 to 2008. Higher levels of education tend to be associated with higher health literacy and greater health awareness, which may lead to higher rates of chronic disease detection.[24] Meanwhile, higher levels of education are usually associated with higher socioeconomic status and wealthier living conditions, which could lead to behavioral changes associated with a greater risk of chronic diseases, such as sedentary lifestyles and unhealthy diets.[25] Moreover, the overall advancements in medical technology may likely have led to higher screening rates, resulting in more individuals being diagnosed with chronic conditions. Lastly, the better survival rates of older persons with medical advancement in China may also contribute to this reversed trend.

Among all chronic diseases, we confirmed that hypertension was the most prevalent among older adults in China, with a prevalence rate reaching 45.27% in 2018. It is worth noting that the prevalence of hypertension rose by 6.44% from 2008 to 2018, but fell by 2.35% from 2018 to 2022, which was the most significant changing trend. The rising prevalence of hypertension is inextricably linked to lifestyle changes brought by urbanization. Factors such as high salt intake, insufficient exercise, and obesity are all important contributors to hypertension.[26] Moreover, the Outline of the Healthy China 2030 Plan issued in 2016 suggested that full coverage of hypertension management and intervention should be realized, which has also significantly increased the screening rate for hypertension.[27] However, the prevalence of hypertension reversed during the COVID-19 pandemic. A key reason is that management and intervention measures for hypertension have begun to be effective, and the prevalence of hypertension has been under control. Another important reason is the restriction of medical screening and outpatient services, which may result in a "decline" in statistics, because some potential hypertension patients were not detected.[21]

Besides, the prevalence of lung disease among older adults in China has improved significantly. Lung disease is the only disease in this study that consistently decreased over the past 2 decades, with the prevalence of 22.19% and 8.73% in 2002 and 2022, respectively. This positive trend reflects the effectiveness of lung disease intervention and treatment strategies implemented in China, and it may also be related to the reduction of air pollution in China.[28] The overall decreasing trend in lung disease prevalence over the past 2 decades offers compelling evidence of the preventability and controllability of chronic diseases and also reveals the success of lung disease intervention in China.

The study examined differences in the prevalence of chronic diseases between 2 age groups across different periods, clearly suggesting the necessity to pay more attention to the oldest-old in the near future. Notably, the prevalence of lung disease among the oldest-old was 7.52% higher than among the young-old in 2002; however, this gap widened to 20.29% in 2008 and further to 52.39% in 2018. Likewise, the prevalence of stroke among the oldest-old surpassed that of the young-old beginning in 2008, and the same pattern applied to heart disease and hypertension in 2018. Behind these findings could be the fact that the onset of chronic diseases of the young-old had been postponed in China, and even with these diseases, the young-old could survive into older ages in China.[29]

The study also analyzed the gender and rural–urban differences. On the one hand, the prevalence of diabetes and heart disease was higher in women than in men, and this trend continued to grow. This is because women are more likely to suffer from obesity, which is closely linked to diabetes and heart disease.[30] It is also typical that the prevalence of lung disease was higher in men, closely related to the higher probability of smoking among men in China. On the other hand, the prevalence of all 6 chronic diseases was consistently higher in urban areas than rural areas, associated with higher screening rates in cities. Notably, the rural–urban gap in lung disease was increasing consistently from 2002 to 2018, which could be attributable to China's rural–urban disparity in air quality.[31] By contrast, the rural–urban gaps in prevalence of hypertension, diabetes, stroke, cancer, and heart disease were all narrowed in 2018. This reflects reduced rural–urban health inequalities in China, benefiting from continuing efforts in expanding health care service coverage.[15]

We also examined the regional disparities. The prevalence of lung diseases was generally lowest in the eastern regions. In terms of urbanization, the level of urbanization in the eastern regions is generally higher, and more cities have completed industrial transformation, resulting in a lower proportion of heavy industry, better air quality, and a lower baseline of lung disease prevalence.[32] Besides, the most significant downward trend in lung disease prevalence in the northeastern regions could be attributed to the adjustment of industrial structure brought by the revitalization strategy of the old industrial regions implemented in 2003.[33] Factors such as the westward shift of the center of economic gravity and the relative lag in prevention and treatment may have led to the highest prevalence of lung disease in the midwestern regions in 2018.[34] Furthermore, the prevalence of hypertension and cancer was relatively higher in the eastern regions, which is inextricably linked to the fast-paced lifestyle and work pressure, as well as higher screening prompted by better health care. In addition, the prevalence of stroke, diabetes, and heart disease was consistently highest in the northeast regions, which was related to differences in climatic conditions, diet, and rates of obesity.[35]

There are also some limitations in this study. For example, this study focused on only a few major chronic diseases. Although the measure of chronic diseases was self-reported doctor's diagnosis by respondents, changes in diagnosis procedures over time for these chronic diseases were not considered. The sample loss across adjacent waves of the CLHLS attributable to deaths, refusals, and losses to follow up may also bring in bias, though the CLHLS has recruited new participants with identical gender and similar ages to compensate for such sample attrition. In addition, the aim of this study was to report trends in 6 common chronic diseases among older Chinese adults; therefore, the specific factors that might influence these trends have not been examined, but these will be studied in our future research.

This study revealed the important changes in the prevalence of common chronic diseases among older Chinese adults. Significantly, the study provided crucial evidence of China's progress in the prevention and treatment of chronic diseases among older adults, especially lung disease, and meanwhile revealed that the downward trends observed in the prevalence of most chronic diseases in the early 10 years of the new century were reversed recently. In particular, it is imperative to pay more attention to the prevention and control of hypertension, which has become the most prevalent chronic disease among older Chinese individuals. Considering the cost and generalizability of hypertension interventions, diet and exercise interventions are the most basic and effective measures at the individual level.[26] Similarly, these are very significant factors in the prevention and intervention of other chronic diseases as well. At the national level, the government should also achieve full coverage for the treatment of hypertension and diabetes, and strengthen the screening of chronic diseases such as cancer, stroke, and heart disease.[27] Furthermore, by showing the substantial disparities across age groups, genders, rural or urban residences, and regions, this study also emphasized the importance of implementing specified intervention measures targeting various subpopulations. AJPH

ABOUT THE AUTHORS

Kai Cao and Wenxin Tian are with the Key Lab of Geographic Information Science (Ministry of Education), School of Geographic Sciences, East China Normal University, Shanghai, China. Qiushi Feng and Minhui Liu are with the Department of Sociology and Anthropology, Center for Family and Population Research, National University of Singapore, Singapore. Daisheng Tang is with the School of Economics and Management, Beijing Jiaotong University, Beijing, China. Taojin Feng and Xinyu Sun are with the Chinese PLA General Hospital, Beijing, China. Yi Zeng and Zhenglian Wang are with the Population Think Tank Corporation, Zhejiang, China.

CORRESPONDENCE

Correspondence should be sent to Zhenglian Wang or Yi Zeng, Population Think Tank Corporation, 1399 Liangmu Road, Cangqian Sub-district, Yuhang District, Hangzhou, China (e-mail: wangzhenglian8886@163.com) Reprints can be ordered at https://ajph.org by clicking the "Reprints" link.

PUBLICATION INFORMATION

Full Citation: Cao K, Feng Q, Tian W, et al. The prevalence of chronic diseases among older Chinese adults in the past 2 decades: a study based on the Chinese Longitudinal Healthy Longevity Survey, 2002–2022. *Am J Public Health*. 2025;115(12):2053–2061.

Acceptance Date: July 4, 2025.

DOI: https://doi.org/10.2105/AJPH.2025.308245

ORCID iDs:

Kai Cao https://orcid.org/0000-0002-8043-1462

Qiushi Feng https://orcid.org/0000-0002-3572-4442

Daisheng Tang https://orcid.org/0000-0002-4149-7696

CONTRIBUTORS

Z. Wang designed the study, performed the statistical data analysis, and drafted the article. K. Cao, Q. Feng, W. Tian, M. Liu, and D. Tang performed the statistical data analysis and worked with Z. Wang to draft the article. Z. Wang, Y. Zeng, Q. Feng, and all other authors discussed and contributed to the theoretical framework and interpretation of the results and gave final approval of this article. K. Cao and Q. Feng contributed equally to the work as co-first authors.

ACKNOWLEDGMENTS

K. Cao was supported by the National Natural Science Foundation of China (grants 42471462, 13901-41211D-22002). Q. Feng was supported by the MOE Tier 2 grant, Analyses and Projections of Households and Living Arrangements in Six ASEAN Countries (MOE-T2EP40222-0002). Z. Wang was supported by the National Natural Science Foundation of China (grant 72274039).

CONFLICTS OF INTEREST

The authors have no conflicts of interest to declare.

HUMAN PARTICIPANT PROTECTION

Publicly available data sets were used, and the research was therefore exempt from institutional review board review.

REFERENCES

1. Fang EF, Xie C, Schenkel JA, et al. A research agenda for ageing in China in the 21st century: focusing on basic and translational research,

long-term care, policy and social networks. *Ageing Res Rev.* 2020;64:101174. https://doi.org/10.1016/j.arr.2020.101174

2. Liu S, Li Y, Zeng X, et al. Burden of cardiovascular diseases in China, 1990–2016: findings from the 2016 Global Burden of Disease study. *JAMA Cardiol.* 2019;4(4):342–352. https://doi.org/10.1001/jamacardio.2019.0295
3. Chen W, Ma Y, Yu C. Unmet chronic care needs and insufficient nurse staffing to achieve universal health coverage in China: analysis of the Global Burden of Disease Study 2019. *Int J Nurs Stud.* 2023;144:104520. https://doi.org/10.1016/j.ijnurstu.2023.104520
4. Qi J, Li M, Wang L, et al. National and subnational trends in cancer burden in China, 2005–20: an analysis of national mortality surveillance data. *Lancet Public Health.* 2023;8(12):e943–e955. https://doi.org/10.1016/S2468-2667(23)00211-6
5. Zhou M, Wang H, Zeng X, et al. Mortality, morbidity, and risk factors in China and its provinces, 1990–2017: a systematic analysis for the Global Burden of Disease Study 2017. *Lancet.* 2019; 394(10204):1145–1158. https://doi.org/10.1016/S0140-6736(19)30427-1
6. Prince MJ, Wu F, Guo Y, et al. The burden of disease in older people and implications for health policy and practice. *Lancet.* 2015;385(9967): 549–562. https://doi.org/10.1016/S0140-6736(14)61347-7
7. Zeng Y, Lu J, Lei X, Shi X. *Trends and Determinants of Healthy Aging in China.* Beijing, China: Springer; 2022.
8. Shilian H, Jing W, Cui C, Xinchun W. Analysis of epidemiological trends in chronic diseases of Chinese residents. *Aging Med (Milton).* 2020;3(4): 226–233. https://doi.org/10.1002/agm2.12134
9. Institute for Health Metrics and Evaluation. Global Burden of Disease results. Available at: https://vizhub.healthdata.org/gbd-results. Accessed May 30, 2025.
10. Hacker K. The burden of chronic disease. *Mayo Clin Proc Innov Qual Outcomes.* 2024;8(1): 112–119. https://doi.org/10.1016/j.mayocpiqo.2023.08.005
11. Xiong S, Jiang W, Wang Y, et al. Using routinely collected data to determine care cascades of hypertension and type-2 diabetes management in China: a cross-sectional study. *Lancet Reg Health West Pac.* 2024:45:101019. https://doi.org/10.1016/j.lanwpc.2024.101019
12. Liu Y, Xiao S, Yin X, et al. Nation-wide routinely collected health datasets in China: a scoping review. *Public Health Rev.* 2022;43:1605025. https://doi.org/10.3389/phrs.2022.1605025
13. Zhang Y. *Social Development and Social Changes in China: From 1949 to 2019.* Singapore: Springer Nature; 2024.
14. Peng W, Chen S, Chen X, et al. Trends in major non-communicable diseases and related risk factors in China 2002–2019: an analysis of nationally representative survey data. *Lancet Reg Health West Pac.* 2024:43:100809. https://doi.org/10.1016/j.lanwpc.2023.100809
15. Yang G, Wang Y, Zeng Y, et al. Rapid health transition in China, 1990–2010: findings from the Global Burden of Disease Study 2010. *Lancet.* 2013;381(9882):1987–2015. https://doi.org/10.1016/S0140-6736(13)61097-1
16. Yang G, Kong L, Zhao W, et al. Emergence of chronic non-communicable diseases in China. *Lancet.* 2008;372(9650):1697–1705. https://doi.org/10.1016/S0140-6736(08)61366-5
17. Zeng Y, Feng Q, Hesketh T, Christensen K, Vaupel JW. Survival, disabilities in activities of daily living, and physical and cognitive functioning among the oldest-old in China: a cohort study. *Lancet.* 2017;389(10079):1619–1629. https://doi.org/10.1016/S0140-6736(17)30548-2
18. Gu D, Feng Q, Chen H, Zeng Y. Chinese Longitudinal Healthy Longevity Survey (CLHLS). In: *Encyclopedia of Gerontology and Population Aging.* Cham, Switzerland: Springer; 2022:957–970.
19. Kroeber AR. *China's Economy: What Everyone Needs to Know.* New York, NY: Oxford University Press; 2020.
20. National Bureau of Statistics of China, Department of Household Survey. Main Data of the China Household Survey. 2022. Available at: https://www.stats.gov.cn/english. Accessed August 25, 2024.
21. Xiao H, Dai X, Wagenaar BH, et al. The impact of the COVID-19 pandemic on health services utilization in China: time-series analyses for 2016–2020. *Lancet Reg Health West Pac.* 2021; 9:100122. https://doi.org/10.1016/j.lanwpc.2021.100122
22. Meng Q, Tang S. Universal coverage of health care in China: challenges and opportunities. World Health Report, Background Paper, No. 7. World Health Organization. 2010. Available at: https://cdn.who.int/media/docs/default-source/health-financing/whr-2010-background-paper-7.pdf. Accessed September 10, 2024.
23. Yip WC-M, Hsiao WC, Chen W, Hu S, Ma J, Maynard A. Early appraisal of China's huge and complex health-care reforms. *Lancet.* 2012; 379(9818):833–842. https://doi.org/10.1016/S0140-6736(11)61880-1
24. Mei X, Zhong Q, Chen G, Huang Y, Li J. Exploring health literacy in Wuhan, China: a cross-sectional analysis. *BMC Public Health.* 2020;20(1):1417–1419. https://doi.org/10.1186/s12889-020-09520-9
25. Su B, Li D, Xie J, et al. Chronic disease in China: geographic and socioeconomic determinants among persons aged 60 and older. *J Am Med Dir Assoc.* 2023;24(2):206–212.e205. https://doi.org/10.1016/j.jamda.2022.10.002
26. Lu J, Lu Y, Wang X, et al. Prevalence, awareness, treatment, and control of hypertension in China: data from 1.7 million adults in a population-based screening study (China PEACE Million Persons Project). *Lancet.* 2017;390(10112): 2549–2558. https://doi.org/10.1016/S0140-6736(17)32478-9
27. The State Council, The People's Republic of China. The Central Committee of the CPC and the State Council print and issue the outline of the "Healthy China 2030" plan. 2016. Available at: https://www.gov.cn/gongbao/content/2016/content_5133024.htm. Accessed September 2, 2024.
28. Yin P, Brauer M, Cohen AJ, et al. The effect of air pollution on deaths, disease burden, and life expectancy across China and its provinces, 1990–2017: an analysis for the Global Burden of Disease Study 2017. *Lancet Planet Health.* 2020;4(9):e386–e398. https://doi.org/10.1016/S2542-5196(20)30161-3
29. Wang H, Chai K, Du M, et al. Prevalence and incidence of heart failure among urban patients in China: a national population-based analysis. *Circ Heart Fail.* 2021;14(10):e008406. https://doi.org/10.1161/CIRCHEARTFAILURE.121.008406
30. Ong KL, Stafford LK, McLaughlin SA, et al. Global, regional, and national burden of diabetes from 1990 to 2021, with projections of prevalence to 2050: a systematic analysis for the Global Burden of Disease Study 2021. *Lancet.* 2023; 402(10397):203–234. https://doi.org/10.1016/S0140-6736(23)01301-6
31. Wang Y, Wang Y, Xu H, Zhao Y, Marshall JD. Ambient air pollution and socioeconomic status in China. *Environ Health Perspect.* 2022;130(6): 67001. https://doi.org/10.1289/EHP9872
32. Tian W, Cao K, Kwan M-P, Chiu MYL, Chen H. How does urbanization affect the cognitive function among older adults: a geospatial analysis in China. *Health Place.* 2024;88:103259. https://doi.org/10.1016/j.healthplace.2024.103259
33. Fan H, Zhao C, Yang Y. A comprehensive analysis of the spatio-temporal variation of urban air pollution in China during 2014–2018. *Atmos Environ.* 2020;220:117066. https://doi.org/10.1016/j.atmosenv.2019.117066
34. Liang L, Chen M, Luo X, Xian Y. Changes pattern in the population and economic gravity centers since the reform and opening up in China: the widening gaps between the South and North. *J Clean Prod.* 2021;310:127379. https://doi.org/10.1016/j.jclepro.2021.127379
35. Yang J, Yin P, Zhou M, et al. The burden of stroke mortality attributable to cold and hot ambient temperatures: epidemiological evidence from China. *Environ Int.* 2016;92-93:232–238. https://doi.org/10.1016/j.envint.2016.04.001

Temporal Trends in Sexual Identity and Sociodemographic Disparities in Stockholm, Sweden, 2010–2021

Willi Zhang, MD, PhD, Per Tynelius, MSc, Maya B. Mathur, PhD, Matteo Quartagno, PhD, Gunnar Brandén, PhD, Fredrik Liljeros, PhD, and Kyriaki Kosidou, MD, PhD

Objectives. To examine temporal trends in sexual identity and sociodemographic disparities in Sweden after gender-neutral marriage legislation in 2009.

Methods. We analyzed 3 cross-sectional surveys from the Stockholm Public Health Cohort (2010, 2014, 2021) that included 76 083 participants 16 years or older. Weighted Poisson regression was used to estimate associations between sexual identity and sociodemographic covariates. Survey weights and multiple imputation addressed sampling design and nonresponse.

Results. Bisexual identity doubled between 2010 and 2021, from 2.1% (95% confidence interval [CI] = 1.8%, 2.4%) to 4.3% (95% CI = 3.8%, 4.7%) among females and from 1.0% (95% CI = 0.8%, 1.2%) to 1.9% (95% CI = 1.6%, 2.3%) among males. In 2021, 15.1% (95% CI = 12.5%, 17.7%) of Generation Z (1997–2012) females and 6.9% (95% CI = 5.8%, 8.0%) of Millennials (1981–1996) identified as bisexual; the figures for males were 4.2% (95% CI = 2.8%, 5.7%) and 2.4% (95% CI = 1.7%, 3.1%). Bisexual identity was associated with lower income and never-married status, although the strength of the associations decreased over time.

Conclusions. The rise in bisexual identity, particularly among younger generations, likely reflects shifting societal and cultural norms. Income and marital disparities persist but have narrowed.

Public Health Implications. Public health should support bisexual individuals as part of broader efforts to promote equity amid evolving norms. (*Am J Public Health*. 2025;115(12):2062–2071. https://doi.org/10.2105/AJPH.2025.308202)

AJPH December 2025, Vol. 115, No. 12

Sexual identity refers to "personally selected, socially and historically bound labels attached to the perceptions and meanings individuals have about their sexuality," such as lesbian, gay, or bisexual (LGB).[1] Although these identities can be sources of pride and community, lived experiences are shaped by structural, social, and cultural environments, including sociocultural norms and stigma.[2,3] For decades, it has been documented that lesbian, gay, bisexual, transgender, or queer (LGBTQ+) individuals experience various health inequalities relative to their heterosexual peers.[4] Furthermore, numerous studies have highlighted socioeconomic inequalities (e.g., inequalities in income or occupation) affecting LGBTQ+ individuals.[5–10] The minority stress framework posits that these inequalities are often rooted in LGBTQ+ individuals facing multiple levels of stigma[11]: structural (e.g., discriminatory policies and community attitudes), interpersonal (e.g., discrimination and victimization), and individual (e.g., concealment of sexual orientation and internalized stigma).

In recent decades, many countries have seen positive shifts in the legal and social climates surrounding LGBTQ+ communities.[12,13] In Sweden, legal recognition of same-sex unions (termed "registered partnerships") was introduced in 1995.[12] In the late 20th and early 21st centuries, a series of laws were enacted to protect against discrimination and hate crimes based on sexual orientation.[14] In 2009, gender-neutral marriage legislation was adopted, legalizing marriage regardless of sex or gender.[12] Concurrently, public support for same-sex marriage reached 90% in 2015, up from 71% in 2006, and has remained above this level since then.[15] Yet despite these advances, peer stigma and health disparities still affect the lived experiences of many young LGBTQ+ individuals in Sweden.[16]

Over the past decade, Sweden has seen a significant rise in the proportion of people identifying as LGB (there are no comparable data for gender-diverse groups).[17] Similar trends have been observed in the United Kingdom and the United States, particularly among younger age groups.[18–20] Interestingly, recent surveys show that men in the United Kingdom are more likely than women to identify as LGB, whereas the opposite is true in the United States.[18,19]

However, in Sweden, it remains unclear how this rise in LGB identity is distributed across different sociodemographic groups (e.g., different age and sex groups) and how these distributions have evolved over time.[14] Furthermore, although substantial evidence links multilevel stigma to disparities affecting LGBTQ+ populations,[11,21] little is known about how sociodemographic disparities have evolved during the recent decade of increasing LGB identification in Sweden (e.g., have income or partnership/marriage rates increased among LGB communities?). Understanding these trends is crucial not only for identifying vulnerable groups to inform targeted public health interventions but for supporting LGB communities by strengthening visibility and awareness, especially in marginalized settings. In this study, we aimed to analyze temporal trends in sexual identity and sociodemographic disparities in Sweden's Stockholm County between 2010 and 2021, subsequent to the 2009 gender-neutral marriage legislation.

METHODS

In the sections to follow, we present an overview of the methods, with comprehensive details available in the Appendix (available as a supplement to the online version of this article at http://www.ajph.org).

Study Population

The Stockholm Public Health Cohort (SPHC) is a prospective, population-based cohort funded by Region Stockholm for health and risk factor surveillance in Stockholm County.[22] It consists of 5 baseline surveys conducted in 2002, 2006, 2010, 2014, and 2021 (Appendix Figures A and B). Stockholm County is Sweden's most populous region, with approximately 2.5 million residents in 2024 (about 23% of the national population). Area-stratified random samples of approximately 50 000 individuals aged 18 years or older (16 years or older from 2014 onward) were drawn from Statistics Sweden's Total Population Register for each survey, representing roughly 3% of the county population at the time. No incentives were provided for participation.

For simplicity, we use "SPHC-B + year" for baseline surveys. Because data collection on sexual identity began in 2010, we analyzed data from SPHC-B 2010, 2014, and 2021. In total, 55 340 individuals were sampled in 2010, 53 037 in 2014, and 47 885 in 2021, of whom 30 767 (55.6%) in 2010, 22 250 (42.0%) in 2014, and 23 066 (48.2%) in 2021 responded.

Sexual Identity

Sexual identity was measured via postal or web-based self-administered questionnaires in 2010, 2014, and 2021. Participants were asked "How do you define your sexual orientation?" The response options were "heterosexual," "homosexual," "bisexual," and "uncertain" (in 2010) or "none of the above" (in 2014 and 2021).

Sociodemographic Factors

In Sweden, each individual registered as a resident is assigned a unique personal identity number, enabling linkage to Swedish national and regional registers. Data on age, sex (female or male, as assigned at birth or legally registered), country of birth (Sweden, Europe excluding Sweden, or outside Europe), and marital status (currently married [same- or opposite-sex marriage or registered partnership], never married, or other [widowed, separated, or divorced]) were retrieved from the Total Population Register. Years of education (≤ 9, 10–12, or ≥ 13) and individual disposable income (2500 or less, 2501–3500, 3501–4500, or ≥ 4501, in units of 100 Swedish kronor per year adjusted via the Consumer Price Index) were sourced from the Longitudinal Integrated Database for Health Insurance and Labor Market Studies. Data on occupation (manual and field trades, service and support, or expertise and leadership), living status (living alone or with others), and social support (yes [personal support during life challenges] or no) were obtained from the survey questionnaires. All variables were measured in their respective survey years except for education and income in the 2021 survey, which were obtained from 2020 registry data.

Statistical Analyses

Initially, we quantified the proportions or counts of individuals identifying as heterosexual, homosexual, bisexual, or other sexual identities in Stockholm County overall and across various sociodemographic groups (e.g., age, sex). Then we applied weighted Poisson regression models with robust variance estimators to estimate the associations between each sexual identity (as the outcome variable) and sociodemographic covariates (e.g., education, income, marital status).[23] We fit 3 models: a bivariate model; multivariable model 1, including age, sex, and country of birth; and model 2, also including education, income, and marital status (Appendix Table B). The association estimates are presented as proportion ratios (PRs) with 95% confidence intervals (CIs).[23] Our analyses were conducted separately for each survey year to capture potential temporal trends.

To address missing data, we applied calibrated weights to account for unequal selection probabilities and unit nonresponse bias[24] and 2-level multivariate normal imputation for item nonresponse bias.[25] In the 2-level multivariate normal imputation, calibrated weights were stratified to define level 2 clusters (n = 25). We used multivariate normal imputation with the latent normal variable approach to impute missing values in categorical variables.[26] Given the different proportions of missing data, we imputed 80 data sets for SPHC-B 2010, 60 for SPHC-B 2014, and 20 for SPHC-B 2021. As a sensitivity analysis, we conducted complete-case analyses; that is, we restricted the analyses to individuals who had complete data for the respective research questions. We analyzed the data using R version 4.3.1 (R Foundation for Statistical Computing, Vienna, Austria), and the R scripts are publicly available at GitHub (https://github.com/willizhang/Temporal-Trends-in-Sexual-Identity-and-Sociodemographic-Disparities-in-Stockholm-County-2010-to-2021).

RESULTS

Of the 156 262 individuals sampled, 76 083 (48.7%) were included in our analysis (mean age = 51.4 years [SD = 18.4]; 54.9% female [n = 41 739]). Appendix Tables G through I present participant characteristics in SPHC-B 2010, 2014, and 2021, respectively. Briefly, relative to individuals identifying as heterosexual, those identifying as bisexual were more likely to be female, younger, and never married; to lack social support; to work in service and support occupations; and to have lower education and income. Those identifying as homosexual were more likely to be male, younger, and never married; to live alone; to have higher education; and to work outside manual and field trade occupations. Individuals with missing sexual identity data were more likely to be born outside Sweden, have lower education and income, work outside expertise and leadership occupations, live alone, and lack social support than those who reported their identity. In the following sections, we present the key results with a focus on homosexual and bisexual identities from multiple imputation analyses, unless otherwise indicated.

Trends by Sex

Bisexual identity was consistently more common than homosexual identity among females, whereas homosexual identity was more common among males (Figure 1). Bisexual identity doubled from 2010 to 2021, increasing from 2.1% (95% CI = 1.8%, 2.4%) in 2010 and 3.3% (95% CI = 2.8%, 3.7%) in 2014 to 4.3% (95% CI = 3.8%, 4.7%) in 2021 among females and from 1.0% (95% CI = 0.8%, 1.2%) in 2010 and 1.8% (95% CI = 1.4%, 2.2%) in 2014 to 1.9% (95% CI = 1.6%, 2.3%) in 2021 among males. By contrast, homosexual identity remained relatively stable, ranging from 2.2% (95% CI = 1.9%, 2.6%) in 2010 to 2.5% (95% CI = 2.1%, 2.8%) in 2021 among males and from 1.1% (95% CI = 0.9%, 1.4%) to 1.5% (95% CI = 1.2%, 1.7%) among females.

Overall, the percentage of individuals identifying as homosexual or bisexual increased from 3.2% (95% CI = 2.9%, 3.6%) in 2010 and 4.6% (95% CI = 4.0%, 5.1%) in 2014 to 5.8% (95% CI = 5.2%, 6.3%) in 2021 among females and from 3.2% (95% CI = 2.8%, 3.6%) in 2010 and 4.0% (95% CI = 3.4%, 4.6%) in 2014 to 4.4% (95% CI = 3.9%, 4.9%) in 2021 among males. The estimated total populations of individuals identifying as homosexual or bisexual were 51 917 in 2010, 75 322 in 2014, and 92 929 in 2021.

Trends by Age

Bisexual identity decreased with increasing age across all 3 survey years, particularly among females (Figure 2 and Appendix Figure H). From 2010 to 2021, bisexual identity showed the largest increase among females 16 to 29 years of age, rising from 5.6% (95% CI = 4.5%, 6.6%) in 2010 and 8.3% (95% CI = 6.8%, 9.8%) in 2014 to 13.1% (95% CI = 11.2%, 14.9%) in 2021. Among males, it increased from 1.4% (95% CI = 0.7%, 2.0%) in 2010 and 3.3% (95% CI = 2.1%, 4.5%) in 2014 to 3.9% (95% CI = 2.8%, 5.1%) in 2021. Among individuals 30 to 44 years of age, bisexual identity increased from 1.9% (95% CI = 1.4%, 2.4%) in 2010 and 3.4%

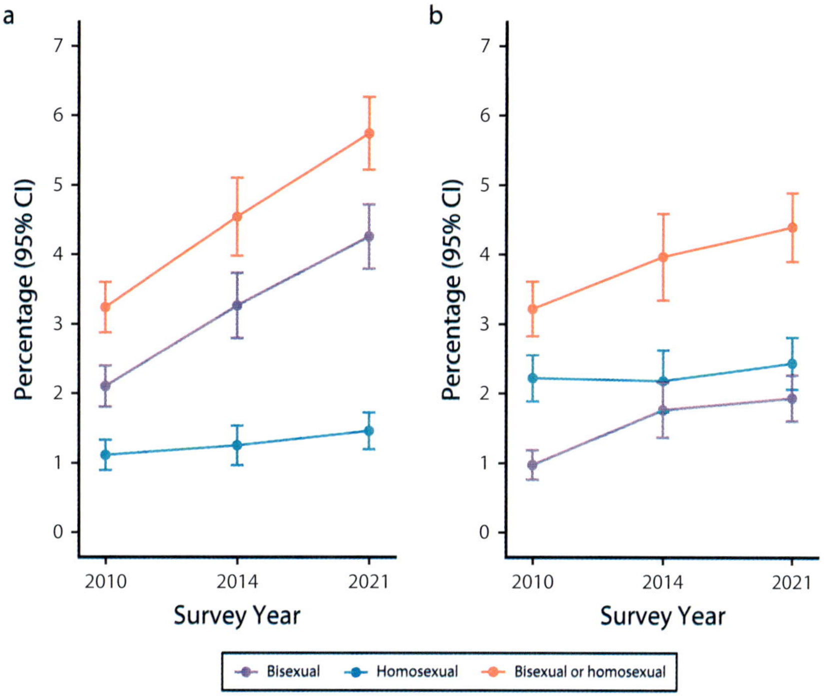

FIGURE 1— Percentages of Homosexual and Bisexual Identities Among (a) Females and (b) Males: Stockholm County, Sweden, 2010–2021

Note. CI = confidence interval. The results were based on multiple imputation analyses incorporating calibrated weights to account for the stratified random sampling design and potential unit nonresponse bias.

(95% CI = 2.6%, 4.3%) in 2014 to 4.8% (95% CI = 3.9%, 5.8%) in 2021 among females and from 0.8% (95% CI = 0.5%, 1.2%) in 2010 and 1.6% (95% CI = 0.9%, 2.2%) in 2014 to 1.9% (95% CI = 1.3%, 2.5%) in 2021 among males.

Overall, the percentage of females 16 to 29 years of age identifying as homosexual or bisexual reached 15.7% (95% CI = 13.7%, 17.7%) in 2021, up from 10.0% (95% CI = 8.4%, 11.7%) in 2014 and 7.0% (95% CI = 5.8%, 8.2%) in 2010. Among males, the percentage rose from 3.3% (95% CI = 2.4%, 4.3%) in 2010 and 6.4% (95% CI = 4.7%, 8.1%) in 2014 to 6.7% (95% CI = 5.2%, 8.2%) in 2021.

Trends by Generation

Bisexual identity increased with younger generations, with the most notable generational differences observed among females in 2021 (Figure 3). By 2021, bisexual identity reached 15.1% (95% CI = 12.5%, 17.7%) among Generation Z (1997–2012) females, up from 9.4% (95% CI = 4.8%, 14.0%) in 2014. Among Generation Z males, it rose slightly from 3.5% (95% CI = 0.8%, 6.3%) in 2014 to 4.2% (95% CI = 2.8%, 5.7%) in 2021. Bisexual identity was 5.6% (95% CI = 4.5%, 6.6%) in 2010, 7.2% (95% CI = 6.0%, 8.5%) in 2014, and 6.9% (95% CI = 5.8%, 8.0%) in 2021 among Millennial (1981–1996) females and 1.4% (95% CI = 0.7%, 2.0%) in 2010, 3.0% (95% CI = 2.0%, 4.0%) in 2014, and 2.4% (95% CI = 1.7%, 3.1%) in 2021 among Millennial males.

By 2021, the percentages of Generation Z and Millennial individuals identifying as homosexual or bisexual were, respectively, 17.6% (95% CI = 14.9%, 20.4%) and 9.3% (95% CI = 8.0%, 10.5%) among females and 6.9% (95% CI = 5.0%, 8.7%) and 6.2% (95% CI = 5.1%, 7.4%) among males. Among Generation X (1965–1980), Baby Boomers (1946–1964), and the Silent Generation (1928–1945), the percentages ranged from 0.8% to 3.1% among females and 1.8% to 3.7% among males.

Associations With Sociodemographic Factors

Across all 3 survey years, bisexual identity was positively associated with being female and younger, having a lower income, and never having been married (Figure 4). The magnitude of the association with younger age consistently increased from 2010 to 2021, whereas

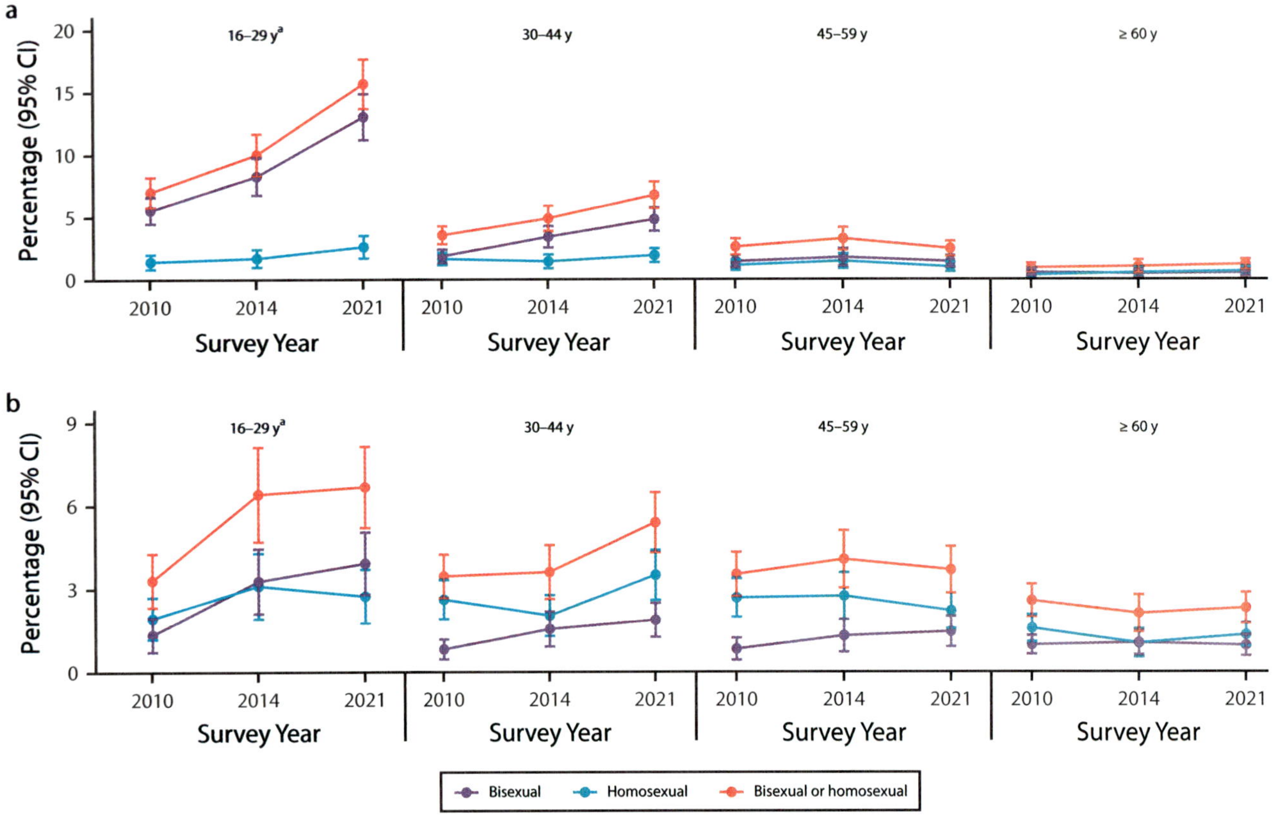

FIGURE 2— Percentages of Homosexual and Bisexual Identities by Age Group Among (a) Females and (b) Males: Stockholm County, Sweden, 2010–2021

Note. CI = confidence interval. The results were based on multiple imputation analyses incorporating calibrated weights to account for the stratified random sampling design and potential unit nonresponse bias.
[a]The minimum age was 18 years in the 2010 survey and 16 years in the 2014 and 2021 surveys.

the associations with lower income (2500 or less vs more than 4500 in units of 100 Swedish kronor per year [model 2]: 2010 PR = 2.46; 95% CI = 1.39, 4.33; 2014 PR = 1.99; 95% CI = 1.34, 2.96; 2020 PR = 1.44; 95% CI = 1.10, 1.88) and never-married status (vs currently married: 2010 PR = 2.00; 95% CI = 1.46, 2.74; 2014 PR = 1.68; 95% CI = 1.18, 2.37; 2021 PR = 1.53; 95% CI = 1.18, 1.99) consistently decreased. Subgroup analyses by sex suggested that the associations with age (Appendix Figure K) and income (complete-case analysis; Appendix Figure L) were more pronounced among females than males.

Homosexual identity was inversely associated with being female and positively associated with living alone (vs living with others: 2010 PR = 1.64; 95% CI = 1.22, 2.22; 2014 PR = 1.75; 95% CI = 1.23, 2.48) and never-married status (2010 PR = 3.23; 95% CI = 2.31, 4.51; 2014 PR = 2.57; 95% CI = 1.75, 3.77; 2021 PR = 2.95; 95% CI = 2.13, 4.08; Appendix Figure J). In addition, homosexual identity was inversely associated with lower education in 2010 (9 years or less vs 13 years or more: PR = 0.46; 95% CI = 0.29, 0.71) and 2020 (PR = 0.56; 95% CI = 0.38, 0.83) and lower income in 2020 (PR = 0.64; 95% CI = 0.46, 0.91).

Subgroup analyses by sex suggested that the association with income was more pronounced among males than females (complete-case analysis; Figure L).

DISCUSSION

Bisexual identity doubled among both females and males in Stockholm County from 2010 to 2021, with the most significant increases observed among females 16 to 29 years of age and Generation Z females. Cross-sectional age and generational differences in bisexual identity were more pronounced among females than males, especially in 2021. Bisexual identity was associated with

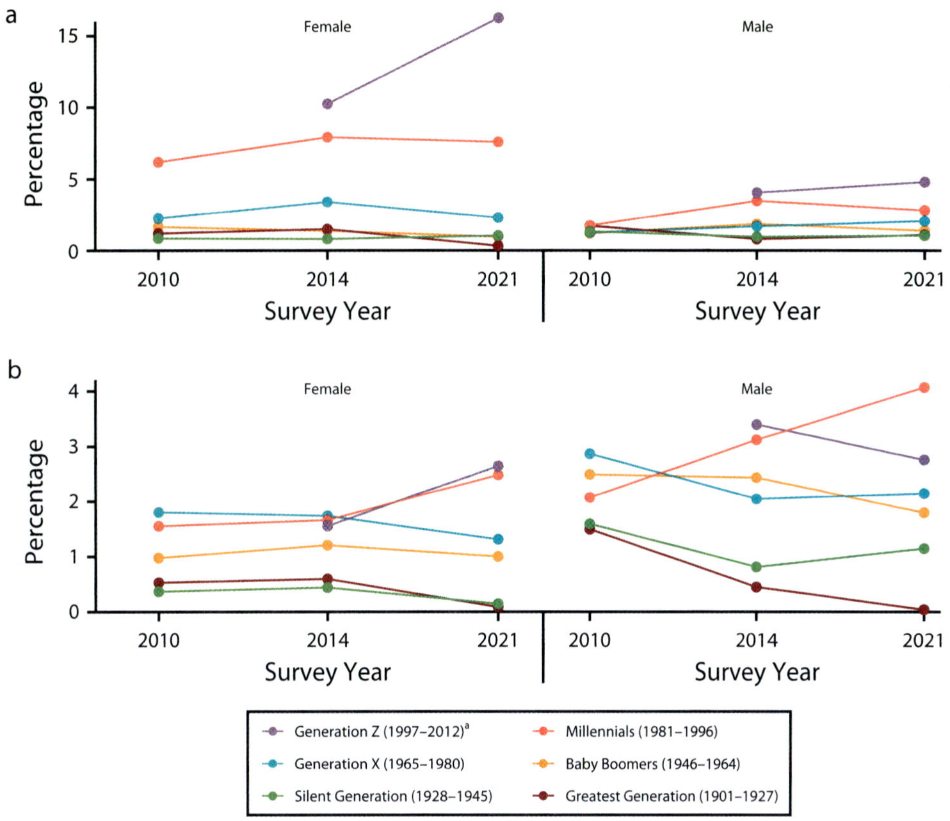

FIGURE 3— Percentages of (a) Bisexual Identity and (b) Homosexual Identity by Sex and by Generation: Stockholm County, Sweden, 2010–2021

Note. The results were based on multiple imputation analyses incorporating calibrated weights to account for the stratified random sampling design and potential unit nonresponse bias.
[a]No participants from Generation Z were included in the 2010 survey.

being female and younger, having a lower income, and never having been married during the study period, although the strength of associations with lower income and never-married status decreased over time. Homosexual identity remained relatively stable over the study period and was associated with being male, having a higher education, having a higher income, living alone, and never having been married in certain years.

Age, Generation, and Period Effects

The concepts of age, generation (or cohort), and period effects are inherently interrelated, making them impossible to distinguish unless certain simplifying assumptions are made.[27] In our study, we found that the percentages of bisexual identity varied across age groups, generations, and time periods. Notably, the age-related differences within each survey year were based on comparisons of individuals of different ages at a single time point. These differences may reflect the effects of being born at different times and having distinct formative sexual identity experiences (i.e., generation effects) rather than or in addition to the effects of growing older (i.e., age effects).[27] Likewise, the differences by generation within the same survey year may be (partly) attributable to age effects and those by time period within the same age or generation group to generation or age effects.

We analyzed follow-up data from approximately 35 000 SPHC participants from 2010 to 2021 and found that bisexual identity increased from 1.1% to 1.6%.[17] The increase was more pronounced among younger individuals: from 3.9% to 5.4% among those 18 to 29 years of age and from 1.6% to 2.8% among those 30 to 44 years of age.

Given the relatively stable social and legal acceptance of LGBTQ+ individuals in Sweden since 2010,[13–15] it might be reasonable to assume that there

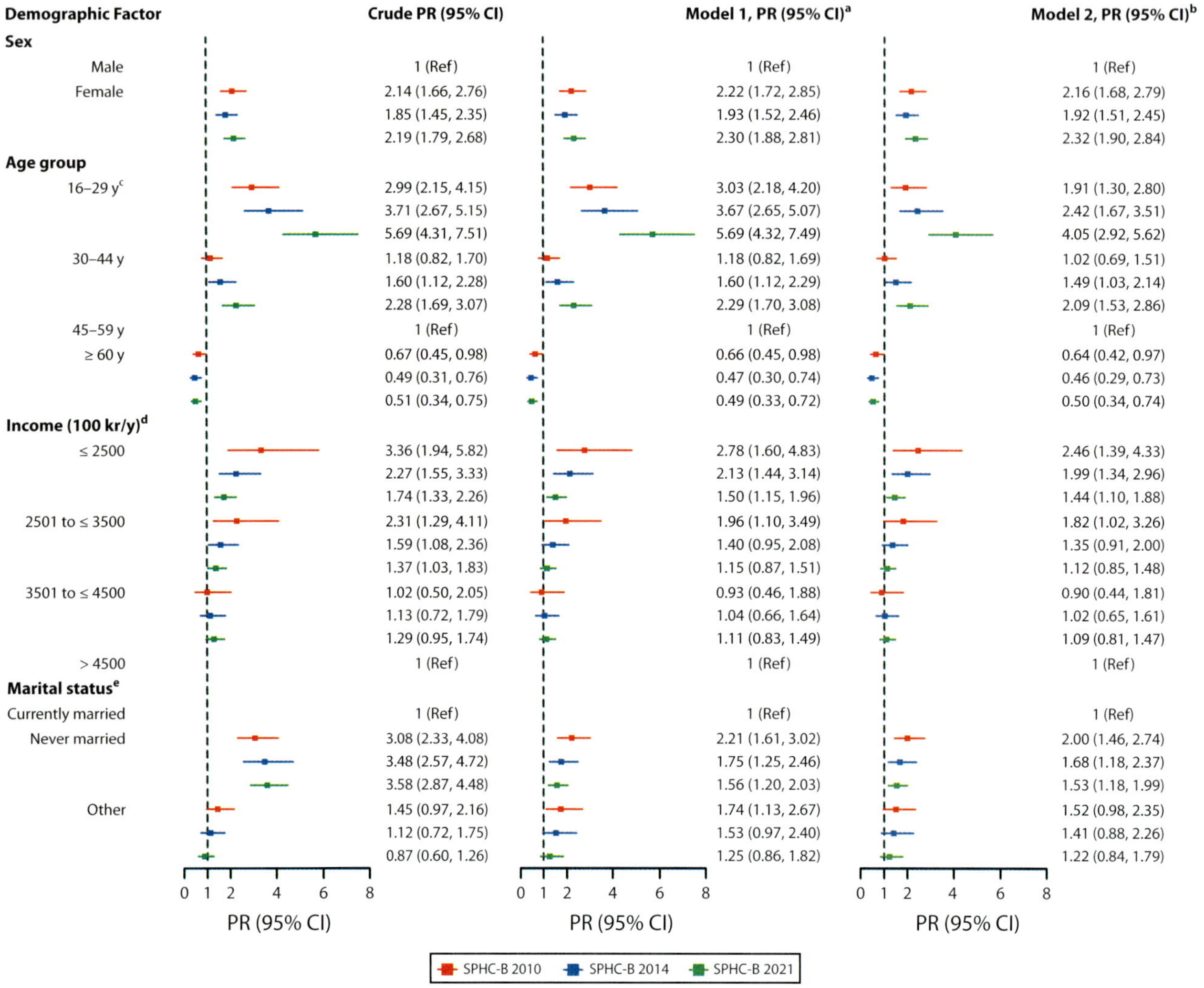

FIGURE 4— Associations Between Bisexual Identity and Sociodemographic Factors in Stockholm County, Sweden, 2010–2021

Note. CI = confidence interval; PR = proportion ratio; SPHC-B = Stockholm Public Health Cohort baseline survey. Models 1 and 2 were multivariable models with bisexual identity as the outcome and different sets of sociodemographic covariates. The results were based on multiple imputation analyses incorporating calibrated weights to account for the stratified random sampling design and potential unit nonresponse bias. Sociodemographic variables were retrieved from Swedish registry data for each survey year (2010, 2014, and 2021) except that income in the 2021 survey was sourced from 2020 registry data.
[a]Model 1 included age, sex, and country of birth.
[b]Model 2 included age, sex, country of birth, education, income, and marital status.
[c]The age range was 18–29 years in the 2010 survey and 16–29 years in the 2014 and 2021 surveys.
[d]Consumer Price Index adjusted income with 2021 as the reference year in units of 100 Swedish kronor per year.
[e]"Currently married" includes same- and opposite-sex marriages and registered partnerships; "other" includes widowed, separated, and divorced.

were minimal period effects on sexual identity during the study period. This assumption may suggest age effects wherein self-identification as bisexual increases as younger individuals grow older.[17] However, this was contradicted by cross-sectional age differences in bisexual identity, which showed a decreasing trend with increasing age, particularly among females. This contradiction appeared to be driven by generation effects in which older generations were much less likely to identify as bisexual than younger generations, thereby reversing the increasing trend associated with age effects.[17] Such reasoning aligns well with our observations that percentages of bisexual identity consistently decreased in older generations, with these generational differences being much more pronounced among females than males.

Interestingly, a similar trend has been observed in the United States, where by 2023 bisexual identity reached 20.7% among Generation Z females (vs 9.0% among Millennials) and 6.9% among Generation Z males (vs 2.5% among Millennials).[19] Taken together, under the assumption of minimal period effects during the study period, our data suggest that generation effects on bisexual identity are more prominent among females than males.

The underlying mechanisms remain unclear. Evolving societal and cultural norms may have shaped the understanding of bisexual identity and facilitated its exploration, adoption, and reporting among younger generations. The sex difference may reflect a higher propensity for bisexual attractions among females,[28] along with greater social acceptance of female bisexuality than male bisexuality.[29] Further research is needed to better understand the underlying factors driving generational differences by sex.

Income Disparity by Sexual Identity

We found that homosexual identity was associated with higher income in 2020, particularly among males. This contrasts with previous reports from Sweden that gay males face an earnings disadvantage relative to heterosexual males, whereas lesbians earn more than heterosexual females.[7,8] Two key differences may explain these findings: the earlier studies[7,8] were conducted in 2003 and 2007, when social acceptance of LGBTQ+ individuals was relatively low,[6,13,15] and they analyzed selected samples, defining homosexual individuals as those living in registered partnerships and heterosexual individuals as those being married. In addition, "gay glass ceilings" (i.e., gay males are less likely than heterosexual males to attain top-level positions and the highest earnings) have been documented in Sweden[8] and elsewhere.[9,10] Further studies are warranted to investigate whether glass ceilings continue to exist in recent years and whether the observed income advantage among homosexual males in our study reflects a true reversal of previous disparities or is instead influenced by a disclosure bias in which males with lower incomes are less likely to disclose their homosexual identity.

We found that bisexual identity was persistently associated with lower income during our study period. This aligns with a recent meta-analysis of 24 studies across multiple countries conducted from 1991 to 2018.[5] Notably, the income disparity in our study was more pronounced among females than males. The underlying mechanisms are likely multifaceted. Bisexual individuals often face additional forms of stigma based on sexual orientation (e.g., biphobia, monosexism), above and beyond those (e.g., homophobia, heterosexism) experienced by homosexual individuals.[30,31] Bisexual-specific workplace discrimination may limit career advancement or earning potential.[32] In addition, some individuals may pursue work at community-based or nonprofit professions that, although affirming, tend to offer lower pay.

Furthermore, recent systematic reviews report that bisexual individuals have a higher prevalence of depression and anxiety,[30] suicide ideation and attempts,[31] and substance use[33,34] than homosexual individuals, with greater disparities among females. Although poorer health may also contribute to labor market challenges,[32] additional research is needed to better understand the structural and social drivers of income inequality among bisexual individuals in Sweden.

Strengths and Limitations

There are several strengths of our study. First, the SPHC surveys recruited representative samples of Stockholm County residents. In addition, we applied survey weights and multiple imputation to address potential biases resulting from unit and item nonresponse, enhancing the robustness and generalizability of our findings. Second, by linking to Swedish national registers, we accessed high-quality sociodemographic information with minimal missing data. Third, the consistent survey methodologies and statistical approaches across survey years enabled reliable comparisons over time.

Several limitations should be considered in the interpretation of our findings. First, the sexual identity question offered limited response options (e.g., homosexual, bisexual) and did not include more contemporary terms (e.g., gay, lesbian, queer). In addition, shifting societal and cultural norms may have shaped individuals' understanding of sexual identity in ways not fully captured by the available terms and may also have influenced their willingness to disclose a minority identity over time. Second, some individuals may experience changes in their sexual identity over time,[17] and our analyses captured identity at only one time point.

Third, the lack of comparable gender identity data limited our ability to examine how gender identity (e.g., transgender, nonbinary) may have affected the interpretation or reporting of sexual identity. Fourth, because of computational constraints, certain analyses were limited to complete-case analyses, and the multiple imputation diagnostics for the SPHC-B 2014 data set were suboptimal. Nonetheless, the results from the complete-case and multiple imputation analyses were generally consistent. Some bias may remain if nonresponse was strongly associated with unobserved sexual identity.

Fifth, we used common social generations primarily based on the context in the United States. This categorization may not be applicable to Swedish society with its distinct social, historical, and cultural trajectories. In addition, the generation effects within a given generation grouping may not be uniform. Sixth, although we investigated sociodemographic factors associated with sexual identity, we did not attempt to establish causal relationships.

Public Health Implications

Since 2014, bisexual individuals have outnumbered homosexual individuals in Stockholm County, making them the largest sexual minority group.[17] A similar trend has been reported in the United States, where bisexual identity has constituted the largest proportion of LGB identity since 2016.[19,20] By 2021, approximately 1 in 7 to 8 females 16 to 29 years of age and Generation Z females identified as bisexual in Stockholm County.

Given generation effects, it can be expected that the proportion of bisexual individuals, particularly among females, will continue to grow in Sweden and potentially in other high-income countries in the near future. Despite growing visibility, bisexual individuals continue to face health and socioeconomic inequalities resulting from structural and sociocultural factors across various contexts.[5,30,31,33–35] Targeted public health policies are warranted to address these disparities, and future studies should prioritize identifying their underlying mechanisms. Conversely, the income disparity among bisexual individuals persists in Stockholm County, despite narrowing over the past decade. This ongoing disparity, even with antidiscrimination policies in place in Sweden,[14] suggests that bisexual-specific workplace guidelines may help promote fair pay and address work-related inequalities based on sexual orientation.

Sexual orientation is a multidimensional construct comprising at least 3 dimensions—identity, attraction, and behavior—that overlap only partially.[2,28] Future studies are warranted to characterize population sizes and potential disparities by each dimension, because different dimensions may relate to different pathways to inequality.[3,35] This will help capture a broader picture of the disadvantages faced by sexual minorities and facilitate efforts to reduce disparities among specific groups. AJPH

ABOUT THE AUTHORS

Willi Zhang, Per Tynelius, Gunnar Brandén, and Kyriaki Kosidou are with the Department of Global Public Health, Karolinska Institutet, and the Centre for Epidemiology and Community Medicine, Region Stockholm, Stockholm, Sweden. Maya B. Mathur is with the Quantitative Sciences Unit, Stanford University, Palo Alto, CA. Matteo Quartagno is with the MRC Clinical Trials Unit, University College London, London, England. Fredrik Liljeros is with the Department of Sociology, Stockholm University, and the Department of Global Public Health, Karolinska Institutet, Stockholm, Sweden.

CORRESPONDENCE

Correspondence should be sent to Willi Zhang, MD, PhD, Solnavägen 1E, 6th Floor, Region Stockholm, 10 431 Stockholm, Sweden (e-mail: willi.zhang@ki.se). Reprints can be ordered at https://www.ajph.org by clicking the "Reprints" link.

PUBLICATION INFORMATION

Full Citation: Zhang W, Tynelius P, Mathur MB, et al. Temporal trends in sexual identity and sociodemographic disparities in Stockholm, Sweden, 2010–2021. *Am J Public Health*. 2025; 115(12):2062–2071.

Acceptance Date: May 18, 2025.

DOI: https://doi.org/10.2105/AJPH.2025.308202

ORCID iDs:

Willi Zhang https://orcid.org/0009-0006-9087-479X

Per Tynelius https://orcid.org/0000-0001-8155-7406

Gunnar Brandén https://orcid.org/0000-0002-9144-2247

Kyriaki Kosidou https://orcid.org/0000-0002-1165-9455

CONTRIBUTORS

W. Zhang drafted the article. W. Zhang, M. B. Mathur, and M. Quartagno contributed to the statistical analyses. W. Zhang, F. Liljeros, and K. Kosidou contributed to the conception and design of the study. P. Tynelius, G. Brandén, and K. Kosidou provided administrative, technical, or material support. M. B. Mathur and M. Quartagno contributed equally to the article. All of the authors contributed to acquisition, analysis, or interpretation of data and critically reviewed and revised the article for important intellectual content.

ACKNOWLEDGMENTS

This study was funded by the Swedish Research Council for Health, Working Life and Welfare (grant 2022-00159 to Kyriaki Kosidou) and Region Stockholm. Portions of the findings were presented at a public seminar during Stockholm Pride House 2025.

We thank the participants for their valuable contributions to the study.

CONFLICTS OF INTEREST

The authors have no relevant financial or nonfinancial interests to disclose.

HUMAN PARTICIPANT PROTECTION

This study was approved by the Stockholm Regional Ethical Review Board. Written informed consent was obtained from all study participants.

REFERENCES

1. Savin-Williams RC. Who's gay? Does it matter? *Curr Dir Psychol Sci.* 2006;15(1):40–44. https://doi.org/10.1111/j.0963-7214.2006.00403.x
2. Barry C, Barry J, Chivers ML. Dimensions of sexual orientation. In: Lykins AD, ed. *Encyclopedia of Sexuality and Gender.* Springer International Publishing; 2020:1–7.
3. Beaulieu-Prévost D, Fortin M. The measurement of sexual orientation: historical background and current practices. *Sexologies.* 2015;24(1):e15–e19. https://doi.org/10.1016/j.sexol.2014.05.006
4. Zeeman L, Sherriff N, Browne K, et al. A review of lesbian, gay, bisexual, trans and intersex (LGBTI) health and healthcare inequalities. *Eur J Public*

Health. 2019;29(5):974–980. https://doi.org/10.1093/eurpub/cky226

5. Drydakis N. Sexual orientation and earnings: a meta-analysis 2012–2020. *J Popul Econ.* 2022;35(2):409–440. https://doi.org/10.1007/s00148-021-00862-1
6. Hammarstedt M, Ahmed AM, Andersson L. Sexual prejudice and labor market outcomes for gays and lesbians: evidence from Sweden. *Fem Econ.* 2015;21(1):90–109. https://doi.org/10.1080/13545701.2014.937727
7. Ahmed AM, Hammarstedt M. Sexual orientation and earnings: a register data-based approach to identify homosexuals. *J Popul Econ.* 2010;23(3):835–849. https://doi.org/10.1007/s00148-009-0265-4
8. Ahmed A, Andersson L, Hammarstedt M. Sexual orientation and full-time monthly earnings, by public and private sector: evidence from Swedish register data. *Rev Econ Household.* 2013;11(1):83–108. https://doi.org/10.1007/s11150-012-9158-5
9. Aksoy CG, Carpenter CS, Frank J, Huffman ML. Gay glass ceilings: sexual orientation and workplace authority in the UK. *J Econ Behav Organ.* 2019;159:167–180. https://doi.org/10.1016/j.jebo.2019.01.013
10. de Vries L, Steinmetz S. Sexual orientation, workplace authority and occupational segregation: evidence from Germany. *Work Employ Soc.* 2024;38(3):852–870. https://doi.org/10.1177/09500170231158513
11. Frost DM, Meyer IH. Minority stress theory: application, critique, and continued relevance. *Curr Opin Psychol.* 2023;51:101579. https://doi.org/10.1016/j.copsyc.2023.101579
12. International Lesbian, Gay, Bisexual, Trans and Intersex Association. Legal frameworks: same-sex marriage and civil unions. Available at: https://database.ilga.org/same-sex-marriage-civil-unions. Accessed March 31, 2025.
13. Flores AR. Social acceptance of LGBTI people in 175 countries and locations, 1981 to 2020. Available at: https://williamsinstitute.law.ucla.edu/wp-content/uploads/Global-Acceptance-Index-LGBTI-Nov-2021.pdf. Accessed March 31, 2025.
14. Bränström R. The health and situation of young LGBTQ people in Sweden—what do we know and where is more research needed? Available at: https://forte.se/en/news/publications/the-health-and-situation-of-young-lgbtq-people-in-sweden. Accessed March 31, 2025.
15. European Commission. Eurobarometer surveys: Eurobarometer. Available at: https://europa.eu/eurobarometer/surveys/browse/all/series/20803. Accessed March 31, 2025.
16. Westerlund U, Sevedag V, Hård V, Karlsson K, Lidmark J. The living conditions of young LGBTQI people. Available at: https://www.mucf.se/sites/default/files/2023/02/MUCF-RAPPORT-eng-HBTQI.pdf. Accessed March 31, 2025.
17. Zhang W, Tynelius P, Mathur MB, et al. Population trends and individual fluidity of sexual identity among Stockholm County residents. *JAMA Netw Open.* 2024;7(12):e2447627. https://doi.org/10.1001/jamanetworkopen.2024.47627
18. Office for National Statistics. Sexual orientation, UK: 2023. Available at: https://www.ons.gov.uk/peoplepopulationandcommunity/culturalidentity/sexuality/bulletins/sexualidentityuk/2023. Accessed March 31, 2025.
19. Gallup. LGBTQ+ identification in US now at 7.6%. Available at: https://news.gallup.com/poll/611864/lgbtq-identification.aspx. Accessed March 31, 2025.
20. Bridges T, Moore MR. Young women of color and shifting sexual identities. *Contexts.* 2018;17(1):86–88. https://doi.org/10.1177/1536504218767125
21. Hatzenbuehler ML, Lattanner MR, McKetta S, Pachankis JE. Structural stigma and LGBTQ+ health: a narrative review of quantitative studies. *Lancet Public Health.* 2024;9(2):e109–e127. https://doi.org/10.1016/S2468-2667(23)00312-2
22. Region Stockholm. Hälsa Stockholm: Stockholm Public Health Cohort data. Available at: https://www.ces.regionstockholm.se/projekt-och-uppdrag/halsa-stockholm/SPHC-data. Accessed March 31, 2025.
23. Tamhane AR, Westfall AO, Burkholder GA, Cutter GR. Prevalence odds ratio versus prevalence ratio: choice comes with consequences. *Stat Med.* 2016;35(30):5730–5735. https://doi.org/10.1002/sim.7059
24. Lundström S, Särndal C. Calibration as a standard method for treatment of nonresponse. *J Off Stat.* 1999;15(2):305–327.
25. Quartagno M, Carpenter J, Goldstein H. Multiple imputation with survey weights: a multilevel approach. *J Surv Stat Methodol.* 2020;8(5):965–989. https://doi.org/10.1093/jssam/smz036
26. Quartagno M, Carpenter JR. Multiple imputation for discrete data: evaluation of the joint latent normal model. *Biom J.* 2019;61(4):1003–1019. https://doi.org/10.1002/bimj.201800222
27. Glenn ND. Distinguishing age, period, and cohort effects. In: Mortimer JT, Shanahan MJ, eds. *Handbook of the Life Course.* Kluwer Academic Publishers; 2002:465–476.
28. Diamond LM. Sexual fluidity in male and females. *Curr Sex Health Rep.* 2016;8(4):249–256. https://doi.org/10.1007/s11930-016-0092-z
29. Manalastas EJ, Blumenau HS, Feinstein BA. Gender differences in attitudes toward bisexual people and bisexuality: a systematic review and meta-analysis. *Psychol Sex Orientat Gend Divers.* 2025;12(1):42–55. https://doi.org/10.1037/sgd0000624
30. Ross LE, Salway T, Tarasoff LA, MacKay JM, Hawkins BW, Fehr CP. Prevalence of depression and anxiety among bisexual people compared to gay, lesbian, and heterosexual individuals: a systematic review and meta-analysis. *J Sex Res.* 2018;55(4–5):435–456. https://doi.org/10.1080/00224499.2017.1387755
31. Salway T, Ross LE, Fehr CP, et al. A systematic review and meta-analysis of disparities in the prevalence of suicide ideation and attempt among bisexual populations. *Arch Sex Behav.* 2019;48(1):89–111. https://doi.org/10.1007/s10508-018-1150-6
32. Mize TD. Sexual orientation in the labor market. *Am Sociol Rev.* 2016;81(6):1132–1160. https://doi.org/10.1177/0003122416674025
33. Shokoohi M, Kinitz DJ, Pinto D, et al. Disparities in alcohol use and heavy episodic drinking among bisexual people: a systematic review, meta-analysis, and meta-regression. *Drug Alcohol Depend.* 2022;235:109433. https://doi.org/10.1016/j.drugalcdep.2022.109433
34. Shokoohi M, Salway T, Ahn B, Ross LE. Disparities in the prevalence of cigarette smoking among bisexual people: a systematic review, meta-analysis and meta-regression. *Tob Control.* 2021;30(e2):e78–e86. https://doi.org/10.1136/tobaccocontrol-2020-055747
35. Dyar C, Taggart TC, Rodriguez-Seijas C, et al. Physical health disparities across dimensions of sexual orientation, race/ethnicity, and sex: evidence for increased risk among bisexual adults. *Arch Sex Behav.* 2019;48(1):225–242. https://doi.org/10.1007/s10508-018-1169-8

Crash-Related Protective and Risky Behaviors Among Micromobility Riders: A Nationally Representative Survey

Nan Ni, MPH, MUP, Michelle Duren, PhD, and Johnathon P. Ehsani, PhD

Objectives. To examine protective and risky behaviors among micromobility users, including bicyclists, moped riders, and e-scooter users.

Methods. We analyzed data from a nationally representative survey (conducted May–June 2022) of 1523 US adults who reported using a bicycle, e-scooter, or moped. We calculated the weighted prevalence of habitual protective and risky riding behaviors across these 3 modes.

Results. Micromobility users were primarily male and skewed toward younger age groups. Although engagement in protective behaviors was similar across modes, risky behaviors varied significantly. Moped users exhibited the highest prevalence of risky behaviors (59.6%), followed by e-scooter users (50.9%) and bicyclists (39.4%). E-scooter users had the highest self-reported lifetime crash rate (44.6%), followed by bicyclists (24.6%) and moped users (15.9%).

Conclusions. Micromobility users exhibit distinct, mode-specific behavioral profiles.

Public Health Implications. Cities should implement mode-specific safety measures, such as targeted campaigns and infrastructure improvements, to address the elevated crash risk among moped and e-scooter users. (*Am J Public Health*. 2025;115(12):2072–2076. https://doi.org/10.2105/AJPH.2025.308256)

AJPH December 2025, Vol. 115, No. 12

Since the introduction of electric scooters (e-scooters) in 2017,[1] micromobility has rapidly become a fixture in US urban transportation systems. With 133 million micromobility trips in 2023, primarily on e-scooters and shared bikes,[2] cities face challenges sustaining this growth while safeguarding public health and road safety. Injuries, especially from e-scooters, have increased with usage,[3] with men and frequent users accounting for most injuries.[4]

Various factors influence micromobility users' risk perception and crash risk, including infrastructure, substance use, and safety knowledge.[5–7] However, few studies compare users across different micromobility modes, such as bicycles and e-scooters. Most research focuses on a single mode and offers little insight into how mode choice relates to safety.[8] E-scooter users are often perceived as more reckless and risk seeking than cyclists, but findings focus on localized samples and lack generalizability.[6] Emerging evidence highlights differences in alcohol and helmet use among injured micromobility users admitted to hospital emergency departments.[9] However, there is limited understanding of behavior profiles before injury occurs.

We present insights from nationally representative survey data on micromobility. We describe the prevalence of protective and risky behaviors by bicyclists, moped users, and e-scooter riders and discuss policy and research implications for improving micromobility safety in jurisdictions across the United States.

METHODS

We conducted a cross-sectional survey of a nationally representative sample of

US adults. The University of Chicago's National Opinion Research Center fielded the survey in English and Spanish between May 4 and June 10, 2022. Detailed methodology, including sampling strategy, weighting, and response rate, is provided in the supplemental material (available as a supplement to the online version of this article at http://www.ajph.org).

The survey yielded responses from 1523 respondents who had used a personal or shared e-scooter, moped, or bicycle within the preceding 6 months. For each applicable mode, we asked respondents about the frequency with which they engaged in a range of protective and risky riding behaviors (Table 1). We operationalized habitual behavior by creating binary variables in which we coded a positive response only if the respondent answered "usually" or "always." A complete list of the survey questions and precise coding for each variable is available in Table A (available as a supplement to the online version of this article at http://www.ajph.org). Geographic distribution of survey respondents by state of residence is available in Table C (available as a supplement to the online version of this article at http://www.ajph.org).

We calculated a weighted prevalence with an SE estimate for each behavior. We used a design-adjusted χ^2 test to assess for significant differences across user groups. To address the potential confounding from multimode use, we conducted a sensitivity analysis excluding multimode users, repeating all analyses among the 1396 single-mode users. We report results from these single-mode users as the primary findings (Table 1), as the sensitivity analysis revealed significant differences in behavioral estimates when multimode users were included (Table B, available as a supplement to the online version of this article at http://www.ajph.org). We conducted all analyses using R version 4.3.1 (RStudio, Boston, MA).

RESULTS

Among the 1396 single-mode micromobility users, 1264 were bicyclists, 101 were e-scooter users, and 31 were moped users. Micromobility users were predominantly male, with significant differences observed in age, race and ethnicity, and household income (Table 1). Demographic comparisons between users and nonusers are available in Table D (available as a supplement to the online version of this article at http://www.ajph.org).

Bicyclists and moped users were significantly more likely than e-scooter users to engage in all protective behaviors except wearing reflective clothing. Helmet use was the most common protective behavior across all groups, with most bicyclists and moped users reporting regular use (Table 1).

Most users reported at least 1 risky behavior, although no single behavior was reported by a majority across all modes. The overall prevalence of any risky behavior did not differ significantly by mode ($P = .11$). However, individual behaviors did vary. Moped users were most likely to ride downhill without braking (38.1%; 95% confidence interval [CI] = 14.0, 62.1), with headphones (39.0%; 95% CI = 13.9, 64.1), or on a highway (29.5%; 95% CI = 4.2, 54.3). E-scooter users most commonly reported riding at night (18.5%; 95% CI = 6.6, 30.3), using a smartphone while riding (18.0%; 95% CI = 7.2, 28.7), or riding with another person (15.5%; 95% CI = 6.0, 24.9). Bicyclists had the lowest prevalence of most risky behaviors, although 14.0% (95% CI = 11.6, 16.5) reported riding with headphones and 13.3% (95% CI = 10.7, 15.9) reported riding into oncoming traffic.

Crash history also varied significantly by mode. A quarter of bicyclists reported a crash (24.6%; 95% CI = 21.4, 27.7) compared with 15.9% (95% CI = 1.8, 30.0) of moped users and 44.6% (95% CI = 28.9, 60.2) of e-scooter users ($P = .007$). Near-miss prevalence was higher overall but did not differ significantly by mode (bicyclists: 59.3%; 95% CI = 55.6, 63.0; moped users: 54.8%; 95% CI = 29.6, 79.9; e-scooter users: 47.8%; 95% CI = 32.5, 63.0; $P = .38$).

DISCUSSION

Our study provides new insights into the behavior profiles of micromobility users in the United States that can inform future research and policy. Specifically, our findings highlight differences in protective and risky behaviors across bicyclists, moped users, and e-scooter users. Although engagement in protective behaviors was generally higher among bicyclists and moped users than e-scooter users, we observed significant variation in risky behaviors, with moped and e-scooter users displaying a higher prevalence of several risky riding practices. Notably, e-scooter users reported the highest crash rates, followed by moped users and then bicyclists. These findings contribute to the growing literature on micromobility safety by offering nationally representative data on user behaviors so that researchers do not need to rely solely on localized injury reports or emergency department data.

Our results align with previous findings in that e-scooter users exhibited a greater tendency to ride after alcohol consumption than bicyclists.[9] However, unlike previous literature, we found

TABLE 1— Demographic Characteristics, Crash History, and Frequent Behaviors of Single-Mode Micromobility Users by Mode: United States, May–June 2022

Characteristic	Bicycle (n = 1278), % (95% CI)	Moped (n = 27), % (95% CI)	E-Scooter (n = 91), % (95% CI)	P
Demographics				
Sex				.47
Male	61.5 (58.0, 65.1)	74.1 (56.1, 92.1)	62.3 (48.6, 75.9)	
Female	38.5 (34.9, 42.0)	25.9 (7.9, 43.9)	37.7 (24.1, 51.4)	
Age, y				< .01
18–29	17.7 (14.4, 21.0)	40.1 (14.9, 65.4)	38.0 (21.8, 54.1)	
30–44	27.7 (24.8, 30.7)	19.6 (3.2, 36.0)	47.7 (32.7, 62.7)	
45–59	24.9 (22.0, 27.8)	15.2 (< 0.1, 29.6)	5.1 (1.3, 8.9)	
≥ 60	29.6 (25.8, 33.5)	25.0 (1.2, 48.9)	9.3 (0.8, 17.7)	
Race/Ethnicity				< .01
Non-Hispanic White	66.5 (62.9, 70.1)	49.1 (24.0, 74.2)	49.5 (34.2, 64.9)	
Non-Hispanic Black	9.5 (7.3, 11.6)	9.2 (< 0.1, 22.9)	24.8 (11.6, 38.0)	
Non-Hispanic Asian	5.2 (3.4, 7.0)	< 0.1 (< 0.1, < 0.1)	2.8 (< 0.1, 6.9)	
Hispanic	14.2 (11.5, 16.9)	41.7 (16.6, 66.8)	18.5 (8.3, 28.7)	
Non-Hispanic with ≥ 2 races	3.2 (2.0, 4.5)	< 0.1 (< 0.1, < 0.1)	4.1 (< 0.1, 8.8)	
Non-Hispanic, other	1.4 (0.5, 2.2)	< 0.1 (< 0.1, < 0.1)	0.2 (< 0.1, 0.6)	
Household income, $				.01
< 30 000	23.6 (20.0, 27.1)	41.5 (16.5, 66.5)	43.1 (27.9, 58.3)	
30 000–59 999	20.7 (17.6, 23.8)	23.8 (5.8, 41.8)	30.1 (17.1, 43.2)	
60 000–99 999	23.2 (20.1, 26.2)	8.8 (< 0.1, 19.1)	8.1 (2.5, 13.6)	
≥ 100 000	32.6 (29.2, 36.0)	25.8 (1.6, 50.1)	18.7 (5.7, 31.8)	
Residential area				.49
Urban	27.2 (23.8, 30.7)	24.8 (< 0.1, 49.0)	34.9 (20.5, 49.3)	
Suburban	52.1 (48.3, 55.9)	40.4 (17.2, 63.6)	48.2 (32.8, 63.6)	
Rural	20.5 (17.4, 23.5)	34.9 (10.7, 59.0)	16.4 (7.1, 25.7)	
Crash and behavioral outcomes				
Crash and near-miss history				
Lifetime crash history	24.6 (21.4, 27.7)	15.9 (1.8, 30.0)	44.6 (28.9, 60.2)	.01
Lifetime near-miss history	59.3 (55.6, 63.0)	54.8 (29.6, 79.9)	47.8 (32.5, 63.0)	.38
Protective behaviors				
Any protective behavior	69.8 (66.4, 73.2)	63.1 (40.4, 85.8)	41.3 (26.4, 56.1)	< .01
Wears a helmet	51.9 (48.1, 55.7)	63.1 (40.4, 85.8)	22.6 (10.4, 34.8)	< .01
Signals turns[a]	47.8 (43.9, 51.6)	NA	21.0 (9.2, 32.7)	< .01
Wears reflective clothing	22.1 (18.6, 25.3)	20.3 (3.4, 37.2)	16.6 (4.6, 28.6)	.7
Risky behaviors				
Any risky behavior	39.4 (35.8, 43.0)	59.6 (34.4, 84.8)	50.9 (35.8, 66.2)	.11
Rides into oncoming traffic[a]	13.3 (10.7, 15.9)	NA	9.0 (2.2, 15.9)	.66
Rides on a highway	5.7 (3.9, 7.4)	29.5 (4.2, 54.3)	11.3 (2.5, 20.1)	.01
Uses smartphone while riding	7.6 (5.6, 9.5)	9.3 (< 0.1, 20.9)	18.0 (7.2, 28.7)	.04
Rides with others on vehicle	4.3 (2.8, 5.9)	17.7 (2.2, 33.2)	15.5 (6.0, 24.9)	< .01
Rides with headphones	14.0 (11.6, 16.5)	39.0 (13.9, 64.1)	9.7 (4.7, 18.9)	.01
Rides at night	4.0 (2.8, 5.3)	14.7 (< 0.1, 30.1)	18.5 (6.6, 30.3)	< .01

Continued

TABLE 1— Continued

Characteristic	Bicycle (n = 1278), % (95% CI)	Moped (n = 27), % (95% CI)	E-Scooter (n = 91), % (95% CI)	P
Rides while impaired	3.0 (1.9, 4.1)	10.5 (<0.1, 24.5)	8.2 (0.9, 15.5)	.04
Rides downhill without braking	13.0 (10.5, 15.4)	38.1 (14.0, 62.1)	10.7 (3.9, 17.4)	<.01

Note. CI = confidence interval; NA = not applicable. Behavior variable percentages represent the weighted prevalence of respondents who reported performing a behavior "usually" or "always."
[a]We did not ask moped users the questions for "signals turns" and "rides into oncoming traffic."

helmet usage was particularly low among e-scooter users and substantially higher among moped users and bicyclists. This suggests that previous studies based on hospital-admitted riders, which often use convenience samples, may not fully represent the general riding population. The discrepancy underscores the need for future research on factors influencing protective behaviors before injury events.

Although our study offers valuable contributions, several limitations should be considered. First, reliance on self-reported data introduces the potential for recall and social desirability biases, which may lead to underreporting risky behaviors or overestimating protective practices.[10] Additionally, our survey does not capture contextual details such as infrastructure differences, enforcement policies, or environmental factors that may influence safety practices.[11] Despite these limitations, the study highlights significant gaps in safety practices and offers a foundation for future research. Future research should explore how social norms, psychosocial factors, legal regulations, and urban design affect user safety. Longitudinal studies evaluating injury outcomes among different user groups could further inform evidence-based policy decisions to enhance micromobility safety nationwide. Although this study is descriptive, future research could apply multivariable or causal modeling approaches to examine predictors of crash risk and mechanisms underlying behavioral disparities.

PUBLIC HEALTH IMPLICATIONS

From a public health perspective, our findings underscore the importance of targeted safety interventions tailored to specific micromobility users. Given the high rates of risky behaviors among moped and e-scooter users, interventions should be tailored to mode-specific risks and may include infrastructure improvements, such as dedicated lanes and traffic-calming measures, to enhance rider safety.[8,11] Although education campaigns alone have limited long-term impact, they are valuable for increasing public awareness and building support for the implementation of more effective policies.[12] A multifaceted approach combining targeted education with evidence-based infrastructure design may be needed to create safer environments for micromobility users and to mitigate the risks associated with these growing transportation modes. AJPH

ABOUT THE AUTHORS

All authors are with the Johns Hopkins Bloomberg School of Public Health, Baltimore, MD.

CORRESPONDENCE

Correspondence should be sent to Nan Ni, 615 N Wolfe St, Baltimore, MD 21205 (e-mail: nni6@jhu.edu). Reprints can be ordered at https://www.ajph.org by clicking the "Reprints" link.

PUBLICATION INFORMATION

Full Citation: Ni N, Duren M, Ehsani JP. Crash-related protective and risky behaviors among micromobility riders: a nationally representative survey. *Am J Public Health*. 2025;115(12):2072–2076.
Acceptance Date: July 19, 2025.
DOI: https://doi.org/10.2105/AJPH.2025.308256
ORCID iDs:
Nan Ni https://orcid.org/0009-0003-0885-2996
Michelle Duren https://orcid.org/0000-0002-7681-9050

CONTRIBUTORS

N. Ni revised the article critically for important intellectual content. N. Ni and M. Duren analyzed and interpreted the data and drafted the article. M. Duren and J. P. Ehsani obtained funding and collected the original data. All authors made substantial contributions to the conceptualization and design of the work and gave final approval of the version to be published.

ACKNOWLEDGMENTS

This work was supported by the National Center for Injury Control and Prevention, Centers for Disease Control and Prevention (grant 1R49CE003090).

No entity that could benefit from the findings of this study was involved in funding the research. The principal investigator had full access to all the data in the study and takes responsibility for the integrity and accuracy of the data and the data analysis.

CONFLICTS OF INTEREST

The authors have no conflicts of interest to disclose.

HUMAN PARTICIPANT PROTECTION

The Johns Hopkins Bloomberg School of Public Health institutional review board deemed this study not human participants research, as the authors received only anonymized, de-identified data. We obtained digital informed consent.

REFERENCES

1. Price J, Blackshear D, Blount W, Sandt L. Micromobility: a travel mode innovation. *Public Roads*. 2021;85(1):8–12. Available at: https://rosap.ntl.bts.gov/view/dot/55708. Accessed September 26, 2025.
2. National Association of City Transportation Officials. Shared micromobility in 2023. 2024. Available at: https://nacto.org/publication/shared-micromobility-report-2023. Accessed November 30, 2024.
3. Aizpuru M, Farley KX, Rojas JC, Crawford RS, Moore TJ, Wagner ER. Motorized scooter injuries in the era of scooter-shares: a review of the national electronic surveillance system. *Am J Emerg Med*. 2019;37(6):1133–1138. https://doi.org/10.1016/j.ajem.2019.03.049
4. Tian D, Ryan AD, Craig CM, Sievert K, Morris NL. Characteristics and risk factors for electric scooter-related crashes and injury crashes among scooter riders: a two-phase survey study. *Int J Environ Res Public Health*. 2022;19(16):10129. https://doi.org/10.3390/ijerph191610129
5. Gioldasis C, Christoforou Z, Seidowsky R. Risk-taking behaviors of e-scooter users: a survey in Paris. *Accid Anal Prev*. 2021;163:106427. https://doi.org/10.1016/j.aap.2021.106427
6. Useche SA, O'Hern S, Gonzalez-Marin A, Gene-Morales J, Alonso F, Stephens AN. Unsafety on two wheels, or social prejudice? Proxying behavioral reports on bicycle and e-scooter riding safety—a mixed-methods study. *Transp Res Part F Traffic Psychol Behav*. 2022;89:168–182. https://doi.org/10.1016/j.trf.2022.06.015
7. Pourfalatoun S, Ahmed J, Miller EE. Shared electric scooter users and non-users: perceptions on safety, adoption and risk. *Sustainability*. 2023;15(11):9045. https://doi.org/10.3390/su15119045
8. Fonseca-Cabrera AS, Llopis-Castelló D, Pérez-Zuriaga AM, Alonso-Troyano C, García A. Micromobility users' behaviour and perceived risk during meeting manoeuvres. *Int J Environ Res Public Health*. 2021;18(23):12465. https://doi.org/10.3390/ijerph182312465
9. Burford KG, Itzkowitz NG, Rundle AG, DiMaggio C, Mooney SJ. The burden of injuries associated with e-bikes, powered scooters, hoverboards, and bicycles in the United States: 2019–2022. *Am J Public Health*. 2024;114(12):1365–1374. https://doi.org/10.2105/AJPH.2024.307820
10. Bound J, Brown C, Mathiowetz N. Measurement error in survey data. In: Heckman JJ, Leamer E, eds. Handbook of Econometrics. Amsterdam, Netherlands: Elsevier; 2001:3705–3843. https://doi.org/10.1016/S1573-4412(01)05012-7
11. Hossein Sabbaghian M, Llopis-Castelló D, García A. A safe infrastructure for micromobility: the current state of knowledge. *Sustainability*. 2023;15(13):10140. https://doi.org/10.3390/su151310140
12. Yannis G, Petraki V, Crist P. Safer micromobility. International Transport Forum Policy Papers. 2024;129:32. Paris, France: OECD Publishing. Available at: https://doi.org/10.1787/0d2e0dd5-en. Accessed June 20, 2025.

Erratum In: "Emergency Food Support Preference and Usage During COVID-19: A Neighborhood Study of Low-Income Black Mothers' Use of School-Based Food Distribution and P-EBT"

In: Fern SE, Kimbro RT, Hill ME, Hughes CC. Emergency food support preference and usage during COVID-19: a neighborhood study of low-income Black mothers' use of school-based food distribution and P-EBT. *Am J Public Health*. 2023;113(S3):S227–S230.

When originally published, the title of the article was listed incorrectly in the XML causing it to display incorrectly on indexing sites such as PubMed. The title should read: "Emergency Food Support Preference and Usage During COVID-19: A Neighborhood Study of Low-Income Black Mothers' Use of School-Based Food Distribution and P-EBT." The title appeared correctly in the published PDF.

This change does not affect the article's conclusions. AJPH

https://doi.org/10.2105/AJPH.2023.307458e

Erratum In: "Navigating Dual-Harm: Integrating Self- and Other-Harm Into Public Health Inquiry"

In: Díaz-Faes DA, Rajan S, Branas CC. Navigating dual-harm: integrating self- and other-harm into public health inquiry. *Am J Public Health*. 2025;115(4):596–604.

When originally published, incorrect terminology was used on p. 599 in the first sentence of the "Harm Groups" section.

The sentence should read:

Once the behaviors are identified, cross-tabulation allows for the identification of individuals who engage in harmful behaviors and classify them into the following groups: no-harm, single-harm, and dual-harm. AJPH

https://doi.org/10.2105/AJPH.2024.307940e

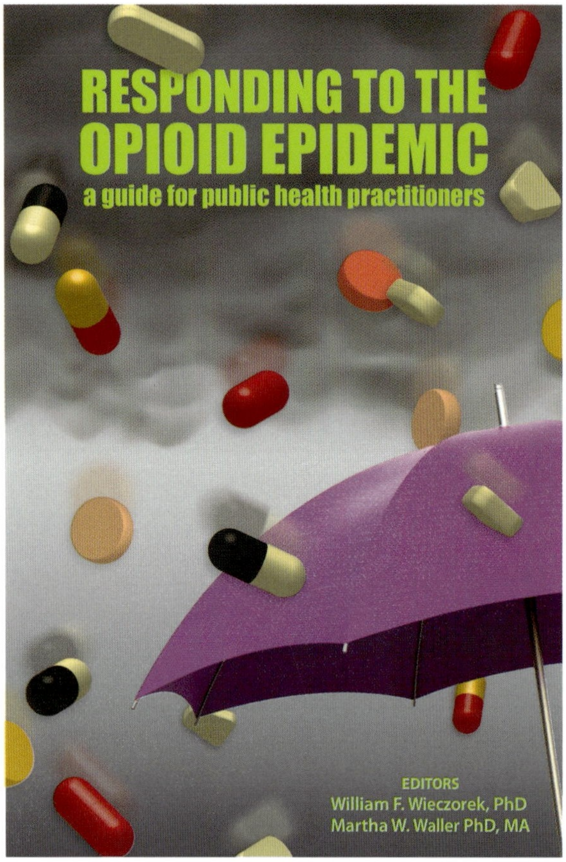

ISBN 978-0-87553-344-5, 400 PP., 2024,
SOFTBOUND/PRINT-ON-DEMAND

Responding to the Opioid Epidemic: A Guide for Public Health Practitioners

Edited by: William F. Wieczorek, PhD and Martha W. Waller PhD, MA

It's impossible to completely prevent the substance misuse defining the opioid epidemic, and it's impossible to treat the problem away. This reality requires a continuum of care (COC) approach, which includes promotion, prevention, case-finding, treatment, and recovery. This book presents research-informed interventions aligned with the COC approach to guide how communities, first responders, lay persons, medical providers, policymakers, treatment providers, and others can respond to the opioid epidemic at an individual, community, state, and national level.

APHABOOKSTORE.ORG

APHA PRESS

AN IMPRINT OF AMERICAN PUBLIC HEALTH ASSOCIATION